THE IMPACT OF DEMOGRAPHICS ON HEALTH AND HEALTH CARE: RACE, ETHNICITY AND OTHER SOCIAL FACTORS

RESEARCH IN THE SOCIOLOGY OF HEALTH CARE

Series Editor: Jennie Jacobs Kronenfeld

Recent Volumes:

Volume 17: Health Care Providers, Institutions, and Patients: Changing Patterns of Care Provision and Care Delivery, 2000

Volume 18: Health, Illness, and Use of Care: The Impact of Social Factors, 2000

Volume 19: Changing Consumers and Changing Technology in Health Care and Health Care Delivery, 2001

Volume 20: Social Inequalities, Health, and Health Care Delivery, 2002

Volume 21: Reorganizing Health Care Delivery Systems: Problems of Managed Care and Other Models of Health Care Delivery, 2003

Volume 22: Chronic Care, Health Care Systems, and Services Integration, 2004

Volume 23: Health Care Services, Racial and Ethnic Minorities, and Underserved Populations, 2005

Volume 24: Access, Quality and Satisfaction with Care: Concerns of Patients, Providers, and Insurers, 2007

Volume 25: Inequalities and Disparities in Health care and Health: Concerns of Patients, Providers, and Insurers, 2007

Volume 26: Care for Major Health Problems and Population Health Concerns: Impacts on Patients, Providers, and Policy, 2008

Volume 27: Social Sources of Disparities in Health and Health Care and Linkages to Policy, Population Concerns and Providers of Care, 2009

RESEARCH IN THE SOCIOLOGY OF HEALTH CARE
VOLUME 28

THE IMPACT OF DEMOGRAPHICS ON HEALTH AND HEALTH CARE: RACE, ETHNICITY AND OTHER SOCIAL FACTORS

EDITED BY

JENNIE JACOBS KRONENFELD

*Sociology Program, School of Social and Family Dynamics,
Arizona State University, Tempe, AZ, USA*

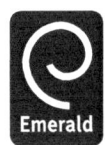

United Kingdom – North America – Japan
India – Malaysia – China

Emerald Group Publishing Limited
Howard House, Wagon Lane, Bingley BD16 1WA, UK

First edition 2010

Copyright © 2010 Emerald Group Publishing Limited

Reprints and permission service
Contact: booksandseries@emeraldinsight.com

No part of this book may be reproduced, stored in a retrieval system, transmitted in any form or by any means electronic, mechanical, photocopying, recording or otherwise without either the prior written permission of the publisher or a licence permitting restricted copying issued in the UK by The Copyright Licensing Agency and in the USA by The Copyright Clearance Center. No responsibility is accepted for the accuracy of information contained in the text, illustrations or advertisements. The opinions expressed in these chapters are not necessarily those of the Editor or the publisher.

British Library Cataloguing in Publication Data
A catalogue record for this book is available from the British Library

ISBN: 978-1-84950-714-1
ISSN: 0275-4959 (Series)

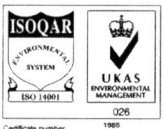

Emerald Group Publishing Limited, Howard House, Environmental Management System has been certified by ISOQAR to ISO 14001:2004 standards

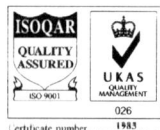

Awarded in recognition of Emerald's production department's adherence to quality systems and processes when preparing scholarly journals for print

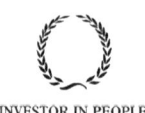

INVESTOR IN PEOPLE

CONTENTS

LIST OF CONTRIBUTORS   ix

SECTION I: SOCIAL FACTORS LEADING TO DIFFERENCES IN HEALTH AND HEALTH CARE

SOCIAL FACTORS LEADING TO DIFFERENCES IN HEALTH AND HEALTH CARE: THE INFLUENCE OF FACTORS SUCH AS RACE/ETHNICITY, GEOGRAPHY, AND GENDER
Jennie Jacobs Kronenfeld   3

SECTION II: RACIAL AND ETHNIC FACTORS IN DIFFERENCES IN HEALTH AND HEALTH CARE

RACIAL DISPARITIES IN KNOWLEDGE OF HEPATITIS C VIRUS (HCV)
Alicia Suarez   21

MEDICARE AND RACIAL DISPARITIES IN HEALTH: FEE-FOR-SERVICE VERSUS MANAGED CARE
Noah J. Webster   47

HOW MUCH TIME DO AMERICANS SPEND SEEKING HEALTH CARE? RACIAL AND ETHNIC DIFFERENCES IN PATIENT EXPERIENCES
Deborah Carr, Yoko Ibuka and Louise B. Russell   71

CAN THE BEHAVIORAL MODEL EXPLAIN
IMMIGRANT STATUS AND ETHNIC
DIFFERENCES IN U.S. ADULTS'
COMPLEMENTARY AND ALTERNATIVE
MEDICINE (CAM) USE?
Georgiana Bostean   *99*

CLASS AND RACE HEALTH DISPARITIES
AND HEALTH INFORMATION SEEKING
BEHAVIORS: THE ROLE OF SOCIAL CAPITAL
Cirila Estela Vasquez Guzman, Gilbert Mireles,   *127*
Neal Christopherson and Michelle Janning

RACIAL DISPARITIES IN STILLBIRTHS
Vicki Dryfhout   *151*

SECTION III: GEOGRAPHIC AND COMMUNITY FACTORS IN DIFFERENCES IN HEALTH AND HEALTH CARE

HABILITATIVE THERAPY AMONG
PRESCHOOL CHILDREN: REGIONAL
DISPARITIES IN THE EARLY INTERVENTION
POPULATION
Richard Lee Rogers   *177*

CONSUMER-DIRECTED HEALTH INSURANCE
VS. MANAGED CARE: ANALYSIS OF
HEALTHCARE UTILIZATION AND
EXPENDITURES INCURRED BY EMPLOYEES
IN A RURAL AREA
Cecilia M. Watkins, John White, David F. Duncan,   *197*
David K. Wyant, Thomas Nicholson, Jagdish
Khubchandani and Lakshminarayana Chekuri

SECTION IV: GENDER DIFFERENCES IN HEALTH AND HEALTH CARE

SOME CONSIDERATIONS REGARDING GENDER WHEN A HEALTHCARE INTERPRETER IS HELPING PROVIDERS AND THEIR LIMITED ENGLISH PROFICIENT PATIENTS
    Stergios Roussos, Mary-Rose Mueller, Linda Hill, Nadia Salas, Melbourne Hovell and Veronica Villarreal   *217*

HIDDEN GENDER INEQUALITIES IN OLD AGE: EQUAL TREATMENT DOES NOT MEAN EQUAL RESULTS
    Sally Bould   *231*

SECTION V: LIFE COURSE FACTORS IN DIFFERENCES IN HEALTH AND HEALTH CARE

MOTHERS' PERSPECTIVES ON ENHANCING CONSUMER ENGAGEMENT IN BEHAVIORAL HEALTH TREATMENT FOR MATERNAL DEPRESSION
    Sandraluz Lara-Cinisomo, Ellen Burke Beckjord and Donna J. Keyser   *249*

MEDIATING HOSPICE CARE: MAPPING RELATIONS OF RULING IN THE INTERDISCIPLINARY GROUP MEETING
    Maria DiTullio and Douglas MacDonald   *269*

LIST OF CONTRIBUTORS

Ellen Burke Beckjord	RAND Corporation, Pittsburgh, PA, USA
Georgiana Bostean	University of California, Irvine, Irvine, CA, USA
Sally Bould	University of Delaware, Newark, DE, USA; University of Massachusetts, Boston, MA, USA
Deborah Carr	Rutgers University, New Brunswick, NJ, USA
Lakshminarayana Chekuri	University of North Texas, Denton, TX, USA
Neal Christopherson	Whitman College, Walla Walla, WA, USA
Maria DiTullio	LeMoyne College, Syracuse, NY, USA
Vicki Dryfhout	University of Cincinnati, Cincinnati, OH, USA
David F. Duncan	Duncan & Associate, Bowling Green, KY, USA; Brown University, Providence, RI, USA
Cirila Estela Vasquez Guzman	University of New Mexico, Albuquerque, NM, USA
Linda Hill	University of California, San Diego, CA, USA; San Diego State University, General Preventive Medicine Residency, San Diego, CA, USA
Melbourne Hovell	San Diego State University, San Diego, CA, USA

Yoko Ibuka	Yale School of Public Health, New Haven, CT, USA
Michelle Janning	Whitman College, Walla Walla, WA, USA
Donna J. Keyser	RAND Corporation, Pittsburgh, PA, USA
Jagdish Khubchandani	University of Toledo, Toledo, OH, USA
Jennie Jacobs Kronenfeld	Sociology Program, School of Social and Family Dynamics, Arizona State University, Tempe, AZ, USA
Sandraluz Lara-Cinisomo	RAND Corporation, Pittsburgh, PA, USA,; University of North Carolina at Charlotte, Charlotte, NC, USA
Douglas MacDonald	LeMoyne College, Syracuse, NY, USA
Gilbert Mireles	Whitman College, Walla Walla, WA, USA
Mary-Rose Mueller	University of San Diego, San Diego, CA, USA
Thomas Nicholson	Western Kentucky University, Bowling Green, KY, USA
Richard Lee Rogers	Southern Wesleyan University, Central, SC, USA
Stergios Roussos	Alliance for Community Research and Development, Merced, CA, USA; San Diego State University, San Diego, CA, USA
Louise B. Russell	Rutgers University, New Brunswick, NJ, USA
Nadia Salas	San Diego State University, San Diego, CA, USA

List of Contributors

Alicia Suarez	DePauw University, Greencastle, IN, USA
Veronica Villarreal	University of California, San Diego, CA, USA; San Diego State University, General Preventive Medicine Residency, San Diego, CA, USA
Cecilia M. Watkins	Western Kentucky University, Bowling Green, KY, USA
Noah J. Webster	Case Western Reserve University, Cleveland, OH, USA
John White	Western Kentucky University, Bowling Green, KY, USA
David K. Wyant	Western Kentucky University, Bowling Green, KY, USA

SECTION I
SOCIAL FACTORS LEADING TO DIFFERENCES IN HEALTH AND HEALTH CARE

SOCIAL FACTORS LEADING TO DIFFERENCES IN HEALTH AND HEALTH CARE: THE INFLUENCE OF FACTORS SUCH AS RACE/ETHNICITY, GEOGRAPHY, AND GENDER

Jennie Jacobs Kronenfeld

ABSTRACT

This chapter provides an introduction to Volume 28, The Impact of Demographics on Health and Health Care: Race, Ethnicity and Other Social Factors. *This chapter introduces the topic of demographic factors leading to differences and disparities in health and health care by reviewing more recent literature within sociology addressing social factors leading to differences in health and health. This chapter also serves as an introduction to the volume. As such, the chapter explains the organization of the volume and briefly comments on each of the chapters included in the volume.*

This chapter provides an introduction to Volume 28 of the *Research in the Sociology of Health Care* series. This volume is entitled *The Impact of Demographics on Health and HealthCare: Race, Ethnicity, and Other Social Factors*. The overall volume is divided into five sections. The first section is this introductory chapter. The second section "Racial and Ethnic Factors in Differences in Health and Health Care" is the largest section of the book and includes six chapters looking at racial disparities on various topics such as knowledge of hepatitis C virus, health services received and patients' experiences in seeking health care, use of complementary and alternative medicine (CAM) services, and the role of social capital in class and race health disparities in health information-seeking behavior. The third section is focused on geographic and community factors and includes chapters covering preschool children, and employees in rural areas and their health utilization patterns. The fourth section includes two chapters, both linked to gender but focused on different topics within that. One looks at linkages between gender and use of an interpreter for limited English proficient patients, whereas the other looks at hidden gender inequalities in old age. The last section examines life course-related factors, and one chapter focuses on maternal depression as linked to birth experiences, whereas the other focuses on end of life issues of hospice care. The last section of this chapter reviews each of these sections in more detail, following several sections that discuss racial/ethnic, geographic, gender, and other social factors leading to differences in health and health care.

DIFFERENCES AND DISPARITIES IN HEALTH AND HEALTH CARE

One of the more robust areas of research in medical sociology and also in epidemiology, public health, and health services research over the past decade have been studies linked to differences and disparities in health and health care. What do we mean by disparities or differences in health and health care? In an address given at the 2008 annual meeting of the American Sociological Association and later published in *Journal of Health and Social Behavior*, Aneshensel (2009) argued that mental health disparities refer to the disproportionate amount of psychopathology among persons of low social status. Following this definition, we can think of disparities in health status as the disproportionate amount of pathology among people, whether linked to socioeconomic status (SES), to race/ethnicity, to gender, or to other social factors. In that same address, Aneshensel argued that health disparities are due to both biological differences and social inequalities, as Adler and Rehkopf (2008) have also pointed out. In general, social scientists particularly tend to focus more on social inequalities because they may be avoidable and are unjust. They are the focus of this volume. In the article by Aneshensel that is entitled "Toward Explaining Mental Health Disparities," she focuses on mental rather than physical health, but this volume will consider all aspects of health. She makes an important point about research that is examining differences and disparities in health as being somewhat different from research that might focus on improving the mental health of the population overall. She argues that by focusing on how social inequities become health disparities, ultimately research also connects to the design of interventions that might alleviate health disparities, with a focus on mental health disparities in her article.

The growth in research about social differences in health or health disparities has been rapid. A recent review of U.S. disparities in health reported on a study that examined past literature for the term "health disparities" and found that this was a key word in only one article in 1980, fewer than 30 in the 1990s and in more than 400 articles from 2000 to 2004 (Adler & Rehkopf, 2008). If the term "health inequalities" was used instead, the pattern of increase was similar. These authors argue that previously, while there was research examining issues of health disparities, the research was more often framed within the context of specific factors such as poverty or race.

Some of the studies with great interest in differences by social factors were British in origin. In 1980, the Black Report in Great Britain was one of the first in that country to apply the term inequality to an examination of health differences. In this study, the expectations of the authors had been that they would find reductions in social class differences in mortality in Great Britain, due to the provision for almost 30 years of universal health care through the British National Health Service. Instead, they reported that the gap between the health of low and higher social class individuals had widened (Adler & Rehkopf, 2008). Some other studies also conducted within the same time frame in Great Britain found significant differences in cardiovascular disease and mortality by occupational level within a population of office-based workers (Marmot, Rose, Shipley, & Hamilton, 1978; Marmot, Shipley, & Rose, 1984). In these studies, the differences found were not only between the top and the bottom of the occupational scale, but increased at each step down in occupational grade.

Related research was also published in the United States in this same period, often linking together death and health information with information on SES from sources such as the Current Population Study, the U.S. Census, and Social Security Administration records (Kitagawa & Hauser, 1978; Kliss & Scheuren, 1978). These studies reported higher age-adjusted mortality rates for nonwhite, for individuals with less education and lower income, and for certain occupational categories.

These early studies led to the now well-known efforts in the United States to examine and try to eliminate health disparities due to race/ethnicity and SES in the *Healthy People* series. Within the federal government, one of the pushes for more research on healthcare inequalities came from the passage of Public Law 106-129, the Healthcare Research and Quality Act of 1999. That law directed the Agency for Healthcare Research and Quality (AHRQ) to develop two annual reports, one focused on quality and one focused on disparities. AHRQ was to track prevailing disparities in healthcare delivery as they relate to racial and socioeconomic factors among priority populations such as low-income groups, racial and ethnic minorities, women, children, the elderly, individuals with special healthcare needs, the disabled, people in need of long-term care, people requiring end-of-life care, and places of residence (rural communities). The first National Healthcare Disparities Report (2003) built on some previous efforts in the federal government, especially *Healthy People 2010* (U.S. Department of Health and Human Services, 2000) and the IOM 2002 Report, *Unequal Treatment: Confronting Racial and Economic Disparities in Healthcare* (Smedley, Stith, & Nelson, 2003). The elimination of disparities in health was a goal of *Healthy People 2010*. *Unequal Treatment* extensively documented healthcare disparities in the United States and focused on those related to race and ethnicity. One weakness of the report was there was not a focus on disparities related to SES. The Institute of Medicine (IOM) report on *Unequal Treatment* also looked at factors related to providers of care and argued providers' perceptions and, from that, their attitudes toward patients can be influenced by patient race or ethnicity (Smedley et al., 2003).

The National Healthcare Disparities Report (2003) did have a focus on the ability of Americans to access health care and variation in the quality of care. Disparities related to SES were included, along with disparities linked to race and ethnicity. In addition, the report began some exploration of the relationship between race/ethnicity and socioeconomic position. Some key findings from the report are important to review. First, inequality in quality of care continues to exist. These disparities often are particularly true for some more serious healthcare problems such as minorities being diagnosed with cancer at later stages, less often receiving optimal care when hospitalized for cardiac problems, and higher rates of avoidable hospital admissions among blacks and poorer patients. Differential access to health care may lead to disparities in quality of care actually received. In addition, opportunities to provide preventive care are often missed. The report closes with a call for more data, more research, and the linkage of those to policy within the United States.

In 2005, the third National Healthcare Disparities Report (2005) was released. One advantage of continuing reports is that they allow a comparison to previous years. This 2005 report focused on findings from a set of core report measures. The two measures of access covered were facilitators and barriers to care and healthcare utilization. The overall summary indicated that disparities still exist, but some disparities are diminishing, an encouraging result, but one that clearly leaves opportunities for further improvement. Disparities remain in both areas of access, all areas of quality, and across many levels and types of care including preventive care, treatment of acute conditions, and management of chronic disease. This applies to a various specific clinical conditions including cancer, diabetes, end stage renal disease, heart disease, HIV disease, mental health and substance abuse, and respiratory diseases.

Looking at access more specifically, major issues of disparity occur for poor people and Hispanics, with lesser but important issues for blacks, American Indians, and Asians. Poor people have worse access to care than high-income people for all eight core report measures. Hispanics have worse access for 88 percent of the core report measures, whereas blacks and American Indians have worse access on half of the measures. Asian Americans have worse access on 43 percent of the measures. The 2005 report also tracks changes in the core measures over time. For each core report measure, racial, ethnic, and socioeconomic groups were compared with a designated comparison group at various points in time. For racial minorities, more disparities in quality of care were becoming smaller rather than larger, whereas for Hispanics, 59 percent were becoming larger and 41 percent smaller. For poor people, half of disparities were becoming smaller and half were becoming larger.

RACE/ETHNICITY AND SES

Early work in sociology especially focused on social class differences, to the extent that data was available. As differences became redefined as disparities with the growth of the federal government efforts, there was greater focus on race/ethnicity. Partially, this was due to greater data availability and partially a belief, especially in the United States, that a policy focus necessitated more attention to race/ethnicity than to class. In more recent years, however, there has been a growing consensus whether in the United States or Great Britain that looking only at data on race/ethnicity without a consideration of social class differences can be problematic (Adler & Rehkopf, 2008; Smith, 2000; Kawachi, Daniels, & Robinson, 2005). One of the most important problems is the differences in the distribution of racial/ ethnic groups across levels of income, wealth, education, and occupation. If studies look only at race/ethnicity and ignore social class issues, it is too easy to conclude that differences are linked either specifically to race/ ethnicity or even to biological differences that may be linked to race and ethnicity (Issacs & Schroeder, 2004).

Recent studies do tend to examine issues in a more complex way, but this very complexity often makes interpretations of the results more difficult and makes it more difficult to make clear policy-oriented conclusions. For example, two recent articles published in *Journal of Health and Social Behavior* in a section entitled "Unraveling Racial and Ethnic Health Disparities" looked at race/ethnicity in combination with other factors and illustrate some of these complexities. Walton (2009) examined racial and ethnic minorities in the United States and the impact of racial segregation on birth weights. The results from this article will be discussed in more detailed under the section on geographic differences. In the second article in this section of the journal, perceived ethnic discrimination is contrasted with acculturation stress as factors that influence substance use among Latino youth in the southwest (Kulis, Marsiglia, & Nieri, 2009). More than half of the sample of fifth-grade students from the southwestern United States perceived some discrimination and almost half reported some acculturation stress. Spanish-dominant and bilingual youth perceived more discrimination than English-dominant youth. Youth who had been in the United States less time (five or fewer years) perceived more discrimination in the United States than youth with more time in the United States. The most acculturation stress was reported by youth who were Spanish-dominant or more recent arrivals. Because some of these results (such as that youth with less time in the United States perceived more discrimination than those who had lived in the United States longer) are inconsistent with research on Latino adults and because linguistic acculturation and time in the United States did not moderate the effects of perceived discrimination or acculturation stress, the article ends up discussing the need for longitudinal data and a much better understanding of the context of determining adaptation processes among immigrants.

In a commentary article in the *American Journal of Public Health* about the role of acculturation research in advancing science and practice to reduce healthcare disparities among Latinos, Zambrana and Carter-Pokras (2010) argue that despite an impressive body of public health knowledge that has been accumulated over the past decade on healthcare disparities among Latinos, inconclusive and conflicting results on predictors of healthcare disparities remain. If forced to make some conclusions, however, they argue that social and economic determinants are more important predictors than is culture in understanding healthcare disparities. They argue for a rethinking of the limitations of acculturation as both an organizing and theorizing principle in the study of Latino healthcare disparities.

Just a limited discussion of these two recent articles illustrates that the more factors that are considered in trying to understand the complexity between health differences and race/ethnicity and SES, the more confusing and more conflicting results researchers may find. It is not possible to summarize results with a few simple statements. If researchers add in complexities across many different racial/ethnic groups, and not just the consideration of Latinos as in these two studies, the complexities and disagreements only grow. One hope for this volume is that some of the studies will add to the complexity of this confusing literature, even though it is unlikely any one article will be able to be the definitive article on these topics.

A new report from the Institute of Medicine (2009) has recommended that researchers develop more detailed categories for race, ethnicity, and English language proficiency. The work of the IOM on this topic was begun in early 2009, at the request of the AHRQ. A Subcommittee on Standardized Collection of Race/Ethnicity Data for Healthcare Quality Improvement was formed. The subcommittee recommended collection of the existing Office of Management and Budget (OMB) race and Hispanic ethnicity categories as well as more fine-grained categories of ethnicity (referred to as granular ethnicity and based on one's ancestry) and language need (such as a rating of spoken English language proficiency of less than very well and information about one's preferred language for health-related encounters). In addition to these national standards, the committee also recommended that locally relevant categories of granular ethnicity and languages be made available and that individuals should be given the opportunity to self-identify their ethnicity or language when it is not listed specifically on local data collection instruments. They argue that to improve the quality of data collected and to be better able to stratify and compare quality performance measures across databases to be able to resolve some of the differences that occur in separate research studies, the importance of standardizing ways to collect data on race and ethnicity and language proficiency is very important. One important aspect of the recommendations from the IOM is that, based on the recommendations of this well-known national group, it is more likely that hospitals, health plans, and physician practices may actually modify the categories they currently use to collect information, and this would then make these applied sources of data more useful for research in the future.

Some of the same concerns about how information is gathered and disparate results depending on the exact ways data are gathered apply to the issue of SES and health disparities. Three traditional ways of measuring SES are occupation, income, and education. Each of these have somewhat different associations with health outcomes (Adler & Rehkopf, 2008; Kitagawa & Hauser, 1978; Kliss & Scheuren, 1978). In the United States, most studies now use income and education more often than occupation, because those questions are much simpler to ask and to code. In addition, in the United States, weaker associations have been found with measures of occupation as compared with income and education, perhaps because of the difficulty of having more standardized measures across studies (Adler & Rehkopf, 2008; Braveman et al., 2005).

Braveman et al. (2005) argue that SES is often implicitly or explicitly equated with income, especially in the United States. There are many problems and limitations with this. Even though researchers all recognize how important it is to obtain income information, many practitioners and some researchers consider income formation to be too sensitive to collect. Instead, information about education (typically measured as years completed or credentials of formal schooling) is more easily obtained and is frequently treated as a proxy for income (or for SES overall). In addition, income itself is a limited measure, and it is better to include measures of wealth as well as income. There is evidence that wealth measures are even more widely varied when racial/ethnic information is examined as linked to SES. Beyond the basic collection of information, in many studies when both income and education were obtained, researchers may hesitate to include both in analytic models because of concerns about colinearity. According to Braveman et al. (2005), both evidence from literature and new analyses they conducted all indicate that while standard measures of education and income are correlated, these correlations are generally not strong enough to justify using education as a proxy for income (or vice versa). Earnings do vary at similar educational levels, and this is even truer if researchers also take into account different social (e.g., racial/ethnic, sex, and age) groups.

Social Factors Leading to Differences in Health and Health Care

GENDER

Gender is an important social factor that has links to differences in health status as well as healthcare services utilization. Generally, women live longer than men, but may actually report poorer health status and especially more disabilities as they age. Women also generally are higher utilizers of the healthcare system. Previous research on gender and health and healthcare utilization also points out that gender differences may also vary by categories considered in the previous section, such as race/ethnicity and SES.

Recent specific studies, whether looking at broader health indicators such as self-rated health (Zheng, 2009) or more specific issues, sometimes in specific age groups such as among adolescents and sometimes with specific health outcomes such as smoking cessation (Castro et al., 2009) or adolescence and obesity (Clark, O'Malley, Schulenberg, & Lantz, 2009; Robinson, Stevens, Kaufman, & Gordon-Larsen, 2010), find complexities in examining issues of gender and health and healthcare disparities. The more general studies point to the need to consider social factors beyond gender to understand health disparities. In a study looking at rising U.S. income inequality and gender and self-rated health, Zheng (2009) finds that most previous research on the effect of income inequality on health has been based on sectional data and often finds mixed results. Using data from 1972 through 2004, Zheng finds that increases in income inequality increase the odds of worse self-reported health by 9.4 percent, but that overall income inequality and gender-specific income inequality harm men's, but not women's, self-rated health. Lack of attention to gender composition may be an important factor in discrepant findings in earlier studies. In a study looking at many indicators of health and healthcare utilization among adolescents, Mulye et al. (2009) argue that young adulthood is a particularly important period of life to examine when interested in health disparities. They find large differences on many different outcomes, after examining areas such as mortality, health-related behaviors, and healthcare access and utilization. They particularly point out that large disparities persist in many areas by race/ethnicity and gender, pointing out the importance of looking at gender but also looking at in along with other social factors such as race/ethnicity.

Recent studies that focus mainly on one or a few health outcomes but include gender as an important social factor in disparities in health and healthcare use also tend to argue that studies need to look at gender in relationship to other social factors. For studies with adolescents, for example, two different studies have looked at obesity and weight-related behaviors. In one study, the authors argue that social disparities in body weight may be due to declining trends in positive weight-related behaviors by black women, Hispanic women, and lower SES men as compared with white young adults of higher SES (Clark et al., 2009). Robinson et al. (2010) examine the differences between black women and men in obesity for young adults. They are particularly interested in whether adolescent behaviors such as hours of television, playing sports with a parent, and amount of physical activity explain the gender differences. Although black females did report less overall physical activity and being less likely to play sports with a parent, these behaviors did not explain the differences in obesity incidence. For whites, there was little gender disparity either before or after adjustments. This study has contrasting results from the previous study and points out the need to consider gender, but also race and the complexity of trying to explain health disparities in even a few health outcome areas and arriving at clear results. The understanding of the underlying mechanism for why black women have more obesity, for example, is not clearly explained well by either study.

GEOGRAPHY AND NEIGHBORHOOD

Another social factor related to differences and disparities in health and healthcare outcomes is geography, including neighborhood. If one looks at mortality as an outcome, for example, there are substantial differences related to geography in the United States, although most researchers believe that socioeconomic factors and race/ethnicity differences are important in explaining these geographic differences. There are some data that indicate that, within metropolitan areas, geographic variation can be explained mostly by these factors (Adler & Rehkopf, 2008). Other data lead to the conclusion that differences in local SES may have a more important impact on African American mortality, as contrasted to white mortality (Subramanian, Chen, Rehkopf, Waterman, & Krieger, 2005). Adler and Rehkopf (2008) conclude that the specific area matters when examining geographic variations in health outcomes and that the confusing relationships often found between geography, race/ethnicity, class, and health are not fixed within specific geographic areas and given periods.

In Walton's (2009) study of residential segregation and birth weight among racial and ethnic minorities in the United States, she finds that the racial segregation of racial and ethnic minorities within metropolitan areas has health consequences. She reports that segregation has a negative effect on the likelihood of having a low birth weight baby for Asian Americans, but that segregation marginally increases the odds of low birth weight babies for African Americans. In looking at a third important racial/ethnic group, Latino Americans, she finds that segregation does not impact birth weight.

Johnson, Call, and Blewett (2010) look at geographic variations with an ethnic group not included in the Walton study, American Indians, and focus on prenatal care as a healthcare outcome. One of their major research interests is whether national data on American Indians/Alaska Natives (AIAN) disparities mask geographic variations in access to care and disparities in access at the subnational levels of states and localities. They found that rates of late prenatal care and inadequate prenatal care utilization did vary by region and by state, and that these variances occurred for both AIANs and for non-Hispanic whites. Patterns were often complex. For example, the Midwest had the highest AIAN-White disparities on both of the indicators; however, it was the only region in which there were no significant changes in disparities over time. If only the 12 states with the largest AIAN birth populations were examined, changes in disparities in prenatal care utilization varied much more, and some states had substantial reductions in disparities but other states had substantial increases in disparities.

One other recent study has pointed out the complexity of looking at neighborhood as a geographic factor along with race (Scribner, Theall, Simonsen, Mason, & Yu, 2009). They found there can be a misspecification of the effect of race in fixed effects models of health inequalities if the issue of individuals being nested in the data within a neighborhood is not taken into account. Using all-cause mortality data from 1989–1991 from Los Angeles County in California, Scribner and colleagues found that single-level models showed blacks having 1.27 times the risk of mortality as compared to whites, but multilevel models demonstrated the importance of between census tract variance in mortality for both blacks and whites and that this was linked to neighborhood poverty. This study, as with several reviewed in this chapter, demonstrates just how complex the consideration of the role of social factors in health and health care can become, and how important it often becomes to consider multiple factors.

REVIEW OF ORGANIZATION OF THE BOOK

As mentioned previously, this volume is divided into five sections, of which the first section includes this introductory chapter. The second section entitled "Racial and Ethnic Factors in Differences in Health and Health

Care" includes six chapters. Several focus on racial differences, whereas some focus on ethnic differences and others look at class and race/ethnicity together in more complex approaches. The first chapter is by Suarez and looks at "Racial Disparities in Knowledge of Hepatitis C Virus (HCV)," which is highly prevalent in the United States, even though it does not receive much public attention. The author has conducted in-depth interviews with over 50 people with this health problem and focused on issues linked to race, of which one of the most important was that minority respondents have lower levels of knowledge about HCV. The second chapter in this section is by Webster and looks at "Medicare and Racial Disparities in Health: Fee-for-Service versus Managed Care." He limits his analyses to people 65 and over and provides evidence that there are racial differences in health services utilization between those on the traditional Medicare plan and those on a managed care Medicare plan. Carr, Ibuka, and Russell examine "How Much Time Do Americans Spend Seeking Health Care? – Racial and Ethnic Differences in Patient Experiences." Using data from the American Time Use Survey, the chapter examines racial differences in the amount of time people spend traveling to, waiting for, and receiving outpatient healthcare services and reports that both blacks and Hispanics spend more time receiving services and spend more time traveling to services. Bostean asks "Can the Behavioral Model Explain Immigrant Status and Ethnic Differences in U.S. Adults' CAM Use?" She reports that recent immigrants use CAM less than do the U.S.-born, partially linked to lack of knowledge. Guzman, Mireles, Christopherson, and Janning examine "Class and Race Health Disparities and Health Information Seeking Behaviors: The Role of Social Capital." They apply the concept of social capital in the examination of the quality of health information-seeking behavior through social networks. They find that social class affects perceived health status more strongly than race. The last chapter in this section by Dryfhout looks at "Racial Disparities in Stillbirths." Very little of the racial gap in stillbirths is explained by the medical or social epidemiological model.

Section III is "Geographic and Community Factors in Differences in Health and Health Care" and includes two chapters, discussing geographic and community factors. The first paper by Rogers looks at "Habilitative Therapy among Preschool Children: Regional Disparities in the Early Intervention Population." He reports the presence of disparities for these various types of therapies (physical therapy, speech therapy, and occupational therapy). Children in the South have low levels of therapy use and northeastern children have the highest rates of use for speech therapy. The second chapter by Watkin, White, Duncan, Wyant, Nicholson, Khubchandani and Chekuri looks at "Consumer-Directed Health Insurance vs. Managed Care: Analysis of HealthCare Utilization and Expenditures Incurred by Employees in a Rural Area." They suggest that consumer-directed healthcare plans may be a way to control healthcare costs in a rural state.

The fourth section on "Gender Differences in Health and Health Care" includes two chapters. Roussos, Mueller, Hill, Salas, Hovell, and Villarreal look at "Some Considerations Regarding Gender When a Healthcare Interpreter is Helping Providers and Their Limited English Proficient Patients." Because most interpreters are female, gender becomes an important issue in interpreted healthcare visits. Rich qualitative data help the researchers to explore this topic. The second gender-related chapter is by Bould and explores "Hidden Gender Inequalities in Old Age: Equal Treatment Does Not Mean Equal Results." This chapter reviews important aspects of data linked to aging and gender and points out that a male model of aging is less and less appropriate as issues are considered for the elderly, because the proportion female tends to increase in each aging decade.

The last section of the book focuses on two studies that deal with life course issues. Each deals with a different part of the life course. The first chapter by Lara-Cinisomo, Beckjord, and Keyser focuses on mothers and their perspectives during childbearing. A focus group approach was used with both women during the prenatal period and during the postpartum period to identify responsive strategies to improve the engagement of low-income and racially diverse mothers at high risk for depression. The second chapter by DiTullio and MacDonald deals with end of life issues, particularly issues of hospice care. Using an institutional ethnography approach in one Northeastern hospice over a six-month period, the authors uncover the linkages between local problems in the delivery of hospice care and extra local sites of power and constraint within the American healthcare system.

REFERENCES

Adler, N. E., & Rehkopf. (2008). U.S. disparities in health: Descriptions, causes and mechanisms. *Annual Review of Public Health, 29*, 235–252.

Aneshensel, C. S. (2009). Toward explaining mental health disparities. *Journal of Health and Social Behavior, 50*(December), 377–394.

Braveman, P. A., Cubbin, C., Egerter, S., Chideya, S., Marchi, K. S., Metzler, M., & Posner, S. (2005). Socioeconomic status in health research – One size does not fit all. *Journal of the American Medical Association, 294*, 2879–2888.

Castro, Y., Reitzel, L. R., Businelle, M. S., Kendzor, D. E., Mazas, C. A., Li, Y., Cofta-Woerpel, L., & Wetter, D. W. (2009). Acculturation differentially predicts smoking cessation among Latino men and women. *Cancer Epidemiology, Biomarkers and Prevention, 18*(12), 3468–3475.

Clark, P. J., O'Malley, P. M., Schulenberg, J. E., & Lantz, P. (2009). Differential treatment in weight-related health behaviors among American young adults by gender, race/ethnicity and socioeconomic status, 1984–2006. *American Journal of Public Health, 99*, 1893–1901.

Institute of Medicine. (2009). *Race, ethnicity, and language data: Standardization for health care quality improvement.* Washington, DC: Institute of Medicine.

Issacs, S. L., & Schroeder, S. A. (2004). Class – The ignored determinant of the nation's health. *New England Journal of Medicine, 351*(11), 1137–1142.

Johnson, P. J., Call, K. T., & Blewett, L. A. (2010). The importance of geographic data aggregation in assessing disparities in American Indian prenatal care. *American Journal of Public Health, 100*(1), 122–128.

Kawachi, I., Daniels, N., & Robinson, D. E. (2005). Health disparities by race and class: Why both matter. *Health Affairs, 24*, 343–352.

Kitagawa, E., & Hauser, P. (1978). *Differential mortality in the United States.* Cambridge, MA: Harvard University Press.

Kliss, B., & Scheuren, F. J. (1978). The 1973 CPS-IRS-SSA exact match study. *Social Security Bulletin, 42*, 14–22.

Kulis, S., Marsiglia, F. F., & Nieri, T. (2009). Perceived ethnic discrimination versus acculturation stress: Influences on substance use among Latino youth in the Southwest. *Journal of Health and Social Behavior, 50*(4), 443–459.

Marmot, M. G., Rose, G., Shipley, M. J., & Hamilton, P. J. S. (1978). Employment grade and coronary heart disease in British civil servants. *Journal of Epidemiology and Community Health, 32*, 244–249.

Marmot, M. G., Shipley, M. J., & Rose, G. (1984). Inequalities in death – Specific explanations of a general pattern. *Lancet, 323*, 1003–1006.

Mulye, T. P., Park, M. J., Nelson, C. D., Adams, S. H., Irwin, C. E., & Brindes, C. D. (2009). Trends in adolescent and young health in the United States. *Journal of Adolescent Health, 45*, 8–24.

National Healthcare Disparities Report. (2003). Agency for Healthcare Research and Quality, Rockville, MD. Available at http://www.ahrq.gov/qual/nhdr03/nhdr03.htm

National Healthcare Disparities Report. (2005). Agency for Healthcare Research and Quality, Rockville, MD, December. AHRQ Publication No. 06-0017. Available at www.ahrq.gov/qual/nhdr05/nhdr05.pdf

Robinson, W. R., Stevens, J., Kaufman, J. S., & Gordon-Larsen, P. (2010). The role of adolescent behaviors in the female-male disparity in obesity incidence in US black and white young adults. *Obesity, 18*(7), 1429–1436.

Scribner, R. A., Theall, K. P., Simonsen, N. R., Mason, K. E., & Yu, Q. (2009). Misspecification of the effect of race in fixed effects models of health inequalities. *Social Science and Medicine, 69*(11), 1584–1591.

Smedley, B. D., Stith, A. Y., & Nelson, A. R. (Eds). (2003). *Unequal treatment: Confronting racial and ethnic disparities in health care.* Institute of Medicine. Washington, DC: National Academies Press.

Smith, G. D. (2000). Learning to live with complexity: Ethnicity, socioeconomic position and health in Britain and the United States. *American Journal of Public Health*, 90, 1694–1698.

Subramanian, S. V., Chen, J. T., Rehkopf, D. H., Waterman, P., & Krieger, N. (2005). Racial disparities in context: A multilevel analysis of neighborhood variation in poverty and excess mortality among black populations In Massachusetts. *American Journal of Public Health*, 95, 260–265.

U.S. Department of Health and Human Services. (2000). *Healthy people 2010: With understanding and improving health and objectives for improving health*, November (2nd ed.). Washington, DC: U.S. Government Printing Office.

Walton, E. (2009). Residential segregation and birth weight among racial and ethnic minorities in the United States. *Journal of Health and Social Behavior*, 50(4), 427–442.

Zambrana, R. E., & Carter-Pokras, O. (2010). Role of acculturation research in advancing science and practice in reducing health care disparities among Latinos. *American Journal of Public Health*, 100(1), 18–23.

Zheng, H. (2009). Rising U.S. income inequality, gender, and individual self-rated health, 1972–2004. *Social Science and Medicine*, 69(9), 1333–1342.

SECTION II
RACIAL AND ETHNIC FACTORS IN DIFFERENCES IN HEALTH AND HEALTH CARE

RACIAL DISPARITIES IN KNOWLEDGE OF HEPATITIS C VIRUS (HCV)

Alicia Suarez

ABSTRACT

Hepatitis C virus (HCV) is highly prevalent in the United States, yet is largely culturally invisible. This study examines what people know about their illness, both before and after diagnosis, and the relationship to race. The data are from in-depth interviews in 2004 with 53 persons, mostly white or African American, with HCV in the southeastern United States. The respondents have varying educational backgrounds, family incomes, and possible modes of transmission of HCV. Regardless of whether the diagnosis of HCV came as a surprise, respondents had a range of reactions including fear, shock, sadness, and ambivalence. Knowledge of the disease postdiagnosis varies as some people have expert knowledge, moderate knowledge, or inaccurate to no knowledge of the disease. Minority respondents have less knowledge of HCV than whites. This racial disparity in knowledge has profound implications for people with HCV and the larger society.

INTRODUCTION

Hepatitis C virus (HCV) is the most common blood-borne pathogen in the United States, affecting an estimated 5 million Americans (Erickson, 2006). In fact, the number of deaths per year from HCV has exceeded deaths from HIV/AIDS since 2000. Similar to other diseases, African Americans have disproportionately high rates of HCV compared to whites and poorer health outcomes (Palmer, 2006). Despite the prevalence rate, HCV remains largely culturally invisible with scant public discourse and awareness campaigns (Suarez & Shindo, 2008).

Given the prevalence yet invisibility of HCV, it is important to ascertain what persons with HCV know about the disease and if this is affected by the race of the patient. According to Bury (1982), chronic illness is often a biographical disruption. Knowledge of one's illness affects the ability to deal with the problem of uncertainty surrounding one's health. Personal knowledge of HCV affects individuals' likelihood to disclose their illness to others and thus access social support or experience discrimination. The content of their disclosure also contributes to the accuracy of information about HCV in the public domain. Finally, accurate knowledge of HCV allows infected individuals to practice self-care, avoid transmission to others, and better their overall health outcomes.

This chapter addresses what persons with a culturally invisible chronic illness, HCV, know about their disease, the implications of that knowledge, and the effects of race. I assess people's experiences with a diagnosis of HCV and their reactions to diagnosis as this will likely affect their subsequent behaviors in terms of knowledge seeking and interactions with healthcare providers. I then address what people know about HCV and how this affects their illness experiences.

LITERATURE REVIEW

Knowledge concerning hepatitis and the liver is poor in the United States. Chronic HCV will lead to serious liver damage, cirrhosis, or liver cancer in approximately 10–25% of those with chronic infection over a 10- to 40-year period, making HCV the leading cause for liver transplants. Yet according to the American Liver Foundation, more than one in four U.S. adults did not know the liver was the primary organ affected by hepatitis (Orr, 2006). In addition, the vast majority of U.S. adults erroneously believe that alcohol abuse is the leading cause of liver disease (Orr, 2006). Nearly one in three persons erroneously thinks that HCV can be spread through fecal-contaminated food or water and does not know that HCV can be spread through any contact with infected blood (AGA, 2003). In fact, intravenous drug use accounts for the preponderance of recent transmissions in the United States. Before blood was routinely screened in 1992, transfusions were the most common method of transmission (Franciscus, 2002; Reddy, 2002). Other means of transmission are less common including needle stick exposures in healthcare settings (less than 10%), mother to infant transmission (less than 5%), and sexual transmission (less than 3%) (Franciscus & Highleyman, 2003).

Knowledge concerning symptoms, disease prevention, and treatment is also lacking. One in five Americans, including 15% of people with HCV, thinks there is a vaccine for HCV (AGA, 2003). Research among primary care residents finds that 66% surveyed would recommend vaccinating for HCV, despite there being no vaccination. Thus, even knowledge among healthcare providers is lacking (Coppola et al., 2004). Treatment usually consists of a combination of pegylated alpha interferon and ribavirin for a period of 24 or 48 weeks. However, response rates are currently around 50% depending on virus genotype, viral load, and several other factors, including race (with whites more responsive to treatment) (Reddy, 2002). In addition, side effects may be severe. Approximately one-third of Americans are unaware that there are prescription treatments for HCV (less than one in five persons with HCV is unaware of this). Many persons will have few to no symptoms for the first 20 years after infection, thus accounting for the many persons who are unaware they are infected and perhaps lack of public awareness of symptoms as only 38% of the public is sure of any of the symptoms (AGA, 2003; Franciscus & Highleyman, 2003). Active symptoms experienced by some with chronic infection include nausea, chronic fatigue, mood swings, loss of appetite, muscle or joint pain, headaches, indigestion, depression, "brain fog," and abdominal pain (Franciscus & Highleyman, 2003).

Evaluating levels of knowledge concerning HCV among people who inject drugs (PWID) is a further reflection of the lack of public awareness as PWID are at such high risks for infection and would presumably have more awareness (Heimer et al., 2002; Rhodes & Treloar, 2008). In one study of PWID, less than half of the sample knew there was no vaccine for HCV and could correctly answer items concerning the transmission of hepatitis through dried blood (Heimer et al., 2002). At least some PWID are aware that their knowledge of HCV is lacking and this causes them anxiety (Davis, Rhodes, & Martin, 2004). Research findings suggest that PWID obtain information about hepatitis from various types of healthcare facilities (Davis et al., 2004; Heimer et al., 2002). Because this population and other nondrug using low-income and minority groups have lower rates of healthcare utilization, their potential for hepatitis knowledge may be less than other groups who have more consistent interactions with healthcare workers (Smaje, 2000).

Attention to race and HCV is especially important as medical researchers have noted differences by race in rates of chronic HCV and responsiveness to treatment. Blacks have disproportionately high rates of HCV compared to whites in the United States with blacks accounting for 22% of the HCV population (Alter, Margolis, Bell, & Bice, 1998; Palmer, 2006). The disease progresses more quickly among blacks (Palmer, 2006; Reddy, 2002). In terms of treatment, whites in general respond better to treatment (Reddy, 2002). Blacks, however, are less likely to receive treatment once diagnosed (Palmer, 2006). Blacks with HCV have a slightly higher history of intravenous drug use (36%) compared to whites (28%) and Hispanics (23%), which may affect experience with the illness (Lepe, Layden-Almer, Layden, & Cotler, 2006). Blacks, generally, are less likely to receive preventative care and are more likely to report low levels of satisfaction with health services (Smaje 2000) (although see (Schnittker, Pescosolido, & Croghan, 2005). Research has found African American parents of children with attention-deficit/hyperactivity disorder (ADHD) have less knowledge of the disorder and less awareness of relevant services than white parents (Bussing, Gary, Mills, & Garvan, 2007). Finally, race and ethnicity have been found to affect the management of stigma for HIV-positive individuals (Tewksbury & McGaughey, 1997). Thus, the need to investigate the actual social experiences is paramount to understand these racial differences in health outcomes with HCV.

One critical component of the social experience of illness begins with diagnosis. Biographical disruption begins, according to Bury (1982), as soon as a person experiences symptoms, seeks help, or is diagnosed with an illness. The cultural invisibility of HCV suggests that the diagnostic experience may be different than for diseases with more cultural visibility. For example, persons with HCV most likely do not have any expectations or understandings about what it means to have HCV unlike persons diagnosed with a mental illness (Link, 1987). Persons with HCV may experience symptoms before they are aware of their infection. Or in contrast, persons may feel perfectly fine and suddenly be diagnosed with HCV. People's experiences of illness are shaped by their diagnostic experiences, interactions with their doctors (and others), as well as influenced by race, class, and gender (Brown, 1995).

Another aspect of biographical disruption involves the emerging disability and problem of uncertainty (Bury, 1982). Not all persons with HCV experience active symptoms, and even for those who have experienced symptoms, there may be times when they have no symptoms. Actual physical experiences of symptoms affect how individuals conceptualize the disease (Albrecht & Levy, 1991). The problem of uncertainty involves the unpredictable course of the illness and also medical discourse. Chronically ill people realize medical knowledge is limited and often combine medical knowledge with their own biographical experiences. Bury notes that, "moral concerns and scientific-based knowledge overlap" (Bury, 1982). Thus, persons do not passively accept expert knowledge, but reinterpret this knowledge along with lay experience. Chronically ill individuals often explain causation through reference to the self, the body, and society (Williams, 1984). Thus instead of persons being disillusioned with medical knowledge, they appropriate it. Medicine can be both a relief and a constraint in making sense of illness.

Given what we know about biographical disruption and chronic illness experience, the lack of cultural imagery about HCV leads to several questions regarding diagnosis, knowledge, and race: *How do people with HCV come to be diagnosed? What are their reactions to diagnosis? What do people with HCV know about their disease? What are the implications of their knowledge about HCV? Does race affect these processes?*

METHODS

Sample

Respondents in this research are 53 men and women over 18 who have or had HCV. The data was collected from May 2004 through July 2004 in a mid-sized metropolitan area in the southeastern United States. The city has nearly a quarter million citizens with African Americans slightly outnumbering Caucasians (U.S. Census Bureau 2000). Potential respondents were located through a public, hepatitis clinic at a teaching hospital that provides care mainly to economically marginalized persons ($N = 21$), the private practice of a hepatologist ($N = 22$), a local support group for HCV ($N = 5$), and through personal contacts in the area ($N = 5$). I used purposive sampling to gain diversity by race as reflected in this locale's demographics (34 respondents identified as white, 16 respondents identified as African American, and 3 respondents identified as Asian).

Respondents met the researcher at a location of their choice. Over half of the interviews took place at the respondents' homes. Other interviews took place in public venues such as public libraries, coffee shops, and diners. A few interviews were conducted in private rooms at the public clinic. Each respondent signed an informed consent sheet acknowledging their rights. All respondents agreed to be tape recorded. Ethical approval was received from the researcher's affiliated institution at that time and the hospital review board for recruitment at the hepatitis clinic. The researcher clearly explained that the research was not in association with their healthcare provider nor would any information received be relayed to their healthcare providers.

Instrument

I conducted all of the interviews, which lasted approximately an hour, using a semistructured interview guide. The guide addressed the following issues: respondents' relationships and lives prediagnosis, the diagnostic experience and subsequent reactions, issues of disclosure, reaction to disclosures, knowledge of HCV before and after diagnosis, current health status including experience with treatment, and the overall meaning(s) of their illness. The guide was pretested to assess the instrument.

Analysis

Each interview was transcribed verbatim and checked for accuracy. All respondents have been assigned pseudonyms. The transcribed interviews were entered into Atlas.ti, a qualitative data analysis program. Each interview was carefully read along with the accompanying field notes. The approach for coding falls between what some see as a technical approach versus an emergent intuitive approach in that the data were approached with regard to specific research questions in mind (Marshall & Rossman, 1999). For example, the data were labeled in terms of broad categories, such as diagnosis. Later, the category of diagnosis was further refined into typologies, such as surprise diagnosis and individual initiated diagnosis (Lofland & Lofland, 1995). Thus, all the transcripts were read with attention to diagnosis; yet, other themes that emerged were also noted. Codes were continuously revised, collapsed, and expanded during the data analysis process. The data were not sorted by race, class, or gender during coding to allow for patterns to emerge rather than forcing any clusters on the data. Only after coding were the data explored with regard to demographics.

Although these data are qualitative and most appropriately analyzed with that methodology in mind, some quantitative comparisons were performed to assess relationships between different variables. The data were quantified using Microsoft Excel and analyzed using STATA. Although there are limited approaches to quantitatively assessing this type of data, the results do strengthen the arguments set forth from the qualitative analysis. Therefore, I do refer to some chi-square analyses in the following sections (tables available upon request).[1]

FINDINGS AND DISCUSSION

Prior Knowledge of HCV

For most diseases, there exists vast cultural imagery and discourse. Once becoming diagnosed, individuals must then come to terms with what that discourse means now that it applies to them. This phenomenon is the crux of modified labeling theory. It is more difficult, however, to apply this theoretical approach to HCV because there is a lack of expectations about what it means to have the disease. Many have never even heard of it. Of the 45 interviews in which I could establish their previous knowledge about HCV, 56% said they had heard of HCV before diagnosis. However, 29% of the sample either admitted to just having heard of it, but not knowing anything about it or gave no indication that they knew anything about the disease. David explained, "I had heard of hepatitis A and B and I heard that there were some other varieties of hepatitis, which I didn't know anything about, I just, was nothing I even thought about really." Daniel said, "I didn't know what it did to you, I didn't know that it, I didn't know it was a liver sickness, nothin'. I didn't know any of that, I just knew that it was, it was hepatitis, and it was a, it was a sickness."

Slightly over a quarter of the sample had information beyond having heard of the disease. Daisy said, "Well, I'd heard of it, but I, you know I never dreamed I'd ever you know have it. I've always heard of A, B, and, and C. I always heard it was the silent disease, killin' disease and all. That's the first thing that goes through a person's mind, you know." Some learned of HCV because of their drug use. Ronald said, "But I had heard of hepatitis C plenty because of bein' part of the drug culture." Samantha adds, "The last time when I went out and really messed up in life, like everybody I was around had hepatitis C and I saw some people die from it, you know." Several others had information because of working in health care and law enforcement. Thus, some respondents did have some previous knowledge about the disease before being diagnosed, albeit not always accurate knowledge. Because there is still such a lack of larger, cultural imagery surrounding HCV, having knowledge about HCV did not necessarily give respondents a sense of what it meant to have HCV.

Diagnosis

For many persons with HCV, their diagnosis came as a complete shock as they had no idea that they were sick in any way. Over half of the respondents found out they had HCV in this fashion.

Routine Screening

Nineteen persons were diagnosed because of results from routine screening. Mark recalled, "Had to take a physical, cuz we were changing the insurances at work, and the liver enzymes showed up high." Jenn was trying to get involved in a research study for her diabetes and was diagnosed as a result. Ronald explained,

> I had insurance, and I thought that I was in real good health, so in – to, to go and just to celebrate my great health, I just, you know, took advantage of the insurance and went in for a physical. A routine, general physical. And that led to this diagnosis. When they did the blood work they said you have elevated enzymes in your liver and we need to kinda, you know, see what that's about, and so I didn't you know, really wasn't thinking about what that meant, but that's what it meant. So it led to the diagnosis.

Several respondents were tested while in rehabilitation centers. Samantha described her experience, "Yeah, and I went to go ahead and you know, they gave me a blood test and all that to make sure, because they were going to put me on Antabuse and make sure my liver all right." Meredith found out while in prison for a drug-related charge, "But while I was there they, right before I left for boot camp they took blood tests and the longer you're there the more they'll do different blood tests. And that's when they found out. And they told me that I had hepatitis C."

Blood Donation/Plasma Center

Donating blood or selling plasma led to a diagnosis for eight respondents. David said, "My mother was havin' surgery and she needed some blood on reserve, and so me and my brother went in." Nick described how he gave blood as a way to get tested for blood-borne diseases because he had been an intravenous drug user. Rick and Charlie were informed about having HCV from letters from the blood donation organizations. Bob found out from a plasma center, "'You have hep C' and I was like, I didn't know what that was and that's pretty much what I said, I was like so what does that mean, do I get the rest of the money or …"

Informed by Hospital
One respondent was informed about possibly having HCV through a letter she received from the military. While in the service, she had a blood transfusion. The hospital went back through the records and contacted anyone who had received blood before a certain year that they may have been exposed to HCV because it was before blood was being screened for it. She was tested and diagnosed.

While many respondents were completely caught off guard regarding their diagnosis, 20 respondents were experiencing symptoms and sought medical attention and 3 other respondents requested or were advised for specific testing for HCV.

Symptoms
Numerous respondents sought care because of fatigue or problems/pain with their stomachs, sides, or backs. It took several months after first seeking care that Sharon was diagnosed:

> It took us till about May to go through all the tests that are natural and normal and I was fine. I mean everything about me was fine, I was just so tired. Uh, and then I got to a point where I would walk in this door and I would on hands and knees crawl upstairs to my bedroom. I could not make it standin' up. And I went back and I said, John [*her physician*] I can't stand this. You know, this is not right. That's when he said, let's try the hepatitis.

Several respondents had severe symptoms, such as profuse vomiting of blood, that led to their diagnoses with HCV. Daisy had a frightening experience. Her husband explained,

> Then one day here she started bleedin' real bad and she went to the bathroom and she was just, full of blood, you know. So we took, I took her and she got weaker and weaker and weaker. So I took her to the doctor, and they, they checked her as to whether there's somethin' wrong you know, they went down into her esophagus, and all that, and checked all that, and found out she was bleedin' from the inside. Come to find out she had varices veins …"

Asymptomatic Testing

Two respondents asked to be tested because of suspicions about HCV. Tari's husband was first diagnosed with HCV and she said,

> Uh huh, and I used to use his razors and stuff, and after, when we got married earlier on, and after he got diagnosed with it, it was always in the back of my mind, you know, cause I kept thinking well I used his razors back then. And we never knew when it happened to him so it was like ... God.

She subsequently asked her doctor to test her. Larry found out a friend died from HCV:

> So I start really researching, and you know, looking into it. I had heard, that you know, hepatitis C could be, is fatal in some cases. And the more and more research I dig in to, I said, well I better go and get tested. Cuz I got it from him, I know I did.

Reaction to Diagnosis

According to Link (1987), once patients are diagnosed, they must now apply what it means to have that label on a personal level. The lack of information regarding HCV or misinformation shaped respondents' reactions.

Fear of the Unknown

A classic reaction to diagnosis is a feeling of uncertainty, according to Bury (1982). Several respondents explicitly discussed how they were fearful because they did not have any knowledge of HCV. Catherine said of first finding out:

> Cuz at first when I, when they first told me, it did scare me, because I didn't have the knowledge that I do have [*now*]. And when they first told me it was like, ok it's like a light that goes off, it's like, you know, you quite don't know what hepatitis is, but you know it's somethin' scary.

Rick explained, "Well, I was inquisitive. I wanted to know what the hell it was ... and that scared me worse, had me freaked out for a long time not knowing what the hell was going on, after I realized they didn't know too much either you know." Thus for Rick, the lack of clarity regarding HCV among healthcare professionals exacerbated his fear.

Shock

Many respondents mentioned feeling shocked by their diagnosis. Sharon relayed information her doctor had told her,

Eventually we'll check you for hepatitis but I know you don't have that cause you didn't do IV drugs. You know and I knew during all that time and he said, anyway, it's a hell of a way to die. And at the time it was, cause there was no Interferon or anything when he had said that, those words stuck in my head. And I probably cried for three solid weeks.

Daisy said upon being diagnosed, "Oh Lord, I thought the world was comin' to an end."

Maruf's shock resulted from the dissonance in his conceptions of self and reality after diagnosis:

> I'm a strong person, and I can't, I don't give up that easy, but I felt bad I mean I couldn't sleep that night knowing that, thinking I'm healthy all my life I'm not ... That I've had something in me for the past ten or twelve years and I didn't even know about.

Fear of Imminent Death

Several respondents mentioned feeling they were going to die. Liz said, "He said, he said I had hepatitis C and I was moderately active cirrhosis, and I thought, I'm gonna die. You know, that's it, I'm gonna die. Y'all just, you know, I guess I better go get myself in order or whatever, you know."

Ronald said,

> Oh, I felt, um ... pretty much devastated. Emotionally pretty much devastated and, and I felt, you know, like, I tend to sort of, I don't know if you call it overreact or what to some circumstances, but I felt like I had been given a death sentence and that my life was basically over.

Sadness

A few respondents specifically mentioned feeling depression as their reaction to diagnosis. Grant said after being diagnosed, "I'm like ooh man, it's just like I'm feelin' depressed – like I went into depression." Sherri, who was all ready suffering from depression at the time of diagnosis, said, "It depressed me more."

Ambivalence

In contrast to respondents who felt shocked, depressed, or fearful, other respondents reported a lackadaisical response to their diagnosis, possibly as a means of denial for some. Daniel explained how he did not really follow up with medical care after diagnosis because of lack of insurance:

> And, and I went and seen the other man one time and he, I did some more tests with him and, to, to, make, you know, clarify that I did have it and I did. And, he wanted to start checkin' into it, but I didn't have insurance ... So I went, I guess I went almost a year without doing anything about it.

David said, "I just didn't, put a lotta seriousness into it, it's hard for me to put serious-seriousness into it right now even, because of the fact that I feel pretty good." Tom also did not place a lot of importance on the initial diagnosis. He said, "Like I had, I had other stuff going on." Sallie Anne said, "I mean when I first found out, when I found out, I was kinda upset, and then when I re-re found out again [*she was diagnosed with non-A, non-B hepatitis years before*], I was really upset, for about 2.5 seconds" (emphasis added). Peggy was concerned about the inconvenience. "Just that it would be a pain in the ass though until you got well, you know with the costs and everything." Unlike respondents who cited the lack of information about the disease as a source of fear, Jamie's lack of knowledge kept her from worrying. Jamie said,

> Well, I mean, well, I was, I was, like I said I didn't know anything about it, and I think I was thinking it was something that could be cured cause he was saying he could put me on this medication and it would help clear up my liver and different things like that. So, I thought it was something that you know that could be cleared up.

Knowledge about HCV

Previous knowledge or lack thereof about HCV may affect the initial reaction to diagnosis. Gaining medical knowledge after diagnosis can be a response to uncertainty (Bury, 1982). It is important to assess respondents' understanding of HCV at the time of the interview to evaluate how current knowledge impacted their illness experience.

Expert Knowledge
Almost one-third of respondents (29%) knew a great deal about HCV. This group of men and women were mostly white except for one Asian woman and one black woman. Their educational backgrounds and income were quite diverse. Over half of this group reported intravenous drug usage as the likely mode of transmission. These respondents understood the disease and the treatment available in a manner commiserate with most healthcare providers' presentation of the disease. While there was a range of knowledge among these respondents, all of the persons accurately discussed numbers such as viral loads and biopsy scores. Isabella said, "He did the viral load which, you know, shows you how many copies per mil–, milliliters is in your blood." Not all of the respondents were familiar with genotypes of the virus in this category but some were.

An overwhelming trend among these respondents was their impetus to seek out information. Melissa said, "And, I remember leaving his office, and the first thing I did, although I don't quite remember it is, I drove straight to Barnes and Nobles book section ... And then just read, you know, devoured them, highlighted, you know." She talked about contacting one of the pharmaceutical companies:

> And spoke with the people in the research department there, and I got information sent to me at the time, which I can't get now. Um, evidently they're really tight about their research, and I didn't tell them who I was, and they didn't ask. So, they sent it to me like I was a doctor [M laughs].

Connie, a Japanese woman, was diagnosed in the early 1980s when little information was available. "So, I wrote to Japan and they send me any of the news that all the information how you contract and how you going to be and how to do those blood tests and those kinda things. There was much more information [*in Japan*]." Sharon said, "I hounded the Internet for information. I ordered books upon books upon books." Catherine, the only African American with this level of knowledge said,

> I just started reading, I started going to the library, I started reading up stuff on it, and just picking up pamphlets everywhere, and every time I would go somewhere, and I would see something about hepatitis I would get it and read it and everything. I just got all the knowledge that I can get off of it, cuz I wanted to know everything there was about it.

Despite the public clinic being very busy, Meredith described her experiences there:

> I have no qualms about asking a million questions and clinics are a good atmosphere. They always have people involved that are just so willing to answer, you know—I mean it's not like they're [*indecipherable*] and just seein' me like cattle, no, if you're articulate and you speak to them and you have, and you have a legitimate question or if they see that like you're, you're writing down your question oh by the way, you know, oh yeah this is what I want to, you know, that sorta thing, they actually like that sorta thing because it's like, well my efforts aren't being wasted, you know.

Meredith discussed how persons being seen at the public clinic can get extensive information, but that they must be proactive and engaged with the staff to do so. Meredith is a white woman with some college who may have the skills necessary to extract this knowledge in that setting. It is unclear, however, whether persons of varied social class and ethnic backgrounds have the same interaction skills available or whether medical personnel would interact with diverse persons in a similar fashion.

Several respondents discussed researching past records as to how or when they were infected. Liz tried to find records from when her child was born and she had a cesarean section. David tried to assess when he might have been infected:

> I went back as far as possible trying to find all lab blood reports that I had, where I had complete blood counts, and, blood work done. In the earliest one I remember was done when I was in my early twenties, twenty, twenty-one, twenty-two years old, and they, they didn't even have a record of it, they had to dig it up on microfilm. Had to pay 'em money to do that, had to research this stuff to find it. But they did locate it ... and the enzymes on the, were elevated.

Moderate Knowledge

Over half of all respondents have what can be conceptualized as moderate knowledge of HCV. Unlike the respondents with expert knowledge, this group is much more racially and ethnically diverse. Again, there does not appear to be a trend regarding educational background, income, reported mode of transmission, and knowledge level. These respondents understand the disease for the most part, but few talk in numbers or are perhaps inaccurate if numbers are mentioned. Some of these persons did, similar to those with expert knowledge, mention researching the disease. Vanessa said,

> I read on the internet about, you know, the facts and that kind of stuff, but then I was, you know, I felt blessed because I wasn't, I guess I wasn't as bad as some of the people that I read about, you know [*with regards to side effects from medication*].

Although Vanessa did not speak in specifics, her understanding of the disease and comparison to others helped her to feel better about her own experience. Not all respondents sought out information as Ronald said,

> I, and I'm still not well-educated. I've been kind of in denial. I've stayed in denial to some degree about it. Now, I mean, you know, I don't study it very much or anything ... I guess they just gave me some general – they gave me some literature to read, a nice booklet that looked real professional and scientifically based, which I haven't read.

Although some respondents did seek out information about HCV, respondents with moderate knowledge were often unfamiliar with the technical language used to describe the disease and tests or discussed results in general terms. For example, Tari said of her biopsy results, which are presented in terms of grading and staging, "I can't remember, there was a one, which it wasn't that, that was like the, it wasn't like stage one. It was more like a percentage." She did mention that "my labs you can't tell that anything is wrong with me." Andrew said of his biopsy, "Then, there wasn't you know, there wasn't too much corrosion, it was lookin fine."

A few respondents seemed to almost have expert knowledge with regard to details such as their viral load or even the genotype of their virus but mentioned other fairly important aspects of the disease that were inaccurate. Derrick understood his liver enzymes were high, which led to his diagnosis. He also knew his liver staging and his genotype. But he added that, "So I mean I knew that there was no cure, that it was really slow, and that you would either need a liver transplant or you're gonna die." HCV is estimated to lead to serious liver disease in roughly 20% of those infected (Franciscus & Highleyman, 2003). Charlie, who catalogued his liver enzyme tests in an Excel file, said of his friend, "He has hepatitis, and he has it bad, like his viral count is at least 8 million. Mine's 825,000." Viral count, however, is not related to prognosis per se. Lauren knows her viral load and understands the medications. Yet, she said no one in her family had a history of hepatitis C, but HCV is not a genetic disease. She also said, "That it's always fatal, and gettin' liver cancer and I think and I don't know, I forgot, 40 percent of people that get liver cancer or 70?". Most research indicates that chances of HCV leading to liver cancer are less than 15% with most citing less than 5% chance (Franciscus & Highleyman, 2003).

Several people discussed a "fast" or "worst" kind of HCV, which was perhaps a reference to genotypes although the genotype of the virus is unrelated to progression of the disease. Genotype is, however, related to responsiveness to treatment and length of treatment, which may be what confused some. Lauren explained,

> I haven't heard any, except the other doctor said that mine must be the very slow kind. I have the worst kind ... .And probably been, all, all different kinds [*of donor blood*], mixed in together, that's how I wound up with the worst kind.

Ronald also mentioned this:

> And that it progresses – there's a slower progressing and a faster progressing and that, you know, depending on your own immune system and your own lifestyle, you know, so what I decided to do was to, was to wait and get another liver biopsy and determine which if it was progressing – how fast it was progressing."

Larry said, "I have genotype 1, which is the worst one. Or, I forget if they call it 1 or A."

In addition to discussing "worse" kinds of HCV, a few respondents compared HCV to other types of viral hepatitis. Although their knowledge of HCV was moderately accurate, their awareness of other types of hepatitis was highly inaccurate. Derrick said, "And they know that A and B are highly contagious and are highly aggressive and can kill you in a week." Charlie explained an interaction with his brother:

> So he fretted all weekend, he finally called me up on Sunday and says, you don't have Hepatitis B, do you? I said, hell no, man, I've got C. Don't – God. Thank God ... Well, he said, yah, because B is worse than C ... With B you're – you've got one foot in the grave and the other one on a banana peel. So he was kinda – because you've got longevity with it, you know, people get hepatitis C and it never jumps up in their face."

Bob said, "I mean he basically told me that it wasn't hepatitis B; so it wasn't, you know, fatal in the immediate sense." These respondents may have been using other types of hepatitis as a deviance exemplar (Ronai & Cross, 2002). In other words, their confusion about the nature of hepatitis B may have allowed them to feel better that they had HCV which was not as severe or bad in their mind.

There was confusion among several respondents regarding sexual transmission. Sexual transmission of HCV is regarded as fairly rare and is associated with less common sexual practices (Franciscus & Highleyman, 2003). Andrew said, "where I got this sexually transmitted disease you know and you got to be very careful and if you date somebody you got to be extra careful and this and that." Mark alludes that he may have got it from promiscuity. It is not unfeasible that persons are confused about sexual transmission, however, as sexual transmission is sometimes listed as a means of transmission despite the improbability.

Little/Inaccurate Knowledge
One-fifth of persons interviewed had either little to no knowledge of HCV or grossly inaccurate information. All but one in the group is black. None of these respondents had a college degree. These respondents often did not know anything about various tests and had a rudimentary understanding of HCV, if any. Ellis understood that his previous experience with treatment kept the virus at bay while on treatment. He talked of having a "spot on his liver." He was on treatment again and said, "and all my blood tests showed up negative I asked them what that meant and they told me that it means that the medicine's workin and I think that's fine." Jerry did not know who diagnosed him with HCV or when he was diagnosed. He said the doctor told him, "And he got the results back and he said my liver's 95% good." While Mack knew he had lower levels of the virus and that doctors did not recommend treatment for him, he did not know if he had a biopsy or not.

The main confusion for this group of respondents was with regard to modes of transmission. Several respondents told me implausible modes of receiving the virus. Although Sparky is knowledgeable with regard to treatment and tests regarding HCV, he told coworkers and believed he may have got it through binge drinking. Sparky explained, "I think I got it from drinking ... I drank, I'd buy a fifth of Wild Turkey, and drink straight whiskey til I'd throw up, and drink some more, and drink some more, and drink some more." Later he revealed "Uh, I did ... I did IV drugs for awhile." He did not offer this as a means of transmission however. Ellis said, "And I think that's why I got the hepatitis, from drinkin' alcohol that's what started that feelin. The other thing only thing I can know, we used to swim in the canal as a kid over there. Back then we drank a lot."

Matthew, who talked mainly of his drug addiction during the interview, added, "And that's anotha thing you know they say that my hepatitis C come from drink."

Little Brother did not know anything about the results of his biopsy or that there could be side effects from the treatment that he was on. Little Brother said about how he might have contracted HCV:

> Yeah, said it could be a earring, could be drinkin' behind somebody. She said it could be a couple a things. Cause in that plant [*chemical plant where he used to work*] you know, you just can't say, she say, you never know, could be a couple a things.

He said of avoiding transmission to others, "Yeah they told me. Uh ... use rubbers and use some other kinda liquid stuff. Don't use, you know, straight out naked, you know what I'm talkin about, you give it to somebody else." Jerry did not know how people get HCV or how he got it.

A few other respondents were aware of how they probably got HCV. Sherri knew that she probably got HCV through a transfusion before a surgery but she knew nothing about treatment or the disease except that it affected the liver. Mack did say he might have gotten HCV through intravenous drug use, but was confused about sexual transmission and kept making comments about homosexual behavior. Although Ann said she was infected from a transfusion, she seemed confused about how it was transmitted:

> Um ... well if in a sense like wanted to know, what could people really do to prevent it. What people could do, I feel sometime a lotta things have to do with the type of food we eat, not being clean. You know, not using the proper utensils, like when you get to doin' something, I mean I just use the example, workin' out in your yard and cleanin' the, the flowers or whatever and some people have a tendency to come in and not wash their hands, and I guess wit me workin' with children, I got in the practice of always washin' your hands. That's a part of sanitary-well if you don't, if your hands are dirty, whatever you touch, your mouth, your, you know if you have a open sore, and that leaves openin'

for other things ta happen to your body. So I guess that part I've always been kinda interested in hearing what I been wantin' to know about that.

Stick told me he had hepatitis B, not C but then accurately described how HCV is transmitted. He said he told his wife. "So, I came back and I told her I had hepatitis B and ... she said somethin like that and I said, well I said you don't catch it, I don't mean you catch it through sex ... You gotta share a needle or something like that." Stick did, however, have HCV as well as HBV.

Ramifications of HCV Knowledge

Knowledge about HCV is variable supporting findings by Heimer and colleagues (2002) as well as Davis et al. (2004). The majority of respondents have a moderate understanding of the disease with some misinformation. A select minority has incorporated physician's terminology into their parlance and can speak eloquently about their disease. Unfortunately, another group has very little understanding of their disease. The most troubling finding regarding HCV knowledge is the strong relationship to racial and ethnic identity whereby minorities are much more likely to have little or inaccurate knowledge ($\chi^2 = 18.38$, $p < .001$). Knowledge does not appear to be related to educational obtainments, income, gender, or mode of transmission. The majority of respondents were patients of one physician or attended the same clinic, thus suggesting that the doctor–patient interactions may be affected by the race of the patient in terms of the cultural relevance of the information discussed.

Knowledge about HCV has both costs and benefits for individuals. Greater knowledge is related to reporting felt stigma ($\chi^2 = 7.77$, $p < .05$) and enacted stigma ($\chi^2 = 6.85$, $p < .05$). Thus, understanding HCV promotes self-labeling and attunement to negative reactions from others. As discussed elsewhere, whites reported experiencing felt and enacted stigma more so than racial and ethnic minorities. Whites also disclosed more openly as discussed elsewhere. HCV knowledge and levels of disclosure are also related to each other ($\chi^2 = 9.06$, $p < .01$). Persons reporting positive reactions from disclosure in the workplace are more likely to have accurate knowledge ($\chi^2 = 7.26$, $p < .05$). Positive reactions from the family are also related to accurate knowledge ($\chi^2 = 6.58$, $p < .05$). Thus, while having an advanced understanding of HCV may lead to greater feelings of stigmatization, it also leads to greater levels of disclosure and accessing positive support in the workplace and from family. Knowledge can be empowering and provide hope for individuals especially as individuals struggle with a tenuous future after diagnosis.

Part of the process of biographical disruption according to Bury (1982) involves the problem of uncertainty. Gaining knowledge about the disease can help alleviate some aspects of the uncertainty. Samantha said, "Knowing how common it is, knowing that a lot of people live productive lives with it, knowing that there's medications for it. I guess that what keeps me not depressed about it. Pretty much, I guess that's helpful." Harold said, "But, I come to realize if you know the education that I've learned and that it's not a death sentence." While ignorance may be bliss in terms of not engaging in felt stigma or recognizing enacted stigma, the risks to physical health, lack of support because of low levels of disclosure, misinformation provided to others by those with little knowledge, and possible transmission because of a lack of knowledge are deleterious and harmful for not only those with little or inaccurate knowledge but also for society as a whole.

CONCLUSION

The process of diagnosis is crucial to the labeling process of having HCV. The manner in which persons came to be diagnosed, either as a surprise or individual initiated diagnosis, appears unrelated to the reactions to diagnosis. Respondents who received letters informing them of their HCV status did often express anger at being informed in this fashion, but had similar reactions to diagnosis as others who were informed in person.

The ensuing reactions of fear of the unknown, shock, fear of imminent death, and sadness are all typical reactions to diagnosis with chronic illness (Bury, 1991, 2000; Charmaz, 1991). The scant research on HCV suggests that persons generally experience a severe and negative reaction to diagnosis (Glacken, Kernohan, & Coates, 2001; Hepworth & Krug, 1999; Hopwood & Southgate, 2003). Hepworth and Krug (1999) note,

> The identities that people have through their relations with others are directly affected by a diagnosis of HCV in that histories and stories about self are challenged, rewritten, and forced to take on new meaning as new discourses intrude into people's lives. (p. 242)

Although I also found that many respondents did have an intense reaction to diagnosis, not all did. As discussed, some respondents had an ambivalent reaction to their diagnosis. For some, the lack of symptoms associated with the diagnosis made it easy to deny the severity or salience of the diagnosis. Bury (2000) discusses how the impact on the body is crucial to understanding identity changes. Other respondents did have symptoms, but still did not describe having an emotional reaction. For Jamie, the ambivalence was related to her lack of knowledge about the disease, but Peggy had fairly accurate knowledge of the disease and was still ambivalent. Perhaps, the respondents who described an ambivalent response are simply organizing their illness account along these lines to minimize disruptions to their identities. Yet, for most, at other points in the interview, they described how HCV did impact them later. Whereas Radley (1989) suggests that indifference to illness increases as social class decreases, there did not seem to be a relationship between an ambivalent reaction and social class, race, or gender in this sample. An ambivalent reaction to diagnosis was linked to practicing reluctant or limited disclosure ($\chi^2 = 4.39$, $p<.05$) most likely because the illness was less salient for these individuals.

The diagnostic process itself may affect knowledge about the disease. Persons may or may not receive testing and subsequent treatment after an initial diagnosis. Most of my respondents were under the care of a physician and had some diagnostic testing done if not also treatment. Although there was diversity in terms of previous knowledge about HCV before diagnosis, we might expect there to be more of a convergence in knowledge after diagnosis, especially for persons receiving care in the same setting. Instead, I found various levels of knowledge about HCV at the time of the interview. Whereas Krug (1995) notes "the impact of an initial positive diagnosis [of HCV] carries with it an almost inevitable desire for information" (p. 312), I found a strong desire for information among persons with expert levels of knowledge and among some with moderate knowledge. Among my sample, there is a connection between attending support groups and expert levels of knowledge. Certainly not all of the respondents in this research described wanting more information, which may be linked to preferring uncertainty than a stark reality (Weitz, 1989).

Most importantly, racial minorities, who in this sample are mostly African American, are more likely to have little or inaccurate knowledge about their disease. Persons of all racial and ethnic backgrounds had different experiences with diagnosis. Most people were largely unaware of HCV before diagnosis or had little knowledge. Initial reactions to diagnosis were undifferentiated by race or ethnicity. The ensuing behaviors were, however, influenced by race.

Knowledge about the disease leads to more open levels of disclosure but also negative self-labeling and reporting experiencing discrimination from others. African Americans relative lack of knowledge may have inhibited more open disclosure practices because of confusion or misunderstandings of their own about HCV. Black respondents' lack of knowledge may reflect the dearth of available information regarding HCV in the larger black community. If there is indeed less information in the black community about HCV, the lack of open disclosure practices among blacks with HCV will only perpetuate the problem. This lack of knowledge represents what Link and Phelan (1995) discuss as a "fundamental cause" of disease as it involves access to resources, specifically knowledge, which can minimize the impact of a disease. Future research must evaluate public knowledge about HCV with attention to sampling various racial and ethnic groups.

Disclosure of health status does allow for support from family, friends, or in the workplace. Social support has profound effects on mental and physical heath status (Thoits, 1995). Thus, while blacks do not experience stigma as much as whites, they miss opportunities for social support. Levels of knowledge were related to positive social support, thus limiting social support for blacks. Positive social support in the workplace was related to higher incomes also disenfranchising blacks, as they are more likely to have lower paying jobs than whites.

Black respondents in this research are clearly experiencing HCV in a different fashion than white respondents. This racial inequality reflects larger trends in health in the United States (Williams & Jackson, 2005). These differences in experiences with HCV do not appear to be attributable to social class supporting research that claims education and income do not explain racial discrepancies in health-seeking behaviors (Schnittker et al., 2005). Instead, racial differences may be an outcome of provider–patient interactions and style.

Numerous researchers have examined provider–patient interactions. Physicians' social class as well as patients' social class affected the informative process (Waitzkin, 1985). Doctors tend to underestimate the amount of information they thought patients wanted (Waitzkin, 1985). The majority of respondents in this research were patients of one physician or one clinic, which was supervised by the same physician. However, a provider does not interact with all patients in exactly the same manner. In fact, providers take on various roles tailored to meet the needs of individual patients (Lutfey, 2005). Lutfey (2005) also found that residents interacted with patients in a different fashion than seasoned physicians. Respondents in this research who were seen at the public clinic were likely to see a different resident at each visit. Thus, these patients do not have the benefits of establishing a long-term relationship with one person possibly affecting information given to them as found by Waitzkin (1985). However, the racial differences in experiences with HCV spanned both recruitment sites, thus limiting the explanatory power of organizational setting.

Style is another factor that influences racial disparities. Style refers to how people present their illness (Bury, 1991). Research has repeatedly found that social class affects style (Anderson, 1991; Blair, 1993; Bury, 1991; Radley, 1989). Middle-class persons focus on the body in a more abstract fashion and are more verbal, whereas lower class persons are concerned with how symptoms affect day-to-day functioning. Anderson (1991) states that what appeared to be racial differences in illness experience were in fact class differences. In this research, however, differences are not linked to educational obtainments or income, which could be due to a relatively small sample. However, there is some support that racial and ethnic minorities experience illness differently regardless of social class (Smaje, 2000). Especially considering the long history of racial oppression in the Deep South, it is feasible that residential segregation and discrimination affect experiences with HCV regardless of socioeconomic status (Mechanic, 2005; Williams & Jackson, 2005).

Other indications that style is linked to race can be seen by the length of the interview process, whites in this sample talked longer about their experiences than minority respondents, perhaps providing a window into their interactions with providers. Although blacks may desire just as much information about HCV as whites, they do not obtain the same levels of knowledge. Blacks' lower levels of knowledge about HCV and more inhibited disclosure patterns are contributing factors to these racial variations in illness experience. These differences are also a result of illness style and subsequent provider and patient interactions. Physicians may unwittingly interact differently with black patients with HCV because they are aware of racial differences in responsiveness to treatment, thus setting up a self-fulfilling prophecy (Lutfey, 2000). Future research should focus specifically on provider and patient interactions among persons with HCV to further explicate racial differences in illness experience.

Despite the lack of ample cultural imagery, respondents found ways to make sense of having HCV. Diagnosis did give rise to trepidation for some. The issue of uncertainty was a salient issue for many as seen in the discussion about fear of the unknown as well as the role that knowledge plays in alleviating uncertainty. Even respondents who reported an ambivalent reaction to diagnosis had to deal with some repercussions regarding interactions with others even if minor. HCV knowledge is quite variable and unequally distributed by race leading to different illness careers for respondents. If HCV education and awareness are promoted, future research should monitor the implications for the illness career of persons with HCV. Public awareness could change an individual's reaction to diagnosis as well as knowledge about the disease thus alleviating some of the current disparities.

NOTE

1. Request can be raised to author at email: asuarez@depauw.edu

REFERENCES

AGA. (2003). *Stigma of hepatitis C stops Americans from getting tested.* Bethesda, MD: American Gastroenterological Association.

Albrecht, G. L., & Levy, J. A. (1991). Chronic illness and disability as life course events. *Advances in Medical Sociology, 2*, 3–13.

Alter, M. J., Margolis, H. S., Bell, B. P., & Bice, S. D. (1998). *Recommendations for prevention and control of hepatitis C virus (HCV) infection and HCV-related chronic disease.* Atlanta, GA: Centers for Disease Control.

Anderson, J. M. (1991). Women's perspectives on chronic illness: Ethnicity, ideology and restructuring of life. *Social Science and Medicine, 33*(2), 101–113.

Blair, A. (1993). Social class and the contextualization of illness experience. In: A. Radley (Ed.), *Worlds of illness: Biographical and cultural perspectives on health and disease* (pp. 27–48). London: Routledge.

Brown, P. (1995). Naming and framing: The social construction of diagnosis and illness. *Journal of Health and Social Behavior, 35*, 34–52. Extra Issue: Forty Years of Medical Sociology: The State of the Art and Directions for the Future.

Bury, M. (1982). Chronic illness as biographical disruption. *Sociology of Health and Illness, 4*(2), 167–182.

Bury, M. (1991). The sociology of chronic illness: A review of research and prospects. *Sociology of Health and Illness, 13*(4), 451–467.

Bury, M. (2000). On chronic illness and disability. In: C. Bird, P. Conrad & A. M. Fremont (Eds), *Handbook of medical sociology.* Upper Saddle River, NJ: Prentice-Hall.

Bussing, R., Gary, F. A., Mills, T. L., & Garvan, C. W. (2007). Cultural variations in parental health beliefs, knowledge, and information sources related to attention-deficit/hyperactivity disorder. *Journal of Family Issues, 28*(3), 291–318.

Charmaz, K. (1991). *Good days, bad days: The self in chronic illness.* New Brunswick, NJ: Rutgers University Press.

Coppola, A. G., Karakousis, P. C., Metz, D. C., Go, M. F., Mhokashi, M., Howden, C. W., Raufman, J.-P., & Sharma, V. K. (2004). Hepatitis C knowledge among primary care residents: Is our teaching adequate for the times? *American Journal of Gastroenterology, 99*, 1720–1725.

Davis, M., Rhodes, T., & Martin, A. (2004). Preventing hepatitis C: 'Common sense', 'the bug' and other perspectives from the risk narrative of people who inject drugs. *Social Science and Medicine, 59*, 1807–1818.

Erickson, D. (2006). By the numbers. *Hepatitis*, 36–37.

Franciscus, A. (2002). Hepatitis C Disclosure. HCV Advocate. Available at http://www.hcvadvocate.org/

Franciscus, A., & Highleyman, L. (2003). A guide to hepatitis C. HCV Advocate. Available at http://www.hcvadvocate.org/

Glacken, M., Kernohan, G., & Coates, V. (2001). Diagnosed with hepatitis C: A descriptive exploratory study. *International Journal of Nursing Studies, 38*, 107–116.

Heimer, R., Clair, S., Grau, L. E., Bluthenthal, R. N., Marshall, P. A., & Singer, M. (2002). Hepatitis-associated knowledge is low and risks are high among HIV-aware injection drug users in three US cities. *Addiction, 97*, 1277–1287.

Hepworth, J., & Krug, G. J. (1999). Hepatitis C: A socio-cultural perspective on the effects of a new virus on a community's health. *Journal of Health Psychology, 4*(2), 237–246.

Hopwood, M., & Southgate, E. (2003). Living with hepatitis C: A sociological review. *Critical Public Health, 13*(3), 251–267.

Krug, G. J. (1995). Discursive domains and epistemic chasms. *Journal of Contemporary Ethnography, 24*(3), 299–321.

Lepe, R., Layden-Almer, J. E., Layden, T. J., & Cotler, S. (2006). Ethnic differences in the presentation of chronic hepatitis C. *Journal of Viral Hepatitis, 13*, 116.

Link, B. G. (1987). Understanding labeling effects in the area of mental disorders: An assessment of the effects of expectations of rejection. *American Sociological Review, 52*(1), 96–112.

Link, B. G., & Phelan, J. (1995). Social conditions as fundamental causes of disease. *Journal of Health and Social Behavior, 35*(Extra Issue: Forty Years of Medical Sociology: The State of the Art and Directions for the Future), 80–94.

Lofland, J., & Lofland, L. H. (1995). *Analyzing social settings: A guide to qualitative observation and analysis.* Belmont: Wadsworth Publishing Company.

Lutfey, K. (2000). *Practitioner assessments of patient compliance with medical treatment regimens: An ethnographic study of two diabetes clinics.* Bloomington: Indiana University.

Lutfey, K. (2005). On practices of 'good doctoring': Reconsidering the relationship between provider roles and patient adherence. *Sociology of Health and Illness, 27*(4), 421–447.

Marshall, C., & Rossman, G. B. (1999). *Designing qualitative research.* Thousand Oaks: Sage.

Mechanic, D. (2005). Policy challenges in addressing racial disparities and improving population health. *Health Affairs, 24*, 335–338.

Orr, T. B. (2006). ALF leader shares goals, vision. *Hepatitis*, 10–13.

Palmer, M. (2006). African-Americans and hepatitis C. *Hepatitis*, 26–28.

Radley, A. (1989). Style, discourse, and constraint in adjustment to chronic illness. *Sociology of Health and Illness, 11*(3), 230–252.

Reddy, K. R. (2002). *Public-health impact, natural history, diagnosis, and clinical management of hepatitis C: Emerging clinical options with interferon-based therapies.* Rete Biomedical Communications Corporation. Available at http://cme.medscape.com/viewarticle/431761

Rhodes, T., & Treloar, C. (2008). The social production of hepatitis C risk among injecting drug users: A qualitative synthesis. *Addiction, 103*, 1593–1603.

Ronai, C. R., & Cross, R. (2002). Stripteasers' management of their deviant identity. In: E. Rubington & M. S. Weinberg (Eds), *Deviance: The interactionist perspective* (pp. 396–408). Boston: Ally and Bacon.

Schnittker, J., Pescosolido, B. A., & Croghan, T. W. (2005). Are African Americans really less willing to use health care? *Social Problems, 52*(5), 255–271.

Smaje, C. (2000). Race, ethnicity, and health. In: C. Bird, P. Conrad & A. M. Fremont (Eds), *Handbook of medical sociology* (pp. 114–128). Upper Saddle River, NJ: Prentice Hall.

Suarez, A. E., & Shindo, A. A. (2008). Silence and stigma: The hepatitis C virus (HCV) epidemic. In: R. Perucci, K. J. Ferraro, J. Miller & G. Muschert (Eds), *Agenda for social justice: Solutions 2008* (pp. 64–68). Knoxville, TN: Society for the Study of Social Problems.

Tewksbury, R., & McGaughey, D. (1997). Stigmatization of persons with HIV disease: Perceptions, management, and consequences of AIDS. *Sociological Spectrum, 17*, 49–70.

Thoits, P. A. (1995). Stress, coping, and social support processes: Where are we? What next? *Journal of Health and Social Behavior, 35*, 53–79. Extra Issue: Forty Years of Medical Sociology: The State of the Art and Directions for the Future.

Waitzkin, H. (1985). Information giving in medical care. *Journal of Health and Social Behavior, 26*(2), 81–101.

Weitz, R. (1989). Uncertainty and the lives of persons with AIDS. *Journal of Health and Social Behavior, 30*(3), 270–281.

Williams, D. R., & Jackson, P. B. (2005). Social sources of racial disparities in health. *Health Affairs, 24*, 325–334.

Williams, G. (1984). The genesis of chronic illness: Narrative reconstruction. *Sociology of Health and Illness, 6*(2), 175–199.

MEDICARE AND RACIAL DISPARITIES IN HEALTH: FEE-FOR-SERVICE VERSUS MANAGED CARE

Noah J. Webster

ABSTRACT

As the size of the U.S. population age 65 and older continues to grow, racial disparities within this population persist despite near universal insurance coverage provided through Medicare. Reform of the government administered program in 2003 has the potential to influence racial disparities due to increased privatization. This study compares racial disparities in health service utilization between Medicare fee-for-service and managed care, the two drastically different ways Medicare administers health care. Data was analyzed from the National Health Interview Survey (NHIS), a nationally representative study of the U.S. civilian, noninstitutionalized, household population. Included in this study were African American and white respondents aged 65 and older who participated in the NHIS in any year from 2004 to 2008 (N = 22,364). Small differences were found in regard to the number of medical office visits, with African Americans reporting fewer visits. However, these differences were significant in only 25% of the analyses conducted.

Across both types of Medicare, significant differences between African Americans and whites regarding consultations with a medical specialist and having surgery were found in 75% of analyses. In all analyses, African Americans were less likely to have interacted with a specialist or have surgery. The greatest difference in racial disparity between fee-for-service and managed care for all three health service use indicators was observed among those who were chronically ill and poor, and the smallest difference was observed among those who were chronically ill and very poor. These racial disparities in health service use may be linked to earlier life disparities in access to health care, higher out-of-pocket costs in Medicare fee-for-service, and the for-profit structure of managed care plans.

INTRODUCTION

Inadequate access to healthcare services is one of many causes of racial health disparities in the United States. Issues of access for some parts of the population are addressed through government-run health insurance programs such as Medicare. When disparities in health service utilization persist despite these programs, researchers, policy makers, and health advocates are forced to look for and address other sources of these disparities.

Medicare, in existence since 1965 (Social Security Administration, 2010), provides health insurance for the majority of adults aged 65 and older in the United States. Without this program, racial health disparities would undoubtedly be much worse than current conditions. Medicare in itself can be viewed as a macro-level institution enacted, maintained, and adjusted at the federal level. This macro-level factor directly influences the health of older adults, but also effects health through interactions with other societal forces, both macro (i.e., socioeconomic inequality) and micro in nature (patient–provider interactions). A current trend in Medicare is increased provision of benefits through managed care or private health plans called "Medicare Advantage" of which the most common is receipt of services through a Health Maintenance Organization (HMO) (Kaiser Family Foundation, 2007) as opposed to the traditional fee-for-service provision of services.

This study compares racial disparities in health service utilization across the two types of Medicare plans using data from the National Health Interview Survey (NHIS). The number of minority adults aged 65 and older is increasing, suggesting these issues examined in this chapter will become increasingly important. Currently, racial and ethnic minorities make up 15% of Medicare enrollees aged 65 and older (Kaiser Family Foundation, 2005a), and this figure is estimated to increase to 26% by 2030 (Kaiser Family Foundation, 2003). Additionally, by 2013, the percentage of Medicare beneficiaries enrolled in "Advantage" plans is expected to rise to anywhere from 16% to 30% (Kaiser Family Foundation, 2005a), stark increases from 4% in 1990 and 11% in 2004 (Kaiser Family Foundation, 2005b).

Racial Health Disparities

Racial disparities exist in many facets of health across the life course (Everson, Maty, Lynch, & Kaplan, 2002). The life expectancy of a newborn in the United States has risen to 77.2 years of age, but African Americans still lag behind whites by over five years (Centers for Disease Control, 2004). African Americans disproportionately experience chronic conditions and have worse outcomes from these conditions compared to whites. For example, African Americans have a 30% higher death rate from cardiovascular disease (U.S. Department of Health and Human Services, Office of Minority Health, 2009), and experience 50% more diabetic complications (Agency for Healthcare Research Quality [AHRQ], 2001). Racial disparities also exist in access to medical procedures and treatments (Agency for Healthcare Research Quality [AHRQ], 2000a) as 20% of African Americans lack a usual source of medical care compared to only 16% of whites (AHRQ, 2000a).

Medicare

Although a single program administered by the government, Medicare offers multiple options for beneficiaries to receive services (Medicare, 2007). The original plan offered under Medicare is called "fee-for-service," which covers the cost for many healthcare services and some prescription drugs and allows beneficiaries to receive care from any physician or hospital that accepts Medicare (Medicare, 2007). Coverage gaps exist with this plan, leading Medicare to encourage beneficiaries to purchase a Medigap policy and add a prescription drug plan, a new provision under the Medicare Modernization Act of 2003 (Medicare, 2007). Approximately 80% of the 44 million Americans eligible for Medicare are enrolled in the fee-for-service program (Kaiser Family Foundation, 2007).

The second major category of plans is Medicare Advantage (Medicare, 2007). These are private plans that before 2003 were referred to as managed care or Medicare+Choice (Kaiser Family Foundation, 2004). Medicare Advantage enrollees do not need to purchase a Medigap policy and may have lower out-of-pocket costs compared to fee-for-service enrollees, but may have restrictions on where they can go for care (Medicare, 2007). Five unique plans fall under this category including HMOs, Preferred Provider Organizations, Private Fee-for-Service, Medicare Special Needs, and Medicare Medical Savings Account Plans (Medicare, 2007). Despite this variability in plans, a large majority (65%) of Medicare Advantage enrollees receive benefits through HMOs (Kaiser Family Foundation, 2007).

In 2003, The Medicare Prescription Drug, Improvement, and Modernization Act was passed into law resulting in the largest overhaul of the program since its inception in 1965. The major provision of the act was that it created a new prescription drug benefit to be administered by private health plans, available to fee-for-service enrollees as a stand-alone plan, but available to Medicare Advantage enrollees through their private plan (Centers for Medicare and Medicaid Services, 2004). The bill increased payments to the managed care/Advantage plans to increase payments to providers, reduce enrollee out-of-pocket costs, and increase benefits (i.e., prescription drug coverage) (Kaiser Family Foundation, 2005a).

Health Disparities within Medicare

One study of Medicare managed care enrollees found that African Americans compared to whites reported lower quality of care (Virnig et al., 2002). Another study compared all Medicare enrollees and found that whites when compared to African Americans used procedures more often for angina, nonangina coronary artery disease, and stroke (Lee, Baker, Gehlbach, Hosmer, & Reti, 1998). Additionally, white Medicare enrollees had a 59% greater likelihood of undergoing angiography than their African American counterparts (Lee et al., 1998). A third study found that African American male Medicare enrollees visited the doctor for ambulatory care 11% less than whites, African American women received 34% fewer mammograms, and African Americans in general received fewer immunizations for the flu (Alva, 1996).

When comparing Medicare fee-for-service and managed care plans, differences in quality have been documented. Studies have shown that referral rates, the rate of inpatient versus outpatient care, and length of hospital visits were all lower in managed care plans (Wong & Hellinger, 2001). One study even found managed care enrollees were less likely to receive needed coronary angiography after the experience of a heart attack (Agency for Healthcare Research Quality [AHRQ], 2000b).

These lower rates of service utilization in managed care are especially important for people with existing chronic conditions who require more services. Ware, Bayliss, Rogers, Kosinski, and Tarlov (1996) compared outcomes among chronically ill Medicare beneficiaries in fee-for-service and managed care plans (Ware et al., 1996) and found managed care enrollees experienced greater declines in physical health compared to fee-for-service enrollees. They also found that those in poverty had better physical and mental health outcomes in fee-for-service plans, and those enrollees not in poverty experienced better outcomes in managed care plans (Ware et al., 1996).

Sociological Perspectives on Preventive Care

Many managed care plans are committed to preventive care, a policy that makes fiscal sense. By preventing future illness and illness-related complications, managed care reduces expenditures and increases profits. Studies have documented the increased attention to preventive care among some Medicare managed care plans (Miller & Luft, 1994; Schneider, Cleary, Zaslavsky, & Epstein, 2001; Greene, Blustein, & Laflamme, 2001; Landon, Zaslavsky, Bernard, Cioffi, & Cleary, 2004).

Preventive medicine usually centers around the identification and modification of individual-level risk behaviors to promote and initiate a healthy lifestyle to prevent the future onset of disease or disease-related complications. There is a certain attractiveness to focus on individual-level risk factors because of the opportunity to see immediate and substantial change. Also, it is easier to tackle one person's behavior at a time rather than eliminating social causes of disease such as poverty and discrimination. This individual-level risk factor paradigm also provides a human face to blame for poor outcomes, as opposed to placing blame on face-less macro structural forces. This ideology of blaming the victim for their poor health grew out of the self-help movement and initiatives to curb rising medical costs by denying medical care to those who do not make the effort to change their behavior (Crawford, 1978). The risk factor paradigm embedded in preventive medicine can also place blame when behavioral risk factors are present in a person's life (Crawford, 1978; Alonzo, 1993; Katz, 2001).

This paradigm can contribute to provider bias and stereotyping, leading to different levels of care (Ahmad, 1989) and does not account for the fact that members of racial minorities tend to be overexposed to risk factors in large part because of disproportionate rates of poverty. With poverty comes overexposure to the associated environmental factors that can alter the success of preventive care. For example, compared to high-income areas, low-income neighborhoods have been found to have a third less supermarkets (Morland, Wing, & Diez-Roux, 2002) and fewer resources and facilities for physical activity (Macintyre, Maciver, & Sooman, 1993; Estabrooks, Lee, & Gyurcsik, 2003).

Providers who blame the victim for their disease status or inability to modify risk behaviors may think of the patient as undeserving of a standard of care. This can become visible in ordering of tests, diagnoses, disregard of patient self-reports, and overall health. This can also lead to a level of perceived racism in the receipt of medical care, which may lead to greater dissatisfaction with the services received, a phenomenon more common among African Americans (LaVeist, Nickerson, & Bowie, 2000).

This study is one of the first to examine and compare racial disparities among Medicare beneficiaries enrolled in Medicare fee-for-service to disparities among those enrolled in private managed care plans. On the basis of the analysis of NHIS data, it is expected that racial disparities in health service utilization will be greater among managed care plan enrollees compared to fee-for-service. Additionally, it is expected that this difference in racial disparity between managed care and fee-for-service plans will be more pronounced among those enrollees who are chronically ill and poor. Generally, it is hypothesized that African American Medicare enrollees compared to whites will report more medical office visits over the past year, but fewer will have seen or talked to a medical specialist and fewer will have undergone surgery in the past year.

METHODS

Data

To answer the research questions, secondary data analysis was conducted on the NHIS, administered by the National Center for Health Statistics at the Centers for Disease Control (CDC). The NHIS is a multipurpose health survey, serving as the primary source of health information on the U.S. civilian, noninstitutionalized, household population (NHIS Survey

Description, 2008). NHIS data is collected using computer-assisted personal interviewing software (NHIS Survey Description, 2008).

The NHIS sample is chosen so that each person in the population (U.S. civilian, noninstitutionalized, household) has a non-zero probability of being selected for participation. Each case in the NHIS dataset is accompanied by a weight that reflects these probabilities for study selection, nonresponse, and 2000 census data on age, sex, and race/ethnicity (NHIS Survey Description, 2008).

Sample

Every year, an adult (over 18 years old) is randomly selected from each of the participating NHIS households to participate in the sample adult portion of the survey (NHIS Survey Description, 2008). The sample used for this study combines all people who participated in the NHIS sample adult survey from 2004 to 2008. The final sample used for analysis includes adults aged 65 or older who are either white or African American ($N = 22,364$); weighted $N = 32,059,576$). As can be viewed in Table 1, the weighted sample used in the analysis has a mean age of 74.6, top-coded at age 85 to ensure confidentiality; 57% female; 91% white; and 9% African American.

Measures

Medicare Type
The question on Medicare type was asked to participants: "Are you under a Medicare managed care arrangement, such as an HMO, that is, a Health Maintenance Organization?" Participants could respond: yes, no, refuse to answer, or don't know. For analysis, this variable was recoded into a dichotomous variable: 1 = fee-for-service, 2 = managed care/HMO, and all other responses set to missing.

Chronic Illness Status
Three variables were used to document the disease status of study participants. The first was if the participant had ever been told by a doctor or health professional that they have diabetes. Participants could respond: yes, no, borderline, refuse to answer, or don't know. For analysis, this variable was recoded into a dichotomous variable: 1 = no, 2 = yes/borderline, and all other responses set to missing. The participants who

Table 1. NHIS Sample Characteristics 2004–2008 (Unweighted $N = 22{,}364$); Weighted $N = 32{,}059{,}576$).

	Mean (SE)[a]	% (Unweighted N)
Age (Range (65–85+))	74.6 (.06)	
Gender (% female)		57.3 (13,670)
Race/ethnicity:		
White		90.6 (19,123)
African American		9.4 (3,241)
Medicare type:		
Managed care/HMO		12.5 (2,485)
Fee-for-service		87.5 (16,955)
Chronic illness status		
Told have diabetes/borderline diabetes		19.2 (4,361)
Told have hypertension		58.3 (13,318)
Told have hypertension *or* diabetes		63.0 (14,319)
Poverty		
Below 200% of poverty level		31.0 (7,498)
Below federal poverty		7.1 (2,009)
Health service utilization		
Total number of medical office visits in past year	3.5 (.02)	
0 – None		6.1 (1,416)
1 – 1		9.6 (2,076)
2 – 2–3		23.6 (5,054)
3 – 4–5		21.0 (4,601)
4 – 6–7		11.5 (2,495)
5 – 8–9		6.4 (1,389)
6 – 10–12		9.4 (2,065)
7 – 13–15		3.5 (743)
8 – 16 or more		8.9 (1,856)
Seen or talked to medical specialist in past year (% yes)		46.5 (9,845)
Had surgery in past year? (% yes)		20.3 (4,296)

[a]Calculated using adult sample weight.

responded they had been told they have borderline diabetes were grouped with those who responded yes because according to the National Institute of Diabetes and Digestive and Kidney Diseases, "borderline" is a former term used to describe type-2 diabetes or impaired glucose tolerance (National Institute of Diabetes and Digestive and Kidney Diseases, 2010). The second variable was if the participant had ever been told by a doctor or health professional that they have hypertension. Participants could respond: yes, no, refuse to answer, or don't know. For analysis, this variable was recoded into a dichotomous variable: 1 = no, 2 = yes, and all other responses set to missing. The third variable, a combination of the first two variables (diabetes and hypertension), documented if participants had ever been told they have diabetes or hypertension, and the values were either: 1 = no, 2 = yes.

Poverty
Two variables were used to measure poverty in this study. The data on income from the NHIS contained a large amount of missing data. The NHIS provides imputed income data for each year of the survey. Specifically multiple imputation was conducted and five separate imputed income datasets were created. For purposes of this study, participants were selected only if all five imputed values matched on the variable to be used for analysis, which occurred for over 85% of the cases in the combined 2004–2008 NHIS data file. The income variable used from the NHIS imputed file documents the ratio of family income to the poverty threshold and ranges from less than .5 to greater than 5. For this study, two variables were computed from this variable. The first indicates the percentage of the sample below 200% of the federal poverty level (FPL) and was coded as 1 = family income is below 200% of FPL; 2 = family income is at or above 200% of FPL. The second variable documents the percentage of the sample below the FPL and was coded as 1 = family income is below FPL; 2 = family income is at or above FDL.

Health Service Utilization
Three variables were used to examine the use of healthcare services over the past 12 months. The first was self-reported total number of medical office visits in the past year. The NHIS codes this variable into eight categories: 0 = none, 1 = 1 visit, 2 = 2–3 visits, 3 = 4–5, 4 = 6–7, 5 = 8–9, 6 = 10–12, 7 = 13–15, and 8 = 16 or more. The second variable documents whether or not the respondent saw or talked to a medical specialist in the past 12 months and was coded as 1 = no, 2 = yes. The last variable indicated whether or not the individual had surgery in the past 12 months and also was coded as 1 = no, 2 = yes.

Data Analytic Procedures

All data analyses were conducted using SPSS 17.0 and the Complex Samples add-on module due to the complex sample design of the NHIS.

which includes stratification, clustering, and multistage sampling (NHIS Survey Description, 2008). In addition, all data were weighted using the NHIS sample adult weight, which includes design, ratio, nonresponse, and poststratification adjustments for sample adults. Even though this chapter and analysis focuses on adults aged 65 and older who were either African American or white, the analyzed dataset included all adults (aged 18 and older) in the NHIS sample adult file to utilize the complex design information of the survey in its entirety.

Descriptive statistics were conducted and presented (population frequencies, unweighted N's, and population means) on Medicare insurance type, chronic illness status, poverty, and health service utilization. Next, a series of bivariate analyses were conducted to examine differences between whites and African Americans on the prevalence of poverty, chronic illness, and health service utilization. For dichotomous measures, cross-tabulation analyses were conducted between race and the variable of interest to obtain the prevalence/frequency within each racial group. Chi-square tests were used to determine if racial differences were significant. To test for mean differences between whites and African Americans on the number of medical office visits, an analysis of variance (ANOVA) was conducted with race as the factor. Due to the large sample size, differences for these analyses were only considered significant when the p-value was less than .001.

The next group of analyses examined the three types of health service utilization by race separately among participants enrolled in Medicare fee-for-service and those in managed care/HMO. This analysis was conducted four times for each measure of health service utilization, using four subsamples. The first analysis included the entire sample, the second included only participants with diabetes or hypertension (the chronically ill), the third participants with diabetes or hypertension and whose family income was less than 200% of the FPL (the chronically ill and poor), and the fourth included those with diabetes or hypertension and whose family income was less than the FPL (the chronically ill and very poor).

To examine the number of medical office visits, eight separate ANOVAs were conducted, and to examine the prevalence of interacting with a medical specialist and having had surgery, cross-tabulation and logistic regression analyses were conducted. In addition to the population mean (and accompanying standard error (SE)) or prevalence for each racial group, the white/African American disparity within each type of Medicare is presented, along with an indication of the significance of the difference/ disparity. Disparities were calculated by subtracting the mean or frequency for whites from that for African Americans; therefore, a negative difference indicates a lower number or frequency for African Americans. Due to the use of smaller subsamples, differences were considered significant when the p-value was less than .05.

ANOVA and logistic regression were used to allow for the inclusion of year of survey completion (coded: 1 = 2004–2005, 2 = 2006–2008) as a control variable. The Medicare Prescription Drug, Improvement, and Modernization Act of 2003 was implemented at the start of 2006, and therefore as of that date, most Medicare enrollees regardless of plan type would have some form of prescription drug coverage. As a result, the 2004–2005 NHIS survey participants may have had a different Medicare experience than the 2006–2008 participants. The inclusion of this control allows the examination of these issues independent of the effect of the prescription drug program.

RESULTS

As can be viewed in Table 1, 12.5% of the respondents indicated they were covered by a managed care plan such as an HMO, and 87.5% were covered by traditional fee-for-service plan. Almost one-fifth (19.2%) had been told they have diabetes, 58.3% hypertension, and 63.0% had either or both conditions. The average number of medical visits over the past 12 months was between four and seven visits (mean category = 3.5; range: 0 = none to 8 = 16+) with just under 40% having gone for three or fewer visits, 21.0% four to five visits, 11.5% six to seven visits, and 28.2% eight or more visits. Just under half (46.5%) had seen or talked to a medical specialist, and 20.3% had surgery in the past 12 months.

As can be viewed in Table 2, over half (54.4%) of African Americans had family incomes below 200% of the FPL, and 22.2% below the FPL, compared to 28.7% and 5.6% for whites. African Americans were much more likely to have diabetes (30.9%), hypertension (73.5%), or have either (77.4%) compared to whites (18.0%, 56.7%, and 61.5%). In terms of medical office visits over the past year, African Americans reported slightly fewer visits (3.4) compared to whites (3.5), but the difference was not significant. African Americans compared to whites were also less likely to have seen a medical specialist (35.1% versus 47.7%) or have surgery in the past year (12.5% versus 21.1%). The results were consistent with the literature on racial disparities in that African Americans disproportionately experience poverty and chronic illness, but are less likely to access health services.

Table 2. Racial Disparities in Poverty and Health.

	White	African American	Significance of Difference
	% (Unweighted *N*)		
Poverty			
Family income<200% of FPL	28.7 (5,820)	54.4 (1,678)	***
Family income<FPL	5.6 (1,257)	22.2 (752)	***
Chronic illness status			
Diabetes	18.0 (3,354)	30.9 (1,007)	***
Hypertension	56.7 (10,925)	73.5 (2,393)	***
Diabetes *or* Hypertension	61.5 (11,802)	77.4 (2,517)	***
Health service utilization			
Seen or talked to medical specialist in past year	47.7 (8,731)	35.1 (1,114)	***
Had surgery in past year	21.1 (3,893)	12.5 (403)	***
	Mean (SE)		
Medical office visits in past year	3.5 (.02)	3.4 (.05)	NS

NS, not significant at $p<.001$.
***Significant difference between whites and African Americans at a level of $p<.001$.

The results presented in Table 3 indicate that within both types of Medicare, significant differences between African Americans and whites regarding the number of medical visits were found in only 25% of the analyses (two of eight), and both findings were found among fee-for-service enrollees. In general, within fee-for-service and across the four samples (full sample, chronically ill, chronically ill-poor, and chronically ill-very poor), whites reported more visits than African Americans. However, the racial disparity/difference was significant only among the chronically ill (−0.2) and chronically ill-poor (−0.4) samples. When comparing African Americans and whites enrolled in managed care plans, there were no significant differences. This may in part be attributable to lower statistical power resulting from fewer people enrolled in managed care. Despite this, the differences were still relatively smaller, with 0.1 being the largest difference

Table 3. Medical Office Visits in the Past Year by Race/Ethnicity and Medicare Type[a].

Medical Office Visits (Mean, SE)	Medicare Type	Fee-for-Service White	Fee-for-Service African American	Managed Care/HMO White	Managed Care/HMO African American
1. Full sample		3.6 (.02)	3.5 (.06)	3.4 (.06)	3.5 (.12)
	Disparity		(−0.1)		(0.1)
2. Have diabetes or hypertension		3.9 (.03)	3.7 (.07)	3.7 (.07)	3.7 (.12)
	Disparity		(−0.2)**		(0.0)
3. Have diabetes or hypertension *and* family income <200% of FPL		4.0 (.05)	3.6 (.09)	3.9 (.12)	3.8 (.17)
	Disparity		(−0.4)***		(−0.1)
4. Have diabetes or hypertension *and* family income <FPL		4.0 (.12)	3.9 (.11)	3.8 (.28)	3.7 (.33)
	Disparity		(−0.1)		(−0.1)

***Significant difference between whites and African Americans at a level of $p < .001$.
**Significant difference between whites and African Americans at a level of $p < .01$.
*Significant difference between whites and African Americans at a level of $p < .05$.
[a]Disparity calculated by subtracting mean for whites from that for African Americans. Negative sign indicates African Americans had fewer visits.

across the four samples, suggesting little racial difference within managed care in terms of office visits.

When comparing the size of the racial disparity between fee-for-service and managed care, the largest difference was observed among the chronically ill-poor sample (−0.4 versus −0.1). This was driven in large part by chronically ill and poor African American fee-for-service enrollees having gone for significantly fewer visits (−0.4) compared to whites. This trend also held true among the chronically ill sample, but was not as pronounced due to a smaller racial disparity among fee-for-service enrollees (−0.2) and no racial difference in managed care/HMO.

The hypothesis that African Americans would report significantly more visits was not supported by the findings. In only one analysis out of eight (full sample-managed care) did African Americans descriptively report more visits, and this finding was not statistically significant. The opposite of the hypothesis was true among fee-for-service enrollees in that African Americans in two analyses reported significantly fewer visits, and in all four analyses, African Americans descriptively reported less. The hypothesis regarding the medical visit racial disparity being larger in managed care was partially supported, mainly due to the significant reverse racial disparity found in two of the fee-for-service samples and lack of differences in managed care.

Table 4 reports that across both types of Medicare, significant differences between African Americans and whites regarding having talked to or seen a medical specialist were found in 75% of the analyses (six of eight), with the majority found among fee-for-service enrollees. In general, within fee-for-service and across the four samples, whites were significantly more likely to have talked to/seen a medical specialist in the past year. The same trend was also found within managed care, but the racial difference was only significant in the full sample and among those who were chronically ill. When comparing the size of the racial disparity between fee-for-service and managed care/HMO, the racial disparity in all four samples was always greater among fee-for-service enrollees. The largest difference in racial disparity between plans was observed among the chronically ill-poor sample (fee-for-service = -11.5 versus managed care = -4.6). Overall, the respondents with the lowest prevalence of medical specialist interaction out of all four samples and both racial groups were chronically ill-very poor African Americans enrolled in fee-for-service (32.6%).

The hypothesis that African Americans compared to whites would be significantly less likely to have had interactions with a medical specialist was upheld in 75% of the analyses. However, the hypothesis that the racial disparity would be greater among managed care enrollees was not true in any of the analyses. In only one sample, the chronically ill-very poor were the racial disparities almost the same (fee-for-service = -12.5 versus managed care/HMO = -12.2).

Table 4 also shows that across both types of Medicare, significant differences between African Americans and whites regarding having had surgery in the past year were found in 75% of the analyses (six of eight), with the majority found among fee-for-service enrollees. In general, within fee-for-service and across the four samples, whites were significantly more likely to have had surgery in the past year. The same trend was also found within managed care/HMO, but the racial difference was only significant in the full sample and among those who were chronically ill. When comparing the size of the racial disparity between fee-for-service and managed care/HMO, the racial disparity in all four samples was always greater among fee-for-service enrollees. These findings parallel those of interaction with a specialist exactly. However, the sizes of the racial disparities were much

Table 4. Medical Specialist Interaction and Surgery in the Past Year by Race/Ethnicity and Medicare Type[a].

	Medicare Type	Fee-for-Service White	Fee-for-Service African American	Managed Care/HMO White	Managed Care/HMO African American
Seen/talked to medical specialist % (unweighted N)					
Full sample		48.8	36.0	45.2	36.7
		(6,901)	(791)	(885)	(168)
	Disparity	(-12.8)***		(-8.5)**	
Have diabetes or hypertension		53.3	38.5	48.7	37.8
		(4,739)	(674)	(589)	(141)
	Disparity	(-14.8)***		(-10.9)**	
Have diabetes or hypertension *and* family income < 200% of FPL		48.1	36.6	45.6	41.0
		(1,409)	(357)	(189)	(76)
	Disparity	(-11.5)***		(-4.6)	
Have diabetes or hypertension *and* family income < FPL		45.1	32.6	48.5	36.3
		(293)	(164)	(27)	(24)
	Disparity	(-12.5)***		(-12.2)	
Had surgery % (unweighted N)					
Full sample		21.5	12.6	20.0	12.0
		(3,058)	(285)	(390)	(55)
	Disparity	(-8.9)***		(-8.0)**	
Have diabetes or hypertension		23.3	13.0%	23.2	13.4
		(2,072)	(235)	(274)	(48)
	Disparity	(-10.3)***		(-9.8)**	
Have diabetes or hypertension *and* family income < 200% of FPL		21.2	11.8	21.7	14.2
		(622)	(127)	(88)	(25)
	Disparity	(-9.4)***		(-7.5)	
Have diabetes or hypertension *and* family income < FPL		18.3	12.9	15.6	10.9
		(116)	(70)	(8)	(8)
	Disparity	(-5.4)*		(-4.7)	

***Significant difference between whites and African Americans at a level of $p<.001$.
**Significant difference between whites and African Americans at a level of $p<.01$.
*Significant difference between whites and African Americans at a level of $p<.05$.
[a]The disparity was calculated by subtracting the percentage for whites from that for African Americans, so a negative sign indicates a lower percentage of African Americans saw/talked to a medical specialist or had surgery.

smaller compared to those observed in the medical specialist analyses, in part due to a general lower prevalence of surgery.

Again paralleling the medical specialist findings, the largest difference in racial disparity between plan types was observed among the chronically ill-poor sample (fee-for-service = -9.4 versus managed care/HMO = -7.5). However, in contrast to specialist visits, the respondents with the lowest prevalence of surgery out of all four samples and both racial groups were chronically ill-very poor African Americans enrolled in managed care/HMO (10.9%).

The hypothesis that a larger percentage of whites compared to African Americans would have surgery was supported in 75% of the analyses. The hypothesis that the racial disparity would be greater in managed care/HMO compared to fee-for-service was not supported and in fact the opposite was found in all analyses.

DISCUSSION

When compared to white older adults, African Americans aged 65 and older were found to be exposed to greater levels of poverty, have higher rates of diabetes and hypertension, and accessed health services (i.e., primary care, specialists, and surgery) less often. A sizeable and growing literature sheds light on causes of these disparities, which include economic and noneconomic discrimination (Williams, Yu, Jackson, & Anderson, 1997), lack of neighborhood resources (Cagney, Browning, & Wen, 2005), and restricted access to medical services over the life course.

Racial Disparities in Primary Care

The goals of this study were to examine racial disparities in health service utilization among Medicare enrollees and to compare the size of the racial disparity between the two drastically different ways Medicare provides services. In terms of access to primary care, measured in this study as medical office visits in the past year, it was hypothesized that African Americans would report more visits based on having worse health and more chronic conditions requiring frequent and consistent care. This hypothesis was not supported in this study as African Americans generally reported slightly fewer visits than whites. However, the hypothesis that the racial disparity (African Americans reporting more visits than whites) would be greater among managed care enrollees was supported. This was due to African American fee-for service enrollees reporting fewer visits and no significant differences found within managed care. This could be indicative of African Americans doing better healthwise in fee-for-service. Alternatively, it could be argued that African American Medicare enrollees go to the doctor less often because of earlier life disparities in insurance coverage. These earlier life disparities disproportionately force African Americans to rely on other sources for medical care (i.e., emergency room). Regardless of how fewer visits are interpreted, the fact that significant racial disparities in medical office visits were found in only 25% of the analyses suggests that both types of Medicare do an efficient job at reducing racial disparities in access to primary care.

Racial Disparities in Access to Specialists and Surgery

In terms of access to more costly medical services such as specialist consultations or having surgery, it was hypothesized that African Americans would report less use of these services. This hypothesis was supported in almost all of the analyses. The hypothesis that racial disparities in access to these more costly services would be greater among managed care enrollees was not supported, and in fact, racial disparities were always greater among fee-for-service enrollees. Fewer consultations with a specialist and not having surgery could indicate less need for these services. However, the consistency of the racial disparity across the samples and the fact that the largest disparities were observed among chronically ill samples suggest this disparity persists independent of need.

It was expected that racial disparities would be greater among managed care enrollees for three interconnected reasons. The first is the way the government pays companies administering the private plans. The companies receive a fixed payment from the government to provide care for a given Medicare enrollee. When care expenditures are less than the fixed rate, profits are made, thus creating a possible incentive to undertreat patients. The second is the gatekeeper structure of Medicare HMO plans that require patients to access services through a single primary care physician who grants further access to specialized care through referrals. The third is the increased emphasis placed on preventive care in managed care plans. The primary intended consequences of preventive care cannot be faulted, rather it is the unintended consequence of blaming individuals for the presence of risk factors or inability to reduce them that can contribute to provider bias, stereotyping, and different levels of care (Ahmad, 1989). The lack of evidence in this study of greater disparities among managed care enrollees does not entirely discount these three factors as contributors to racial health disparities because significant racial disparities were still found within managed care.

In this study, the comparatively larger racial disparities found within fee-for-service were surprising. Poverty or ability to pay Medicare out-of-pocket costs coupled with African Americans being disproportionately exposed to poverty may in part explain these larger disparities. Out-of-pocket costs are generally higher in fee-for-service Medicare compared to managed care plans (Centers for Medicare and Medicaid Services, 2009a), possibly persuading lower income enrollees to forgo medical office visits or more costly services. Medicare enrollees who are very poor and therefore qualify for Medicaid (income at or below 100% of the federal poverty and resources at or below twice the amount allowed by Social Security) receive financial assistance to pay Medicare premiums, deductibles, and coinsurance (Centers for Medicare and Medicaid Services, 2005).

These facts of Medicare provision are consistent with this study's findings that the greatest difference in racial disparity between fee-for-service and managed care for all three health service use indicators was observed in the chronically ill-poor (have diabetes and/or hypertension and family income less than 200% of FPL) sample, and the smallest difference was observed in the chronically ill-very poor (have diabetes and/or hypertension and family income below the FPL) sample, a majority of whom if not all would be covered by Medicaid.

Another potential explanation for larger racial disparities found within fee-for-service is the lack of a case management program (Foote, 2003). In contrast, managed care plans rely heavily on sophisticated case management programs (Cantor, 2008). Case management may be especially important for older adults who up until the age of 65 were without health insurance or had spotty coverage throughout their life and may have had limited experience with primary care physicians, specialists, or the process required to undergo surgery. African Americans have been documented to disproportionately be a part of this population, and therefore, case management could be functioning as a valuable resource to reduce racial disparities resulting from earlier life racial disparities in access to health care.

Policy Implications

Addressing disparities in healthcare access at earlier ages has the potential to mitigate some of the factors that contribute to racial disparities in health service use among older adults. However, the current attempt at healthcare reform in the United States appears it will come up short in terms of guaranteeing all Americans some form of health insurance (i.e., universal coverage). While debate continues, it is useful to consider how Medicare itself can be changed to reduce racial disparities in health service use.

Prescription Drug Benefit and Addressing Coverage Gaps
The changes made to Medicare as of 2006 may have some benefit to all older adults especially poor seniors because of increased access to medications, which can possibly lead to better management of chronic conditions, a reduction in the need for services (i.e., visits with specialists or surgery), and ultimately a reduction in racial health disparities. However, there are gaps in this prescription drug coverage, a phenomenon commonly referred to as the "donut hole." Once a Medicare enrollee's prescription drug expenses reach a certain threshold, Medicare will no longer cover the cost until the enrollee's out-of-pocket spending reaches another threshold, upon which Medicare catastrophic coverage will provide assistance (Centers for Medicare and Medicaid Services, 2009b). According to a recent study, 26% of Medicare enrollees who filled one of more prescriptions had enough prescription drug costs to reach the donut hole, and of this group, 15% had stopped taking needed medications (Hoadley, Hargrave, Cubanski, & Neuman, 2008). Through healthcare reform, the Obama administration is looking to reduce the size of the Medicare prescription drug benefit donut hole and by 2019 completely close the gap in coverage (The White House, 2010).

This policy proposal has great promise to reduce racial disparities in health. However, this study suggests that additional reforms can be put in place to help further reduce these disparities. First, Medicare fee-for-service coverage gaps for other services can be addressed by raising the income threshold required to be eligible for Medicaid assistance from 100% of the FPL to at least 200%.

Second, prescription drug coverage could be provided to Medicare fee-for-service enrollees directly through the government in similar fashion as their other services. Currently, fee-for-service enrollees have to enroll in a stand-alone prescription drug plan to receive the benefit, which may create confusion, whereas managed care enrollees can receive all their benefits under one plan. A government-run prescription drug plan has the potential to reduce overall Medicare costs, as analysis of the current prescription drug plan shows the government could have saved $15 billion in 2007 from cutting the administrative costs of the companies who administer the private drug plans (Freking, 2007). This type of prescription drug coverage has public support as a study conducted before the 2003 reforms found 51% of older adults were opposed to legislation that would offer more generous drug benefits through managed care plans (Harvard School of Public Health, 2003).

Case Management
The Obama administration also proposes through healthcare reform to coordinate Medicare services to help reduce government costs (The White House, 2010). Assistance to Medicare enrollees in navigating the confusing landscape of accessing medical services through case management has the possibility of reducing racial disparities that are the result of earlier life restrictions on access to health services.

Preventive Care
The number of Medicare enrollees accessing preventive care services is likely to increase if older adults continue to switch to private plans as predicted. Also, the Obama administration is looking to reduce barriers in access to preventive care in Medicare through the elimination of co-payments for checkups and wellness visits (Healthreform.gov, 2010). With this greater emphasis on prevention comes the social justice responsibility to ensure that the unintended consequences that are possible when focusing on individual-level risk factors are addressed and eliminated to ensure equal levels of care. One way to address these possible unintended consequences at the micro-level patient–physician encounter is to educate doctors to be understanding of the constraints in lifestyle that come along with poverty. This effort would be important to help reduce provider bias, discrimination, stereo-typing, and victim blaming in regard to personal behaviors. Once doctors are aware of the social context perpetuated by poverty, they may be more understanding of patients living in poverty, thus increasing the effectiveness of the interaction.

Limitations

A limitation of this study is the cross-sectional design. To make stronger causal arguments about the influence of Medicare insurance plan type on racial disparities, longitudinal data would need to be analyzed. Future studies could be undertaken to document changes in health overtime of individuals matched on a range of characteristics enrolled in each type of plan or the transition of enrollees from managed care to fee-for-service or vice versa to observe how the change effects health service utilization. Another limitation is no measures were available that documented need for health services. If any bias is introduced due to this, it would be expected that it may work to deflate disparities observed due to less need among healthier whites to see a specialist or have surgery. Despite these limitations, this study provides a first look at how health service utilization varies by race across Medicare insurance plans.

CONCLUSIONS

Racial health disparities are ever-present among older adults in the United States, resulting from documented social causes such as poverty and racism. This study found that generally African American Medicare enrollees access health services less often, and for more costly services, racial disparities were greater in fee-for-service compared to managed care plans. Proposed reforms to address these racial disparities are likely to increase the cost of Medicare, but would equate to policy that benefits all older adults equally, both rich and poor as well as sick and healthy, keeping in line with its original grounding as a social insurance program.

REFERENCES

Agency for Healthcare Research and Quality. (2000a). Addressing racial and ethnic disparities in health care. Fact sheet. AHRQ Publication No. 00-PO41. Rockville, Maryland. Available at http://www.ahrq.gov/research/disparit.htm. Retrieved on October 15, 2007.

Agency for Healthcare Research and Quality. (2000b). Coronary angiography is underused for both Medicare managed care and fee-for-service heart attack patients. Available at http://www.ahrq.gov/research/nov00/1100RA1.htm. Retrieved on October 15, 2007.

Agency for Healthcare Research and Quality. (2001). Diabetes disparities among racial and ethnic minorities. Available at http://www.ahrq.gov/research/diabdisp.htm. Retrieved on October 15, 2007.

Ahmad, W. I. (1989). Policies, pills, and political will: A critique of policies to improve the heath status of ethnic minorities. *Lancet*, *1*(8630), 148–150.

Alonzo, A. A. (1993). Health behavior: Issues, contradictions and dilemmas. *Social Science and Medicine*, *37*(8), 1019–1034.

Alva, M. (1996). Racial disparities mark care under Medicare, says study. *Contemporary Long Term Care*, *19*(11), 16.

Cagney, K. A., Browning, C. R., & Wen, M. (2005). Racial disparities in self-rated health at older ages: What difference does the neighborhood make? *Journals of Gerontology Series B: Psychological Sciences and Social Sciences*, *60*, S181–S190.

Cantor, M. D. (2008). The value of case management for Medicare Advantage plans. *Managed Care Outlook*, *21*(16), 1–8.
Centers for Disease Control. (2004). National vital statistics reports. 52(14), 18 February. Available at www.cdc.gov/nchs/data/nvsr/nvsr52/nvsr52_14.pdf. Retrieved on August 16, 2010.
Centers for Medicare and Medicaid Services, Department of Health and Human Services. (2004). CMS legislative update. Available at http://www.cms.hhs.gov/MMAUpdate/downloads/PL108-173summary.pdf. Retrieved on October 2, 2007.
Centers for Medicare and Medicaid Services, Department of Health and Human Services. (2005). Medicaid at-a-glance. Available at http://www.cms.hhs.gov/medicaiddatasourcesgeninfo/02_maag2005.asp. Retrieved on January 31, 2010.
Centers for Medicare and Medicaid Services, Department of Health and Human Services. (2009a). Medicare: Overview. Available at http://www.medicare.gov/choices/Overview.asp. Retrieved on January 31, 2010.
Centers for Medicare and Medicaid Services, Department of Health and Human Services. (2009b). Prescription drug plan finder: Glossary of definitions. Available at http://www.medicare.gov/MPDPF/Shared/Static/ResourcesGlossary.asp. Retrieved on January 31, 2010
Crawford, R. (1978). You are dangerous to your health. *Social Policy*, *8*, 10–20.
Estabrooks, P. A., Lee, R. E., & Gyurcsik, N. C. (2003). Resources for physical activity participation: Does availability and accessibility differ by neighborhood socioeconomic status? *Annals of Behavioral Medicine*, *25*, 100–104.
Everson, S. A., Maty, S. C., Lynch, J. W., & Kaplan, G. A. (2002). Epidemiologic evidence for the relation between socioeconomic status and depression, obesity, and diabetes. *Journal of Psychosomatic Research*, *53*(4), 891–895.
Foote, S. M. (2003). Population-based disease management under fee-for-service Medicare. *Health Affairs – Web Exclusive*, *W3*, 342–356.
Freking, K. (2007). More Medicare savings possible. Available at http://www.globalaging.org/health/us/2007/savings.htm. Retrieved on October 15, 2007.
Greene, J., Blustein, J., & Laflamme, K. A. (2001). Use of preventive care services, beneficiary characteristics, and Medicare HMO performance. *Health Care Financing Review*, *22*(4), 141–153.
Harvard School of Public Health. (2003). New survey finds most seniors favor reforms that build on existing Medicare program, but younger adults are more favorable toward private plans. Press Release, Thursday, June 19. Available at http://www.pnhp.org/news/2003/june/younger_adults_are_u.php. Retrieved on October 15, 2007.
Healthcarereform.gov. (2010). Health insurance reform and Medicare: Making Medicare stronger for America's seniors. Available at www.healthreform.gov/reports/medicare/medicare.pdf. Retrieved on January 31, 2010.
Hoadley, J., Hargrave, E., Cubanski, J., & Neuman, T. (2008). The Medicare part D coverage gap: Costs and consequences in 2007. Available at www.kff.org/medicare/upload/7811.pdf. Retrieved on January 31, 2010.
Kaiser Family Foundation. (2003). Key facts: Race, ethnicity & medical care, Update June 2003. Available at http://www.kff.org/minorityhealth/upload/Key-Facts-Race-Ethnicity-Medical-Care-Chartbook.pdf. Retrieved on October 15, 2007.
Kaiser Family Foundation. (2004). Medicare advantage. Available at http://www.kff.org/medicare/upload/Medicare-Advantage-Fact-Sheet.pdf. Retrieved on August 17, 2010.

Kaiser Family Foundation. (2005a). *Medicare chartbook* (3rd ed.). Washington, DC: Kaiser Family Foundation.
Kaiser Family Foundation. (2005b). Trends and indicators in the changing health care marketplace. Available at http://www.kff.org/insurance/7031/ti2004-2-17.cfm. Retrieved on October 15, 2007.
Kaiser Family Foundation. (2007). Fact sheet: Medicare advantage. Available at http://www.kff.org/medicare/upload/2052-10.pdf. Retrieved on October 15, 2007.
Katz, D. (2001). Behavior modification in primary care: The pressure system model. *Preventive Medicine, 32*, 66–72.
Landon, B. E., Zaslavsky, A. M., Bernard, S. L., Cioffi, M. J., & Cleary, P. D. (2004). Comparison of performance of traditional Medicare vs Medicare managed care. *Journal of the American Medical Association, 291*(14), 1744–1752.
LaVeist, T. A., Nickerson, K. J., & Bowie, J. V. (2000). Attitudes about racism, medical mistrust, and satisfaction with care among African American and white cardiac patients. *Medical Care Research and Review* (Suppl. 1), 146–161.
Lee, A. J., Baker, C. S., Gehlbach, S., Hosmer, D. W., & Reti, M. (1998). Do African American elderly Medicare patients receive fewer services? An analysis of procedure use for selected patient conditions. *Medical Care Research and Review, 55*(3), 314–333.
Macintyre, S., Maciver, S., & Sooman, A. (1993). Area, class and health: Should we be focusing on places or people? *Journal of Social Policy, 22*, 213–234.
Medicare. (2007). Medicare plan choices. Available at http://www.medicare.gov/Choices/Overview.asp. Retrieved on October 15, 2007.
Miller, R. H., & Luft, H. S. (1994). Managed care plan performance since 1980. A literature analysis. *Journal of the American Medical Association, 271*(19), 1512–1519.
Morland, K., Wing, S., & Diez-Roux, A. (2002). The contextual effect of the local food environment on residents' diets: The atherosclerosis risk in communities study. *American Journal of Public Health, 92*, 1761–1767.
National Health Interview Survey. (2008). Survey description. Available at ftp://ftp.cdc.gov/pub/Health_Statistics/NCHS/Dataset_Documentation/NHIS/2008/srvydesc.pdf. Retrieved on January 6, 2010.
National Institute of Diabetes and Digestive and Kidney Diseases. (2010). Diabetes dictionary. Available at http://diabetes.niddk.nih.gov/dm/pubs/dictionary/A-E.htm. Retrieved on October 15, 2007.
Schneider, E. C., Cleary, P. D., Zaslavsky, A. M., & Epstein, A. M. (2001). Racial disparity in influenza vaccination: Does managed care narrow the gap between African Americans and whites? *Journal of the American Medical Association, 286*(12), 1455–1460.
Social Security Administration. (2010). The development of medicare. Available at http://www.ssa.gov/history/ssa/lbjmedicare1.html. Retrieved on August 17, 2010.
The White House. (2010). Health care: The Obama plan. Available at http://www.whitehouse.gov/issues/health-care/plan. Retrieved on January 31, 2010.
U.S. Department of Health and Human Services, Office of Minority Health. (2009). African American profile. Available at http://minorityhealth.hhs.gov/templates/browse.aspx?lvl = 2&lvlID = 51. Retrieved on August 17, 2010.
Virnig, B. A., Lurie, N., Huang, Z., Musgrave, D., McBean, A. M., & Dowd, B. (2002). Racial variation in quality of care among Medicare+choice enrollees: African American/white patterns of racial disparities in health care do not necessarily apply to Asians, Hispanics, and native Americans. *Health Affairs, 21*(6), 224–230.

Ware, J. E., Jr., Bayliss, M. S., Rogers, W. H., Kosinski, M., & Tarlov, A. R. (1996). Differences in 4-year health outcomes for elderly and poor, chronically ill patients treated in HMO and fee-for-service systems. Results from the Medical Outcomes Study. *Journal of the American Medical Association, 276*(13), 1039–1047.

Williams, D. R., Yu, Y., Jackson, J. S., & Anderson, N. B. (1997). Racial differences in physical and mental health. *Journal of Health Psychology, 2*(3), 335–351.

Wong, H., & Hellinger, F. (2001). Conducting research on the Medicare market: The need for better data and methods. *Health Services Research, 36*(1 Pt. 2), 291–308.

HOW MUCH TIME DO AMERICANS SPEND SEEKING HEALTH CARE? RACIAL AND ETHNIC DIFFERENCES IN PATIENT EXPERIENCES

Deborah Carr, Yoko Ibuka and Louise B. Russell

ABSTRACT

We use data from the American Time Use Survey (ATUS) to investigate racial differences in the amount of time individuals spend traveling to, waiting for, and receiving outpatient healthcare services on a randomly selected survey interview day. Of the 60,674 participants in the 2003–2006 waves of the ATUS, 2.67% (n = 1,621) reported a clinical encounter on their designated day; this proportion did not differ significantly by race. Among those reporting a clinical encounter, blacks reported spending 30 more minutes than whites in receiving services, and this race gap persisted net of socioeconomic, health, and geographic factors. Hispanics also reported significantly longer visits than whites; yet, this difference was partially accounted for by Hispanics' relatively poorer health status. Hispanics and persons of other ethnicity reported significantly longer wait times than whites, whereas blacks and Hispanics reported significantly longer travel times than did whites; these significant differences did not attenuate in the fully adjusted models. The results show that ethnic minorities spend far more time than whites when traveling to, waiting for, or receiving outpatient services, revealing another aspect of health care where stark racial inequities exist. We suggest that the relatively long wait and transportation times reported by ethnic minorities may reflect overcrowded care sites and the lack of quality care in neighborhoods inhabited largely by blacks and Hispanics, thus impeding the delivery of timely and "patient-centered" medical care.

Health policy experts and practitioners have articulated two core missions: to make the U.S. health care system more patient-centered and to reduce racial and ethnic disparities in care. In its influential report, *Crossing the Quality Chasm*, the Institute of Medicine's Committee on Quality of Health Care in America (2001) recommended that patient-centered medical care should not waste patients' time and should not vary in quality on the basis of patients' personal characteristics such as ethnicity or socioeconomic status. The *Healthy People 2010* initiative, which sets forth the federal government's health objectives for the United States, articulated a similar goal: "to eliminate health disparities that occur by race and ethnicity, gender, education, income, geographic location" and other social characteristics (U.S. Department of Health and Human Services, 2000).

Despite policy makers' lofty aim of eradicating health disparities in the first decade of the 21st century, racial and social class disparities remain a persistent feature of health and health care in the United States. Blacks, Hispanics, and Native Americans are disadvantaged relative to whites in terms of virtually every documented health outcome, including quality of care, insurance coverage, morbidity, and mortality (Institute of Medicine, 2003; Mead et al., 2008). However, we know of no studies that investigate whether these disparities extend to patients' time use when seeking care. We use data from the American Time Use Survey (ATUS) to investigate racial differences in the amount of time individuals spend traveling to, waiting for, and receiving outpatient healthcare services on a randomly selected survey interview day. Documenting racial disparities in the time spent seeking medical care is an important line of inquiry; the opportunity costs involved in seeking care – such as travel time or time taken away from paid employment – may pose obstacles to the receipt of high quality and convenient medical care.

BACKGROUND

Access to timely, efficient, and geographically proximate medical care can reduce mortality and long-term disability, especially from treatable conditions such as stroke, heart attack, and bacterial infections. Ethnic minority patients typically wait longer than white patients to obtain an appointment for health care; they are less likely than whites to get a next day or same day appointment to see a doctor (The Commonwealth Fund, 2006). Data collected from 1997 to 2004 reveal that black patients seeking care in emergency rooms are more likely than white patients to leave without receiving care – a finding that the researchers speculated might be due to long and frustrating wait times (Agency for Healthcare Research and Quality [AHRQ], 2006). Some studies suggest further that blacks and Hispanics are more likely than whites to reside in areas underserved by healthcare providers; thus, they may wait longer for care in crowded, understaffed physician offices or they may travel to more distant yet better served areas to receive care (Guagliardo 2004; Williams, Neighbors, & Jackson, 2003). Ethnic minorities, especially the economically disadvantaged, also may lack efficient transportation to their healthcare providers, often relying on public transit. As such, the extensive travel time required may be an obstacle to seeking timely medical care.

The primary aim of our study is to evaluate racial and ethnic differences in the amount of time spent traveling to, waiting for, and receiving outpatient care. Prior studies have revealed the vast amount of time that Americans devote to receiving outpatient medical care (Russell, Ibuka, & Carr, 2008). Daily diary reports from the ATUS show that the average outpatient visit, including traveling to and from, waiting for, and receiving services, averages two hours for patients, and another two hours for the companions who accompany them. Over the course of a year, for persons aged 15 and older, this amounts to 207 million 40-hour work weeks for outpatient visits alone. However, an important, yet unresolved, question is whether the time burden of seeking care is equivalent for all Americans, or whether racial and ethnic minorities bear a particularly intrusive burden.

Potential Pathways Linking Race and Time Spent on Clinical Encounters

A further aim of our study is to evaluate the extent to which an observed statistical association between race and time spent traveling to, waiting for, and receiving outpatient care is accounted for by socioeconomic, demographic, access, and health characteristics. First, we consider the role of socioeconomic resources. Blacks and Hispanics lag behind whites in educational attainment, income, and assets (U.S. Bureau of the Census, 2008). Socioeconomic resources, in turn, are a widely documented correlate of receiving timely and high-quality care (AHRQ, 2006).

Second, we consider family characteristics, including marital and parental statuses. Marital status varies by race, where blacks are less likely than whites, Hispanics, and Asians to ever marry and to remain married (U.S. Bureau of the Census, 2008). Marital status and parental status, to a lesser extent, are associated with seeking regular health care; persons with close family ties receive health-enhancing supports including encouragement to seek timely care and assistance with transportation (e.g., Waite & Gallagher, 2000).

Third, we consider whether one resides in a metropolitan versus nonmetropolitan area. Persons residing in nonmetropolitan areas travel longer distances to reach healthcare delivery sites, compared to persons in urbanized areas (Larson & Fleishman, 2003). Although an estimated 20% of Americans reside in rural areas today, only 9% of physicians practice in such areas, and this shortage is compounded as hospital closures disproportionately strike rural areas (van Dis, 2002). Persons living in nonmetropolitan areas are disproportionately white non-Hispanics; yet, racial minorities living in rural areas are particularly disadvantaged with respect to seeking and receiving health care (Hartley, Quam, & Lurie, 1994).

Fourth, we consider physical health status, because it may affect the content, duration, and location of clinical encounters (Cherry, Woodwell, & Rechtsteiner, 2007). Persons with serious health conditions may face long travel and wait times when seeking specialist care (Merritt Hawkins & Associates, 2009). Health status also is associated with race/ethnicity, as African Americans and Hispanics tend to have poorer overall health and higher rates of disability and chronic conditions such as diabetes, obesity, and high blood pressure, relative to whites (Centers for Disease Control, 2008). Finally, we consider the role of health insurance, because it is an important pathway to receiving quality and timely medical care; yet, ethnic minorities are less likely than whites to have health insurance, especially employer-provided coverage (Institute of Medicine, 2001).

In sum, building upon prior studies of patients' time use and ethnic disparities in quality of and access to care, we use data from the ATUS to (1) document the amount of time that whites, blacks, Hispanics, and persons of other ethnicities spend traveling to, waiting for, and receiving outpatient medical services; and (2) evaluate the extent to which racial disparities are accounted for by differences in socioeconomic resources, demographic characteristics, health, and access to care.

DATA

We use data from the first four years (2003–2006) of the nationally representative ATUS. The ATUS, conducted by the U.S. Census Bureau for the Bureau of Labor Statistics, is designed to produce "nationally representative estimates of how people spend their time" (Bureau of Labor Statistics [BLS], 2007; Horrigan & Herz, 2004). Households are selected from those that complete their final interview for the Current Population Survey (CPS), the nation's monthly labor force survey. After the CPS's oversampling of small states is corrected, households are stratified by race and Hispanic origin, presence and age of children, and, for childless households, number of adults, and sampled at different rates within each stratum. An individual respondent is randomly selected from persons 15 years or older in each household to participate in the ATUS. In 2003, 3,375 households were selected each month. In 2004–2006, the number was reduced to 2,194 households per month for budgetary reasons.

The ATUS sample is partitioned into four subgroups, one for each week of the month. Within each week, 10% of the sample is assigned to each weekday, 25% to each weekend day. Respondents are randomly assigned a day of the week and phoned the next day. Interviews take place using computer-assisted telephone interviewing (CATI); questions focus primarily on the respondent's activities over the preceding 24-hour period. If interviewers do not reach the respondent, they attempt subsequent contacts on the same day of the week for up to eight consecutive weeks. The 5% of households that do not provide telephone numbers are mailed a request to call the telephone center for the interview.

Response rates declined slightly from 57.8% in 2003 to 55.1% in 2006 (Tai-Seale, McGuire, & Zhang, 2007; Horrigan & Herz, 2004). The ATUS sample weights adjust for differential rates of nonresponse, as well as the oversampling of weekend days and oversampling based on demographic and household characteristics (e.g., ethnicity, presence of children in household). In 2003–2006, 60,674 respondents aged 15 years or older completed the ATUS.

Analytic Sample

Our analysis is limited to the 1,621 persons (1,208 whites, 191 blacks, 179 Hispanics, and 43 persons of other ethnicity) who reported seeking medical care for themselves on their designated survey day. Of the 60,674 participants in the 2003–2006 ATUS, 2.67% ($n = 1,621$) reported an outpatient health encounter; this proportion increased slightly to 3.4% when the full sample was weighted to represent the U.S. population. The proportion of the total sample reporting a health encounter did not differ significantly by race or ethnicity.

MEASURES

Dependent Variables

We focus on three outcomes: the number of minutes spent *receiving, waiting for*, and *traveling to inpatient medical services*. ATUS participants are asked how they spent the 24 hours beginning 4:00 a.m. the previous day (their "designated day") and ending 4:00 a.m. the day of the call. Responses are coded independently by two interviewers who did not conduct the interview; coding differences are resolved by trained adjudicators (Tai-Seale et al., 2007). Each activity is assigned a six-digit code; the first two digits indicate one of 17 major activity categories, the next four signify an intermediate category and specific activity (Abraham, Maitland, & Bianchi, 2006; Shelley, 2005). The ATUS data file shows the times each activity began and ended (see Shelley 2005 for further detail on ATUS codes).

We focus here on activities coded as traveling to, waiting for, or receiving care. We focus solely on care the respondent sought for himself or herself; different codes are used for time spent accompanying others as they seek care. All types of outpatient visits are included in the ATUS. Although inpatient stays are included in the ATUS activity definitions, no respondents reported times long enough to suggest that they were inpatients on their survey day.

Independent Variables

Our key independent variable is *race/ethnicity*. We contrast four categories: non-Hispanic white (reference category); non-Hispanic black; Hispanic; and other ethnicity, three-quarters of whom are Asian/Pacific Islander. All analyses control for *age* and *gender*.

Our goal is to evaluate the extent to which racial differences in time use reflect disparities in socioeconomic resources, physical health, and access to care. First, we consider two indicators of socioeconomic status: *educational attainment* (years of schooling completed) and *total family income*. Education categories include less than a high school degree (reference category), high school degree, some college, college degree, and post-college education. Family income includes income of all members of the household who are 15 years of age or older. Income includes money from jobs; net income from business, farm, or rent; pensions; dividends; interest; social security payments; and any other monetary income received by family members.

Second, we consider family characteristics, including marital status and parental status. *Marital status* refers to whether an individual is never married, married (reference category), separated/divorced, or widowed. *Parental status* refers to the number of children residing in one's household: none (reference category), one, two, or three or more children. Third, we consider potential proximity to care, with an indicator of whether one lives in a *metropolitan* (reference category) versus *nonmetropolitan* geographic area. We also include a dichotomous variable indicating those persons for whom geographic location could not be ascertained.

Fourth, we captured one's *physical health* with a single dichotomous indicator of "ill health." Before 2006, the ATUS did not obtain data on physical health. The only information about health came from questions that asked whether health was a reason for the respondent's employment status. We coded a person as being in ill health if he or she cited ill health or disability as the reason why she/he was for either not working over the last four weeks, working less than full time, not wanting to work full time, leaving their last job, or not participating in the labor force.

Fifth, we considered four indicators of employment status that may be conceptualized as broad (and, admittedly imprecise) proxies for whether one has *health insurance*; we used this approach because the ATUS does not obtain data on health insurance status. Drawing on prior work describing the types of jobs and employers that typically provide health insurance (e.g., Seccombe, 1993), we developed indicators of whether one is an hourly wage earner; class of worker; full-time work; and major occupational group. *Hourly worker* refers to whether people are paid an hourly wage versus an annual salary. Persons not currently working are the reference category. *Class of worker* refers to whether one is a wage and salary (reference category), government, or self-employed worker, or not currently working.

Full-time status captures whether one works 35 or more hours per week (omitted category), less than 35 hours, variable hours, or is not currently working. *Occupational group* refers to whether one works in a management/ business, professional (reference category), service, sales, administrative, or blue-collar occupation. We presume that hourly workers, self-employed persons, part-time workers, and those in nonprofessional occupations will be less likely to have employer-provided insurance and thus may have limited access to care.

Finally, in preliminary analyses, we also included an indicator of one's English language capacity, which can be conceptualized as a cultural barrier to receiving timely, proximate, and efficient care. Persons with limited English capacity may require translation services, which are not available at all healthcare sites (Jacobs et al., 2001) and may require lengthier waits or travel times. We considered a dichotomous variable signifying whether Spanish was the only language spoken by all members of one's household. The variable was not a significant predictor of any of the three outcome variables, nor did it mediate the effect of Hispanic ethnicity; thus, we do not include this measure in our analyses.

RESULTS

Descriptive Statistics

Descriptive statistics are presented in Table 1. The second column shows results for our analytic sample ($n = 1,621$) and the third column provides information on the full ATUS sample ($N = 60,674$). The two samples are very similar in their racial and ethnic composition, although whites are slightly overrepresented and persons of other ethnicity slightly underrepresented in the analytic sample, relative to the full ATUS sample. In our analytic sample, whites account for 74.5% of respondents, whereas blacks and Hispanics comprise roughly 11% each, and other ethnicities account for 2.7%. Our analytic sample includes a disproportionately high number of women and older adults, reflecting the greater tendency of both subgroups to seek health care, relative to men and younger persons. For example, 30% of the analytic sample but just 17% of the full ATUS sample is ages 65 and older. Consequently, members of the analytic sample are more likely than persons in the full sample to be not currently employed (versus employed), widowed versus married, and residing in a household with no children.

Table 1. Frequency Distribution, All Variables Used in Analysis, ATUS 2003–2006.

	Analytic Sample (n = 1,621)	Full Sample (N = 60,674)
Demographic characteristics		
Race		
White (reference category)	74.5	71.9
Black	11.8	11.6
Hispanic	11.0	11.9
Other	2.7	4.5
Age (years)		
15–24	5.7	11.8
25–34	11.0	16.6
35–44	17.9	22.2
45–54 (reference category)	20.2	18.8
55–64	16.0	13.6
65–74	15.9	9.2
75+	13.9	7.8
Female	67.4	56.7
Socioeconomic resources		
Education		
Less than high school (reference category)	16.3	17.5
High school diploma/GED	26.9	27.4
Some college	29.4	26.6
College degree	16.6	36.3
Postcollege	10.8	10.4
Income		
Less than $15,000 (reference category)	16.0	12.3
$15–29,999	15.0	15.6
$30–49,999	17.4	19.1
$50–74,999	17.4	16.9
$75–99,999	17.2	14.6
$100,000+	2.5	8.3
Missing	14.0	13.0
Family characteristics		
Married (reference category)	53.5	53.3
Divorced/separated	16.4	15.1
Widowed	13.1	8.2
Never married	17	23.2
No children in household (reference category)	61.9	52.1
1 child in household	15.4	19.4
2 children in household	13.6	18.3
3+ children in household	9.1	9.3

Table 1. (*Continued*)

	Analytic Sample (n = 1,621)	Full Sample (N = 60,674)
Geographic access		
Lives in metro area (reference category)	73.7	72.7
Lives in nonmetro area	16.8	17.6
Metro status not identified	9.5	9.7
Health		
Ill health	12.8	5.1
Proxies for health insurance status		
Hourly wage worker	22.8	32.5
Salaried worker (reference category)	18.6	24.3
Not working/NA	58.5	43.3
Wage and salary worker (reference category)	36.9	49.9
Government worker	10.9	11.1
Self-employed	4.9	7.0
Not working/NA	47.4	31.9
Full-time worker (reference category)	32.2	47.1
Part-time worker	9.8	10.5
Variable hours at work	3.9	4.8
Not working/NA	54.1	37.5
Occupation		
Business/finance	8.1	10.5
Professional (reference category)	13.5	15.9
Service	9.0	10.6
Sales	4.5	7.4
Administrative	0.2	9.8
Blue collar	9.1	14
Not working/NA	47.4	31.9

Note: Analytic sample includes persons who reported a clinical health encounter on their selected day.
Abbreviations: GED, General Equivalency Diploma; NA, not applicable.

Bivariate Analysis

Our first aim is to investigate whether the average time spent on health encounters differs across racial groups. We conducted analysis of variance (ANOVA) using unweighted data; we contrasted whether whites, blacks, Hispanics, and persons of other ethnicity differed significantly from one another with respect to each healthcare encounter measure. Results are

Table 2. Race/Ethnic Comparison of Clinical Encounter Reports, ATUS 2003–2006.

	Total Sample	White	Black	Hispanic	Other Race/Ethnicity	Significant Subgroup Differences	Valid N
Percentage reporting a clinical encounter	2.67	2.77	2.70	2.47	2.38		60674
Number of minutes, total encounter	123.48	110.07	167.91	161.97	146.59	WB, WH, WO	1621
Number of minutes, travel	33.59	30.79	42.52	43.29	34.65	WB, WH	1621
Number of minutes, receiving services	74.11	66.88	102.62	89.04	88.72	WB, WH	1621
Number of minutes, waiting	45.23	37.16	56.47	73.24	73.76	WB, WH, WO	565

Notes: Unweighted data are presented. Post hoc comparisons of unadjusted means were conducted using ANOVA; significant ($p<.05$) subgroup differences are denoted as WB: white versus black; WH: white versus Hispanic; and WO: white versus other race/ethnicity.

presented in Table 2, and we denote those subgroups that differed significantly from one another at the $p<.05$ level.

We first examined whether the proportion reporting an outpatient encounter differed significantly by race. We did not find a statistically significant difference ($p<.05$); across each of the four ethnic groups, 2–3% reported that they had a clinical encounter on their designated survey day. When we focused on only those reporting the clinical encounter, we found statistically significant differences in the amount of time spent on each of three components of the medical visit, with whites consistently reporting the shortest durations and blacks and Hispanics reporting the longest. The total time spent traveling to, waiting for, and receiving care ranges from just under two hours for whites (110 minutes) to nearly three hours for blacks and Hispanics (168 and 162 minutes, respectively). Persons of other ethnicity report an average of 147 minutes.

Upon examining each of the three components of the encounters, we found that blacks and Hispanics report significantly more time traveling and receiving services than did whites, whereas Hispanics and persons of other ethnicity reported longer wait times than whites. The amount of time spent traveling to health care averaged 30 minutes among whites, but nearly 45 minutes among blacks and Hispanics. The amount of time receiving services was also lowest for whites; 67 minutes compared to 89 minutes for Hispanics and other ethnicities; and 103 minutes for blacks. Only one-third of persons with a healthcare encounter reported waiting, and this proportion did not vary significantly by race. However, whites reported significantly less waiting time than blacks, Hispanics, and other ethnic groups ($M = 37.2$ minutes versus 56.5, 73.2, and 73.8, respectively).

Multivariate Analyses

The ANOVA analyses provide a description of racial differences in time use, based on the unweighted sample. We next evaluate potential explanations for these observed race disparities. We estimated ordinary least squares (OLS) regression models using weighted data, to predict the minutes spent receiving services (Table 3), waiting for services (Table 4), and traveling to and from services (Table 5). Model 1 includes race/ethnicity, age, and gender only; model 2 incorporates socioeconomic status indicators; model 3 adjusts for family characteristics; model 4 controls for region; and model 5 adjusts for health status. Unstandardized regression coefficients and standard errors are presented. We also estimated models that included proxies for health insurance; these are discussed in the text, but not presented in the tables.

Receiving Services

The results in Table 3 reveal that blacks spend roughly 30 minutes more receiving services during their clinical encounters than whites. Models 1 through 4 show a black–white difference of roughly 35 minutes; yet, this effect size declines to 30 minutes when health status is controlled. This slight attenuation reflects the poorer health of blacks in the analytic sample; 28.3% are classified as having ill health, compared to 12% of whites. The black–white gap does not change, however, when socioeconomic, region, and family characteristics are controlled.

By contrast, the gap between whites and both Hispanics and other ethnicities declines and becomes marginally significant when health status is controlled. For example, models 1 through 4 show that Hispanics spend 16–18 more minutes than whites receiving healthcare services ($p < .05$); yet, this gap declines to just 12 minutes and becomes marginally significant ($p = .06$) when health status is controlled. These results suggest that the longer duration of healthcare visits for Hispanics may partly reflect their relatively poorer health; 19.6% of Hispanics, yet just 12% of whites are classified as having ill health in the ATUS.

Table 3. OLS Regression Predicting Minutes Receiving Care, ATUS 2003–2006 ($N = 1621$).

	Model 1	Model 2	Model 3	Model 4	Model 5
Demographic characteristics					
Race					
Black	35.69***	34.54***	35.39***	34.39***	30.34***
	(6.28)	(6.46)	(6.54)	(6.56)	(6.55)
Hispanic	18.36***	18.62***	17.18***	15.78*	12.18
	(6.01)	(6.22)	(6.23)	(6.26)	(6.24)
Other	21.05*	18.92	20	19.84*	17.51
	(10.11)	(10.21)	(10.22)	(10.21)	(10.13)
Age (years)					
15–24	1.94	3.72	14.05	15.76	20.44*
	(7.16)	(7.44)	(9.24)	(9.26)	(9.22)
25–34	−3.67	−4.25	−.34	−.10	4.23
	(6.96)	(7.01)	(7.33)	(7.32)	(7.30)
35–44	−1.14	−1.95	1.38	1.41	3.69
	(6.18)	(6.23)	(6.63)	(6.62)	(6.57)
55–64	10.31	9.22	6.99	7.09	8.17
	(6.17)	(6.22)	(6.39)	(6.39)	(6.33)
65–74	−.62	−1.44	−3.75	−3.15	3.2
	(6.41)	(6.55)	(6.82)	(6.82)	(6.86)
75+	1.05	0.17	−3.26	−3.33	4.25
	(6.40)	(6.67)	(7.23)	(7.22)	(7.29)
Female	−17.46***	−18.87***	−19.65***	−19.45***	−18.25***
	(3.79)	(3.83)	(3.89)	(3.89)	(3.86)
Socioeconomic resources					
Education					
12 years		8.05	8.12	8.55	9.11
		(5.78)	(5.80)	(5.82)	(5.77)
Some college		5.51	5.25	5.24	6.29
		(5.90)	(5.93)	(5.93)	(5.88)
College degree		2.56	1.71	1.88	3.53
		(6.95)	(7.00)	(7.00)	(6.94)
Postcollege		0.20	0.28	0.24	3.45
		(8.11)	(8.16)	(8.16)	(8.11)
Income					
$15–29,000		−9.40	−6.95	−7.41	−4.37
		(7.28)	(7.33)	(7.33)	(7.29)
$30–49,000		−10.87	−6.57	−8.38	−1.55
		(7.09)	(7.28)	(7.32)	(7.37)
$50–74,000		−7.86	−3.76	−5.39	0.64
		(7.13)	(7.34)	(7.37)	(7.39)
$75–99,000		−2.35	2.99	0.55	7.56
		(7.79)	(8.08)	(8.15)	(8.18)

Table 3. (*Continued*)

	Model 1	Model 2	Model 3	Model 4	Model 5
$100,000+		−16.78*	−10.70	−13.17	−4.87
		(8.74)	(9.11)	(9.17)	(9.22)
Missing		−12.15	−8.67	−10.26	−4.16
		(7.07)	(7.27)	(7.29)	(7.32)
Family characteristics					
Divorced/separated			13.56*	13.16*	8.72
			(6.21)	(6.21)	(6.21)
Widowed			11.44	10.92	10.01
			(7.13)	(7.12)	(7.06)
Never married			−6.74	−7.24	−7.21
			(6.44)	(6.44)	(6.38)
1 child			−14.60*	−14.67*	−12.36*
			(6.06)	(6.06)	(6.02)
2 children			−2.50	−2.84	−1.79
			(6.69)	(6.68)	(6.62)
3+ children			−1.63	−1.61	0.23
			(7.72)	(7.71)	(7.65)
Geographic access					
Lives in nonmetro area				−9.79*	−9.90*
				(5.02)	(4.98)
Metro status not identified				−57.09	−51.65
				(45.42)	(45.03)
Ill health					33.60***
					(6.18)
Intercept	76.25***	81.80***	79.06***	82.22***	68.53***
	(4.92)	(8.26)	(8.98)	(9.09)	(9.35)
Adjusted R^2	0.03	0.03	0.04	0.04	0.06

Notes: Unstandardized regression coefficients and standard errors (in parentheses) are presented. Data are weighted to reflect each respondent's share of the noninstitutionalized civilian population age 15 or older.
*$p<.05$; **$p<.01$; ***$p<.001$.

We conducted additional analyses to assess whether the racial gaps would attenuate further when four proxies for health insurance were separately incorporated into model 4. Only one indicator was a statistically significant predictor; part-time workers spent an average of 15 minutes more per visit than did full-time workers. However, the inclusion of this measure did not alter the size or significance levels of the race coefficients.

Few other characteristics were significant predictors of the time spent receiving services. Women reported average visits that are 18 minutes

Table 4. OLS Regression Predicting Number of Minutes Waiting, ATUS 2003–2006 ($N = 565$).

	Model 1	Model 2	Model 3	Model 4	Model 5
Demographic characteristics					
Race					
Black	9.88	3.62	3.31	2.74	2.4
	(6.75)	(6.82)	(6.95)	(6.94)	(6.98)
Hispanic	31.73***	21.77***	22.18***	20.61***	20.63***
	(6.35)	(6.46)	(6.48)	(6.46)	(6.48)
Other	34.01***	33.85***	33.46***	35.20***	35.30***
	(12.01)	(11.82)	(11.85)	(11.82)	(11.83)
Age (years)					
15–24	−3.22	−10.96	−11.67	−7.38	−6.54
	(7.64)	(7.89)	(9.89)	(9.98)	(10.12)
25–34	−13.51	−17.14*	−16.19	−15.47	−14.98
	(8.12)	(7.97)	(8.45)	(8.42)	(8.48)
35–44	−8.40	−11.66	−9.42	−9.22	−9.01
	(7.14)	(7.06)	(7.61)	(7.58)	(7.60)
55–64	−1.10	−6.26	−7.16	−7.47	−7.57
	(6.88)	(6.82)	(7.10)	(7.07)	(7.08)
65–74	0.86	−5.48	−5.29	−3.97	−3.10
	(6.91)	(6.97)	(7.33)	(7.31)	(7.51)
75+	12.36	4.52	6.06	5.87	7.1
	(6.81)	(7.01)	(7.64)	(7.61)	(7.98)
Female	7.67	7.39	8.1	8.4	8.49*
	(4.20)	(4.21)	(4.32)	(4.31)	(4.31)
Socioeconomic resources					
Education					
12 years		−19.66***	−20.42***	−19.80***	−19.58***
		(5.98)	(6.10)	(6.08)	(6.10)
Some college		−8.16	−9.50	−9.39	−9.36
		(6.12)	(6.24)	(6.22)	(6.23)
College degree		−25.29***	−26.07***	−25.49***	−25.22***
		(7.18)	(7.31)	(7.29)	(7.31)
Postcollege		−24.83***	−28.01***	−28.30***	−27.85***
		(8.42)	(8.68)	(8.64)	(8.69)
Income					
$15–29,000		−2.05	−1.45	−1.75	−1.44
		(7.31)	(7.36)	(7.34)	(7.37)
$30–49,000		11.4	11.45	9.48	10.27
		(7.22)	(7.47)	(7.47)	(7.63)
$50–74,000		−8.99	−8.31	−10.14	−9.44
		(7.20)	(7.59)	(7.59)	(7.72)
$75–99,000		−14.41	−12.84	−15.36	−14.38
		(8.27)	(8.78)	(8.79)	(9.00)

Table 4. (*Continued*)

	Model 1	Model 2	Model 3	Model 4	Model 5
$100,000+		−11.45	−10.66	−12.15	−11.31
		(9.53)	(9.88)	(9.85)	(9.99)
Missing		−10.48	−10.18	−12.32	−11.79
		(7.25)	(7.48)	(7.49)	(7.57)
Family characteristics					
Divorced/separated			4.89	4.60	4.07
			(7.14)	(7.11)	(7.19)
Widowed			−8.71	−9.83	−10.17
			(7.34)	(7.32)	(7.35)
Never married			2.36	1.16	1.11
			(6.92)	(6.91)	(6.91)
1 child			−7.11	−8.83	−8.53
			(6.52)	(6.56)	(6.59)
2 children			0.90	−1.05	−.79
			(7.22)	(7.23)	(7.25)
3+ children			−12.23	−13.94	−13.64
			(8.82)	(8.81)	(8.83)
Geographic access					
Lives in nonmetro area				−12.94*	−13.09*
				(5.37)	(5.38)
Metro status not identified				−44.68	−44.03
				(38.76)	(38.80)
Ill health					3.47
					(6.76)
Intercept	32.35***	57.60***	58.93***	62.77***	61.09***
	(5.60)	(9.02)	(9.77)	(9.84)	(10.37)
Adjusted R^2	0.05	0.1	0.1	0.11	0.11

Notes: Unstandardized regression coefficients and standard errors (in parentheses) are presented. Data are weighted to reflect each respondent's share of the noninstitutionalized civilian population age 15 and older.
*$p<.05$; **$p<.01$; ***$p<.001$.

shorter than men's, whereas persons in nonmetropolitan areas reported visits that were roughly 10 minutes shorter than their urban counterparts. Not surprisingly, persons with ill health reported visits that were more than 30 minutes longer than their healthier counterparts. Taken together, these variables explained relatively little variance in amount of time receiving services, however. Even in the fully adjusted models, the adjusted R^2 values never surpassed .06.

Table 5. OLS Regression Predicting Minutes Traveling, ATUS 2003–2006 ($N = 1621$).

	Model 1	Model 2	Model 3	Model 4	Model 5
Demographic characteristics					
Race					
Black	10.94***	9.10***	9.40***	9.45***	8.98**
	(2.73)	(2.80)	(2.84)	(2.85)	(2.87)
Hispanic	11.49***	10.87***	10.98***	10.91***	10.49***
	(2.61)	(2.69)	(2.70)	(2.72)	(2.73)
Other	6.76	6.54	5.72	5.73	5.45
	(4.40)	(4.42)	(4.44)	(4.44)	(4.44)
Age (years)					
15–24	−7.26*	−6.41*	−6.46	−6.34	−5.79
	(3.11)	(3.23)	(4.01)	(4.03)	(4.04)
25–34	−5.93*	−5.67	−3.83	−3.82	−3.31
	(3.02)	(3.04)	(3.18)	(3.18)	(3.20)
35–44	−4.31	−4.71	−2.26	−2.24	−1.98
	(2.69)	(2.70)	(2.88)	(2.88)	(2.88)
55–64	0.27	−.38	−1.97	−1.97	−1.84
	(2.68)	(2.70)	(2.77)	(2.78)	(2.78)
65–74	−2.91	−4.30	−5.77*	−5.62	−4.88
	(2.79)	(2.84)	(2.96)	(2.97)	(3.01)
75+	−.96	−2.73	−3.98	−3.98	−3.09
	(2.78)	(2.89)	(3.14)	(3.14)	(3.20)
Female	−2.64	−2.77	−2.47	−2.41	−2.27
	(1.65)	(1.66)	(1.69)	(1.69)	(1.69)
Socioeconomic resources					
Education					
12 years		−.42	−.96	−1.10	−1.03
		(2.50)	(2.52)	(2.53)	(2.53)
Some college		−.85	−1.73	−1.87	−1.75
		(2.56)	(2.57)	(2.58)	(2.58)
College degree		−3.33	−4.70	−4.82	−4.63
		(3.01)	(3.04)	(3.04)	(3.04)
Postcollege		6.92*	5.65	5.52	5.9
		(3.51)	(3.54)	(3.55)	(3.55)
Income					
$15–29,000		−3.96	−3.37	−3.35	−2.99
		(3.16)	(3.18)	(3.19)	(3.19)
$30–49,000		0.14	0.67	0.6	1.4
		(3.07)	(3.16)	(3.18)	(3.23)
$50–74,000		−4.02	−3.20	−3.29	−2.59
		(3.09)	(3.19)	(3.20)	(3.24)
$75–99,000		−5.83	−4.63	−4.73	−3.91
		(3.38)	(3.51)	(3.54)	(3.59)

Table 5. (Continued)

	Model 1	Model 2	Model 3	Model 4	Model 5
$100,000+		−8.11	−6.72	−6.82	−5.85
		(3.79)	(3.95)	(3.99)	(4.04)
Missing		−1.25	−.95	−1.07	−.35
		(3.07)	(3.15)	(3.17)	(3.21)
Family characteristics					
Divorced/separated			0.81	.80	0.27
			(2.70)	(2.70)	(2.72)
Widowed			−1.65	−1.76	−1.87
			(3.09)	(3.10)	(3.10)
Never married			1.40	1.36	1.36
			(2.79)	(2.80)	(2.80)
1 child			−6.05*	−6.00**	−5.73*
			(2.63)	(2.63)	(2.64)
2 children			−7.07**	−7.10**	−6.98*
			(2.90)	(2.90)	(2.90)
3+ children			−6.84*	−6.87*	−6.66*
			(3.35)	(3.35)	(3.35)
Geographic access					
Lives in nonmetro area				−.31	−.14
				(2.18)	(2.18)
Metro status not identified				−19.61	−18.98
				(19.74)	(19.74)
Ill health					3.95
					(2.71)
Intercept	35.64***	39.78***	41.69***	41.87***	40.26***
	(2.14)	(3.58)	(3.90)	(3.95)	(4.10)
Adjusted R^2	0.02	0.03	0.03	0.03	0.03

Notes: Unstandardized regression coefficients and standard errors (in parentheses) are presented. Data are weighted to reflect each respondent's share of the noninstitutionalized civilian population age 15 and older.
*$p<.05$; **$p<.01$; ***$p<.001$.

Waiting For and Traveling To Services

We next investigate two aspects of the healthcare encounter that do not directly involve the receipt of care: waiting for (Table 4) and traveling to and from (Table 5) outpatient services. We find that Hispanics and persons of other ethnicity report significantly longer wait times than do whites, whereas blacks and Hispanics spend significantly more time traveling than whites – and these racial gaps remain sizeable and statistically significant even when potential confounding factors and mediators are controlled.

The results presented in Table 4 are limited to the 565 respondents (34% of the 1621 persons reporting a healthcare encounter) who indicated that they had to wait. In preliminary analyses, we conducted logistic regression analyses to identify significant predictors of whether one reported any waiting time. We did not find statistically significant ethnic or racial differences in the odds of waiting; similar results emerged in both unadjusted models and models adjusted for all independent variables included in our analyses.

The baseline model (model 1) in Table 4 reveals that Hispanics and persons of other ethnicities report waiting more than 30 minutes longer than whites to receive health care ($p<.001$), although blacks did not differ significantly from whites. The Hispanic–white gap declines from 30 to 22 minutes, after socioeconomic status indicators are controlled (model 2). However, the 22-minute gap persists even after health status, geographic region, and family characteristics are controlled. Likewise, the large gap (34 minutes) between other ethnic groups and whites remains virtually unchanged, net of all other variables adjusted in the model. None of the four proxies for health insurance was a significant predictor of wait time, nor did the inclusion of these indicators alter the race effects. Moreover, health status was not associated with the duration of waiting time.

We found sizeable differences in wait time based on educational attainment, with high school graduates, college graduates, and persons with advanced degrees reporting significantly shorter wait times than persons with less than a high school education. Persons in nonmetropolitan areas also reported shorter wait times than their counterparts in metro areas. The models presented here account for 11% of the explained variance in wait times.

Table 5 indicates that blacks and Hispanics spend roughly 10 minutes more than whites traveling to healthcare services, and this racial gap barely budges when other factors are controlled. Few other characteristics are associated with traveling time, although persons with children in the household report significantly shorter travel times (6–7 minutes) than those with no children in the household. In supplementary analyses, we found that persons working for an hourly wage have significantly shorter travel times ($b = -5.37$, $p<.05$) although the inclusion of this measure did not alter the race effects. Moreover, no other proxy measure for health insurance affected the average travel times. Only 3% of the variance in travel time is explained by the models estimated here.

DISCUSSION

Our analyses reveal that the time spent on outpatient visits is yet another in a long list of health outcomes where blacks, Hispanics, and – to a lesser extent – persons of other ethnicity are disadvantaged relative to whites. Respondents who had a clinical encounter on their designated day reported that the average encounter required roughly two hours of their time; yet, this ranged from just 110 minutes among whites to more than 160 minutes for blacks and Hispanics. How this time was spent varied widely by race as well. Blacks spent a full 30 minutes more receiving services than did whites; yet, neither Hispanics nor other ethnics differed significantly from whites on this indicator. By contrast, Hispanics and persons of other ethnicities reported significantly longer wait times, whereas blacks and Hispanics reported significantly longer travel times than whites. Each of these findings persisted when we controlled for potential pathway and control variables, including socioeconomic status, health, and access to care. We elaborate each of these findings below.

Receiving Services: Why Do Blacks Spend an Additional Half Hour?

Overall, ATUS respondents reported spending an average of 74 minutes receiving services. This figure is considerably higher than the average duration reported by physicians. Data from the National Ambulatory Medical Care Survey (NAMCS), a probability-based sample survey of office-based physicians in the United States, shows that on average physicians spend less than 20 minutes face-to-face with patients (Cherry et al., 2007). The discrepancy in reports between the ATUS and the NAMCS reveals that patients and care providers experience the clinical health encounter very differently.

The main reason for the difference between physicians' and patients' reports of time use is that an outpatient visit includes many components that do not directly involve the physician: check-in, which can require completing short forms for returning patients, longer forms for new patients; insurance verification; the trip to the examination room; time to undress if needed (and dress again afterward); tests and measures done by staff, such as height and weight, blood pressure, recording current symptoms, and vision and hearing checks; preparation for exams such as the Pap smear; having blood drawn; giving a urine sample; receiving a shot; and the delays between these tasks (Russell et al., 2008).

A critically important, yet unresolved, question is why the time spent receiving services is nearly 30 minutes longer for blacks than whites, even when socioeconomic factors, health, and access to care are controlled. We suggest two potential explanations, each of which requires exploration in future research. First, blacks are significantly less likely than whites to have a regular healthcare provider (AHRQ, 2006). As such, each visit to a new practitioner or care site may require a greater amount of time devoted to completing paper work and reporting details of one's medical and medication history. Second, blacks are significantly more likely than whites to have multiple chronic conditions, including hypertension and diabetes (Centers for Disease Control, 2008), and these conditions typically require medication therapy. Discussing multiple conditions and the medications for these conditions may require extensive time – time that the patient presumably spends with a nurse or pharmacist rather than the physician.

We cannot adjudicate which if these explanations is more plausible, because the ATUS does not collect information on whether one is seeking care at one's primary care provider versus an emergency room, clinic, or other site. Moreover, we do not have detailed information on the precise condition(s) for which one is seeking care. Our analysis provides suggestive evidence, however, that the duration of the visit may be shaped by specific health conditions. Persons classified as having ill health, based on our coarse measure of work-related disability, reported spending 33.6 minutes more than their healthier counterparts receiving services – although unhealthy persons did not differ significantly from healthy persons in the analyses predicting wait or travel times. Pinpointing which conditions require the lengthiest visits may help to shed light on the sizeable and persistent black–white gap in the time spent receiving services.

Beyond the Examination Room: Waiting For and Traveling To Services

Our analysis also revealed a considerable race gap in the amount of time spent waiting for and traveling to services. Hispanics and persons of other ethnicities reported wait times that were 20 and 35 minutes longer than whites, respectively, although blacks and whites did not differ significantly on this outcome. By contrast, blacks and Hispanics reported transportation times that were roughly 10 minutes longer than whites, even after socioeconomic status and region of residence were controlled.

As with the race gap in time spent receiving services, our analysis cannot fully explain the race disparities in wait and travel time. However, we propose several explanations, based on prior research on health inequalities. The most obvious explanation for the extensive wait times reported by Hispanics and persons of other ethnicity is that they are seeking care at crowded or understaffed offices. However, if crowds and staffing issues were the primary explanation, then we might expect to see a significant black–white gap in waiting times. We were surprised that blacks did not report longer wait times than whites, given prior research showing that blacks are more likely than whites to receive care at emergency rooms and other crowded or understaffed settings (Baker, Stevens, & Brook, 1996). It is possible that blacks, Hispanics, and persons of other ethnicities use different frameworks when reporting wait times, where blacks counted time spent waiting in the examination room as part of their "receiving services" tally rather than as a component of their wait times.

An alternative explanation for the lengthier wait times of Hispanics and persons of other ethnicities, nearly three quarters of whom are Asian, is that they may be more likely than whites to seek care at sites that provide translation services, or where staff are of similar cultural backgrounds to themselves (Ngo-Metzger, Legedza, & Phillips, 2004). Persons with limited English skills or who are relatively new immigrants also may lack the cultural capital to advocate for themselves or to request immediate attention from care providers. A growing body of research also suggests that persons who speak English as a second language perceive discriminatory treatment on the part of healthcare providers. For instance, Johnson and colleagues (2004) found that blacks, Asians, and Hispanics are significantly more likely than whites to perceive that they would receive better medical care if they belonged to a different race and that the medical staff judged them unfairly or treated them with disrespect because of their race or ability to speak English.

The more extensive travel times reported by blacks and Hispanics likely reflect the shortage of appropriate healthcare providers in areas with large concentrations of ethnic minorities (AHRQ, 2006; Bach, Pham, Schrag, Tate, & Hargraves, 2004), thus requiring patients to travel long distances for care. Studies of residential segregation reveal that blacks and Hispanics reside in neighborhoods that are more racially segregated than do Asians, with Asians more likely to reside in neighborhoods that are majority white (e.g., Reardon et al., 2009). Consistent with this context of high levels of racial residential segregation, recent studies reveal that poor and ethnic neighborhoods not only lack a high number of healthcare providers, they also lack a sufficient number of *high-quality* health providers. As such, persons intent on receiving excellent care, especially in particular subspecialties, may be required to travel long distances. For example, a recent analysis of data from 4,300 primary care doctors in the Community Tracking Study revealed that the geographic distribution of highly qualified doctors affected care of black patients. Clinicians caring for black patients were less likely to be board certified than those caring for white patients, and they were less likely to report that they could "always" or "nearly always" provide access to high-quality subspecialists, diagnostic imaging, and ancillary services (Bach et al., 2004). Consequently, persons requiring particular technologies or services may need to travel extensively for the receipt of appropriate care.

Although differentials of 10–30 minutes in travel and wait times may not appear to be an important indicator of health inequities, we believe that these patterns may ultimately affect the health and well-being of ethnic minority patients. Research has shown persuasively that blacks and Hispanics are more likely than whites to delay seeking medical care until after a serious condition has developed rather than receiving regular preventive care, to be diagnosed with major health conditions at later stages, and to have "avoidable admissions" to hospital, due to the late receipt of care (AHRQ, 2006; Weissman, Stern, Fielding, & Epstein, 2001). If patients view extensive travel and wait times as costly and as interfering with other essential daily activities (especially wage labor), then these perceptions may create an obstacle to seeking preventive care.

LIMITATIONS AND FUTURE DIRECTIONS

Our study has several limitations that potentially weaken the persuasiveness and generalizability of our findings. First, the early waves of the ATUS did not obtain data on the specific symptoms, conditions, or health behaviors that may affect the time spent receiving care. Given widely documented racial differences in physical health, we suspect that at least part of the sizeable and intransigent 30-minute black–white gap in time receiving services may reflect underlying health conditions of African Americans. This study limitation may ultimately be remediable, however. The 2006 and 2007 ATUS data include information on self-reported health status, weight, and height. Several waves of such data will be required to have adequate sample sizes for exploring racial differences in time spent in healthcare encounters, given that less than 3% of the sample reports such encounters on their survey day, however. We look forward to replicating our study in future waves of the ATUS, with more detailed information on respondent health.

Second, we were unable to investigate whether access to care, measured in terms of health insurance, accounts for the racial gap in time spent on health encounters. However, we did control for socioeconomic status and age, which are associated with the receipt of public health insurance such as Medicare and Medicaid. We also constructed several proxies for health insurance, which captured attributes of jobs that are typically associated with employer-provided health insurance (Seccombe, 1993). We found that these proxies did not have direct effects on the time spent on health care, nor did they mediate the large and persistent race gaps in time use. We encourage the ATUS investigators to add a simple indicator of presence and type of health insurance in future waves.

Third, we included only a broad proxy for physical access to care – comparing persons who reside in metropolitan versus nonmetropolitan areas. Future analyses could incorporate area-level indicators of the number of healthcare providers per capita, or hospital and physician capacity in a census tract or county, or hospital referral region. We suspect that the long wait and travel times for ethnic minorities may partly reflect a relatively low ratio of healthcare professionals per potential patient in geographic regions distinguished by low socioeconomic status and high proportions of ethnic minority residents (The Dartmouth Institute for Health Policy and Clinical Practice, 2008). As such, they may be forced to wait in overcrowded settings or travel long distances to receive care.

Fourth, we are unable to distinguish whether the wait times reported vary based on site of care. For instance, prior research suggests that blacks and Hispanics are more likely than whites to use emergency departments for routine medical care (Baker et al., 1996), thus the racial gap in waiting may reflect ethnic minorities' greater tendency to seek care at emergency rooms, clinics, or other sites that typically require long waits.

Finally, it is possible that our analytic sample is biased to include persons who are healthier on average than nonparticipants; thus, the amount of time spent in receiving care may actually be *underestimated*. The response rate for the ATUS has been just under 60% instead of the 70% envisioned when the survey was being developed (Tai-Seale et al., 2007). Because the early waves of the ATUS did not obtain health data, we do not know if unhealthy people or those with particularly complex or time-intensive healthcare regimens are less likely than others to participate. Analyses of response rates reveal that busy people (indicated by work hours and children in the household) were as likely to respond as those less busy, but socially isolated people (indicated by marital status, school-age children, and homeownership) had lower response rates (Abraham et al., 2006). Older persons have higher response rates than younger persons, but those of any age with serious health problems may be less likely to respond. Thus, the ATUS may be best suited for describing routine outpatient visits, rather than more intensive healthcare use.

CONCLUSIONS

Despite these limitations, our study is the first that we know of to document the time spent receiving, traveling to, and waiting for healthcare services among a nationally representative sample of whites, blacks, Hispanics, and persons of other ethnicities. Prior studies have documented the time spent by physicians on outpatient visits (Gottschalk & Flocke, 2005; Lo, Ryder, & Shorr, 2005), but not the time spent by patients. The *patient's perspective* – and disparities in the experiences reported by patients – provides an important yet seldom acknowledged indicator of healthcare effectiveness.

We have shown that whites fare better than ethnic minorities on all dimensions of time use. This is a troubling phenomenon, and one that we have not fully explained using measures from the ATUS. *Healthy People 2010* calls for the elimination of disparities in health, well-being, and access to and quality of health care. We would argue further that time spent receiving, traveling to, and waiting for care also are critical indicators of patient-centered care.

This time may be taken away from other valuable activities including paid employment, household tasks, child care, and other family caregiving. Moreover, the time spent seeking care is compounded by the fact that 40% of persons are accompanied by a family member or friend; these companions spend an average of 124 minutes per encounter (Russell et al., 2008). The time cost of receiving or accompanying others to receive care, in addition to the financial costs, may be onerous – particularly for those working in low-paying hourly positions and who thus lose wages when seeking care. These time investments, particularly with respect to traveling to and waiting for care, may increase in the current economic climate (Associated Press, 2008). Cash-strapped hospitals are closing, especially in poor and underserved areas, forcing local patients to travel greater distances to outpatient clinics and emergency rooms. Such cutbacks also may lead to crowding and longer wait times for patients (Buchmueller, Jacobson, & Wold, 2006).

In its definition of patient-centered care, the Institute of Medicine emphasized that care should be timely and equitable. The ATUS, in particular, could provide new measures to benchmark timeliness, patient-centeredness, and equity of care. These measures could supplement those already used in the influential annual *National Healthcare Quality Report* (AHRQ, 2006). Documenting racial inequities in patients' time use may provide valuable insights to policy makers concerned with reducing disparities in health and health care in the United States.

ACKNOWLEDGMENT

We thank Katharine Abraham for her helpful comments.

REFERENCES

Abraham, K., Maitland, A., & Bianchi, S. (2006). Nonresponse in the American time use survey: Who is missing from the data and how much does it matter? *Public Opinion Quarterly, 70,* 676–703.

Agency for Healthcare Research and Quality. (2006). *National healthcare disparities report.* Washington, DC: Author.

Associated Press. (2008). Bad debt triggers hospital closings around U.S. MSNBC (December 28, 2008). Available at http://www.msnbc.msn.com/id/28394340/. Retrieved on June 12, 2009.

Bach, P. B., Pham, H. H., Schrag, D., Tate, R. C., & Hargraves, J. L. (2004). Primary care physicians who treat blacks and whites. *New England Journal of Medicine, 351,* 575–584.

Baker, D. W., Stevens, C. D., & Brook, R. H. (1996). Determinants of emergency department use: Are race and ethnicity important? *Annals of Emergency Medicine, 28,* 677–682.

Buchmueller, T. C., Jacobson, M., & Wold, C. (2006). How far to the hospital? The effect of hospital closures on access to care. *Journal of Health Economics, 25,* 740–761.

Bureau of Labor Statistics. (2007). American time use survey user's guide: Understanding ATUS 2003 to 2009. Washington, DC: Bureau of Labor Statistics and U.S. Census Bureau, June 2007. Available at http://www.bls.gov/tus/atususersguide.pdf. Accessed on April 15, 2008.

Centers for Disease Control. (2008). Racial/ethnic disparities in self-rated health status among adults with and without disabilities – United States, 2004–2006. *Morbidity and Mortality Weekly Report, 57*(39), 1069–1073.

Cherry, D., Woodwell, D. A., & Rechtsteiner, E. (2007). National ambulatory medical care survey: 2005 summary. *Advanced Data from Vital and Health Statistics, No. 387.* Hyattsville, MD: Centers for Disease Control.

Gottschalk, A., & Flocke, S. A. (2005). Time spent in face-to-face patient care and work outside the examination room. *Annals of Family Medicine, 3,* 488–493.

Guagliardo, M. F. (2004). Spatial accessibility of primary care: Concepts, methods and challenges. *International Journal of Health Geographics, 3*(1), 3.
Hartley, D. L., Quam, L., & Lurie, N. (1994). Urban-rural differences in health insurance and access to care. *Journal of Rural Health, 10,* 98–108.
Horrigan, M., & Herz, D. (2004). Planning, designing, and executing the BLS American time-use survey. *Monthly Labor Review, 127,* 3–19.
Institute of Medicine. (2001). *Coverage matters: Insurance and health care.* Washington, DC: National Academy of Sciences.
Institute of Medicine. (2003). *Unequal treatment: Confronting racial and ethnic disparities in healthcare.* Washington, DC: National Academy of Sciences.
Institute of Medicine's Committee on Quality of Health Care in America. (2001). *Crossing the quality chasm.* Washington, DC: National Academy of Sciences.
Jacobs, E. A., Lauderdale, D. S., Meltzer, D., Shorey, J. M., Levinson, W., & Thisted, R. A. (2001). Impact of interpreter services on delivery of health care to limited-English-proficient patients. *Journal of General Internal Medicine, 16,* 468–474.
Johnson, R. L., Saha, S., Arbelaez, J., Beach, M. C., & Cooper, L. A. (2004). Racial and ethnic differences in patient perceptions of bias and cultural competence in health care. *Journal of General Internal Medicine, 19,* 101–110.
Larson, S. L., & Fleishman, J. A. (2003). Rural-urban differences in usual source of care and ambulatory service use: Analyses of data using urban influence codes. *Medical Care, 41*(Suppl.), 65–74.
Lo, A., Ryder, K., & Shorr, R. I. (2005). Relationship between patient age and duration of physician visit in ambulatory setting: Does one size fit all? *Journal of American Geriatric Society, 53,* 1162–1167.
Mead, H., Cartwright-Smith, L., Jones, K., Ramos, C., Siegel, B., & Woods, K. (2008). *Racial and ethnic disparities in U.S. health care: A chartbook.* Washington, DC: The Commonwealth Fund.
Merritt Hawkins & Associates. (2009). *Survey of physician appointment wait times.* Irving, TX: Author.
Ngo-Metzger, Q., Legedza, A. T. R., & Phillips, R. S. (2004). Asian American's reports of their health care experiences: Results of a national survey. *The Journal of General Internal Medicine, 19,* 111–119.
Reardon, S. F., Farrell, C. R., Matthews, S. A., O'Sullivan, D., Bischoff, K., & Firebaugh, G. (2009). Race and space in the 1990s: Changes in the geographic scale of racial residential segregation, 1990–2000. *Social Science Research, 30,* 55–70.
Russell, L. B., Ibuka, Y., & Carr, D. (2008). How much time do patients spend on outpatient visits? The American time use survey. *The Patient: Patient-Centered Outcomes Research, 1*(3), 211–222.
Seccombe, K. (1993). Employer-sponsored medical benefits: The influence of occupational characteristics and gender. *The Sociological Quarterly, 34,* 557–580.
Shelley, K. J. (2005). Developing the American time use survey activity classification system. *Monthly Labor Review, 128,* 3–15.
Tai-Seale, M., McGuire, T. G., & Zhang, W. (2007). Time allocation in primary care office visits. *Health Services Research, 42,* 1871–1894.
The Commonwealth Fund. (2006). *Health care quality survey.* Washington, DC: Author.
The Dartmouth Institute for Health Policy and Clinical Practice. (2008). *Tracing the care of patients with severe chronic illness.* Hanover, NH: Author.

U.S. Bureau of the Census. (2008). *The 2008 statistical abstract*. Washington, DC: Author.
U.S. Department of Health and Human Services. (2000). *Healthy people 2010, With understanding and improving health and objectives for improving health.* (November, 2nd ed., 2 Vols). Washington, DC: U.S. Government Printing Office.
van Dis, J. (2002). Where we live: Health care in rural versus urban America. *Journal of American Medical Association, 287*, 108.
Waite, L. J., & Gallagher, M. (2000). *The case for marriage*. New York: Doubleday.
Weissman, J. S., Stern, R., Fielding, S. L., & Epstein, A. M. (2001). Delayed access to health care: Risk factors, reasons and consequences. *Annals of Internal Medicine, 114*, 325–331.
Williams, D. R., Neighbors, H. W., & Jackson, J. S. (2003). Racial/ethnic discrimination and health: Findings from community studies. *American Journal of Public Health, 93*, 200–208.

CAN THE BEHAVIORAL MODEL EXPLAIN IMMIGRANT STATUS AND ETHNIC DIFFERENCES IN U.S. ADULTS' COMPLEMENTARY AND ALTERNATIVE MEDICINE (CAM) USE?

Georgiana Bostean

ABSTRACT

Immigrants' access to health services is a widely researched topic, yet few studies examine immigrants' use of complementary and alternative medicine (CAM). This study uses the Behavioral Model to compare overall CAM use and use of acupuncture, chiropractic, herbs, yoga, and relaxation by immigrant status (nativity and time in the United States). It then explains the nativity gap in use by assessing knowledge, cost, and need as potential reasons for not using these modalities. Results show that controlling for predisposing, enabling, and need factors, recent immigrants use CAM less than the U.S.-born. Lack of knowledge of CAM modalities partially explains why some recent immigrants do not use acupuncture, chiropractic, or relaxation, while established immigrants cite lack of need as a reason for not using yoga. Cost does not explain immigrants' lower use of these five modalities. Finally, ethnicity moderates the association between immigrant status and reasons for not using CAM.

INTRODUCTION

Access to health services is among the most important social factors that shape health disparities in the United States (Gortmaker & Wise, 1997). An increasingly popular and rapidly growing sector of health services is complementary and alternative medicine (CAM). Nearly 75% of adults have tried some form of CAM (Barnes, Powell-Griner, Mcfann, & Nahin, 2004) at some point in their lives, and visits to alternative medical practitioners increased by 47.3% between 1990 and 1997 (Eisenberg et al., 1998). Moreover, many immigrants come from countries where health practices that are defined as CAM in the United States are commonplace. For example, acupuncture is used alongside Western medicine in China (Xu & Yang, 2009). Yet, few studies examine immigrants' CAM use and those that do yield conflicting results; some find that immigrants turn to CAM before conventional medicine, others find that immigrants use CAM less than the U.S.-born, and still others find no association between nativity and CAM use.

Understanding whether and why immigrants use CAM less than the U.S.-born will illuminate questions of potential access to health services (Andersen, 1995), provide insight into their health behaviors, and perhaps help explain why they underutilize conventional health care in the early years of their stay in the U.S. (Leclere, Jensen, & Biddlecom, 1994). Immigrants' unequal access to and impact on the U.S. healthcare system, the increasing use of CAM in the United States, and conflicting findings about immigrants' CAM use make it an important area of study for sociologists in the fields of health and health care. Using the most recent nationally-representative data on CAM, the 2007 National Health Interview Survey (NHIS), this study examines immigrants' CAM use (both overall use and use of five specific modalities), focusing on whether immigrants use CAM more, less, or equally to the U.S.-born, and the reasons why immigrants may use CAM less than the U.S.-born. It also examines ethnic differences in the immigrant status–CAM relationship.

THEORETICAL AND EMPIRICAL BACKGROUND

Seemingly paradoxically, research finds that CAM users are not from social groups with the highest health needs, with high rates of health problems, such as minorities and older adults. Overall, African Americans use CAM less than White Americans (Keith, Kronenfeld, Rivers, & Liang, 2005), and older adults less than middle-age adults, despite these groups being in poorer health on average. In fact, many studies find that CAM users are predominantly White, middle-aged, females of relatively high socioeconomic status (SES), who suffer from chronic conditions (Eisenberg et al., 1998; Grzywacz et al., 2007; Barnes & Bloom, 2008). However, age and ethnic differences in CAM use reflect not only differences in need due to health conditions but also the convergence of individual history and age. The middle-aged may be more likely to use CAM than the young and the old because CAM was becoming more popular in the United States when they began to make health decisions in young adulthood.

Similarly, ethnic differences in CAM use reflect both cultural differences in what interventions are deemed appropriate for particular ailments and access to various interventions (Grzywacz et al., 2007). For example, White Americans are the predominant users of manipulative and body-based therapies such as chiropractic care, Hispanics tend to use herbs, and African Americans use self-prayer (prayer for one's own health) more than other racial and ethnic groups (Barnes et al., 2004). Racial and ethnic differences such as these raise questions about the importance of immigrant status, which scholars note is intimately related to ethnicity in the United States (Jasso, Massey, Rosenzweig, & Smith, 2004; Kronenfeld & Ayers, 2009) in CAM use. Despite the overwhelming evidence that life-course and socio-cultural factors impact the decision to seek care and the types of care sought, many studies omit immigrants – a rapidly growing segment of the U.S. population, which is inherently linked to ethnic diversity, and which may be predisposed to using CAM.

Immigrant Status, Ethnicity, and CAM Use

Precisely because ethnicity and immigrant status are so closely linked in the United States, they should be analyzed together. It is likely that in addition to ethnic differences in CAM use, there are immigrant status differences by ethnicity. The monolithic term "immigrants" obscures important cultural and social group differences that affect the immigrant status–CAM use relationship. A significant body of research evidences sociocultural and demographic differences among pan-ethnic and immigrant groups by origin; for example, while Mexicans have a mortality and health advantage compared to White Americans, Puerto Ricans are one of the unhealthiest Hispanic groups and fare much worse than Whites. With regard to CAM, as previously noted, some regions and countries have a long history of use of particular types of CAM. However, although there are heterogeneities even down to ethnic sub-groups, in many cases analysis by country of origin is implausible or impractical due to data constraints; nevertheless, pan-ethnic analysis of CAM, with the caveat that there may be variance even within these pan-ethnic groups, reveals important patterns in use, such as the use of Asian-specific CAM types among Asians (Hsiao et al., 2006). Before I turn to the interaction between ethnicity and immigrant status, I first discuss how immigrant status may be related to CAM use.

A priori, there are reasons to hypothesize both that in general, immigrants are significant CAM users and that immigrants are less likely than the U.S.-born to use CAM. For example, immigrants may have knowledge of certain CAM practices that are common in their homelands. However, they may not have access to these CAM modalities in the United States due to socioeconomic or other barriers. Reflective of these competing possibilities, empirical evidence is mixed. Some studies find CAM use to be prevalent among certain immigrant groups (Ahn et al., 2006; Garcés, Scarinci, & Harrison, 2006), others find that immigrants use CAM less than the U.S.-born (Su, Li, & Pagán, 2008), and still others find no effect of nativity on CAM use (Upchurch et al., 2008).

Immigrants' use of CAM is an important area of study for several reasons. Healthcare providers are increasingly concerned with better serving this segment of the population by making healthcare practices more culturally sensitive, and although widespread CAM use in the United States is a relatively new phenomenon, globally, many countries use treatments that are classified as CAM in the United States alongside conventional medicine (Barnes et al., 2004). For example, the use of homeopathic and natural remedies as a primary step in health self-management in Mexico is widespread (Zolla, 2009), while in China, traditional Chinese medicine is used alongside Western medicine in hospitals (Xu & Yang, 2009). Therefore, some immigrants may be culturally predisposed to using certain CAM modalities.

In fact, several studies find that many ethnic groups use their ethnic-specific types of CAM more than other types of CAM (Najm, Reinsch, Hoehler, & Tobis, 2003; Hsiao et al., 2006), indicating a cultural knowledge of, or belief in, one's own ethnic CAM practices. For example, Asians are most likely users of some Asian-specific CAM modalities, such as acupuncture and use of green tea and soy products in their diets, whereas Latinos are the most likely users of Latino-specific CAM, such as curandero use (Hsiao et al., 2006). Furthermore, immigrants may have access to some CAM therapies due to their availability in immigrant communities and enclaves.

Empirical research provides some support for the hypothesis that immigrants are predisposed to using some forms of CAM. One study of 322 adults living in the Houston, TX, area finds that having an immigrant family history is associated with more than twice the odds of herb use, net of sociodemographic controls (Kuo, Hawley, Weiss, Balkrishnan, & Volk, 2004). In addition, several smaller-scale, qualitative studies find that immigrants are significant CAM users. For example, Poss and Jezewski (2002) interviewed 22 type 2 diabetes patients in El Paso, Texas, and found that the use of CAM remedies such as prayer and herbs was common. Garcés et al. (2006) find that many U.S. Latino immigrants try CAM before they turn to conventional medicine.

On the contrary, although some immigrants may have knowledge of certain culturally specific CAM practices because of use in their countries of origin, they may have little knowledge of, or access to, CAM modalities specific to other cultures. Therefore, while use of one modality may be high, overall CAM use among immigrants may be low. Second, immigrants are healthier than the U.S.-born (Markides & Coreil, 1986; Jasso et al., 2004; Hummer, Powers, Pullum, Gossman, & Frisbie, 2007), decreasing the need for using CAM for treatment of ailments such as pain, limitations, and chronic conditions, which are more prevalent among CAM users. Third, a large proportion of recent immigrants are of low SES which research shows is related to lesser CAM use. These findings suggest that immigrants use CAM less than the U.S.-born.

Some recent large-scale empirical studies, using the 2002 NHIS provide mixed evidence. Su et al. (2008) find that immigrants are less likely to use CAM, even after controlling for factors like immigrants' younger age, lower SES, and better health. Another study, using the same dataset, finds no significant effect of nativity (foreign-born versus U.S.-born); however, the sample was limited to females and only examined acupuncture use (Upchurch et al., 2008).

In summary, studies on immigrant status and CAM use yield conflicting results. Many are limited by small, constricted samples and others by either treating "CAM" as homogeneous or analyzing a single CAM modality, both of which obscure important variations by CAM modality. So, the question remains: is immigrant status related to CAM use (both overall and of specific modalities) and, if so, what determines immigrants' CAM use? The previous literature points to several possibilities: First, immigrants may or may not have knowledge of some CAM practices. Second, they may not have the socio-economic resources to use costly CAM practices. Third, they may not need to use CAM because they are in good health.

Finally, the reasons for using or not using CAM likely vary by ethnicity and CAM modality. I return to the final point in a moment.

Theoretical Background: Behavioral Model of Health Service Utilization

The three potential explanatory factors in immigrant CAM use mentioned in the previous section are all components of the Behavioral Model of health services' utilization (Andersen, 1968; Andersen, 1995). Fundamentally, this model explains the decision to seek care (in this case CAM) as a function of a vector of factors, categorized into three groups – predisposing, enabling, and need – and provides a useful framework for understanding immigrants' use, or nonuse, of CAM. Predisposing factors include health beliefs, such as knowledge and values, and demographic and sociostructural factors, such as ethnicity, gender, age, and education. Factors that impede or enable use include income, health insurance, and region of residence (a measure of availability of services). Lastly, need factors include perceived health such as self-rated health and other measures of health conditions such as pain or activity limitation.

Although it was not specifically designed to address CAM, this framework for understanding healthcare-seeking behaviors may be fruitfully applied to CAM use (Sirois & Gick, 2002). For example, Upchurch et al. (2008), using the 2002 NHIS find associations between predisposing, enabling, and need factors and women's acupuncture use. This model may be especially suited to examine immigrant status differences in CAM use because immigrants may have different predisposing, enabling, and need factors compared to the U.S.-born and compared to immigrants from other ethnic groups. For instance, immigrants' individual histories likely shape their health knowledge, beliefs, and values in distinct ways from the U.S.-born, while their areas of residence such as immigrant enclaves may provide unique enabling resources.

Moreover, predisposing, enabling, and need factors may change over time. It is likely that immigrants' health beliefs and healthcare utilization patterns change over time. Indeed, previous research reveals that immigrants' contact with physicians increases with time in the United States (Leclere et al., 1994), as do adverse health conditions and behaviors, such as poor diet and lack of exercise (Abraído-Lanza, Chao, & Flórez, 2005). With regard to CAM use, immigrants who have lived in the United States the longest are just as likely to use CAM as the U.S.-born, whereas recent immigrants are significantly less likely to do so (Su et al., 2008). It is likely that the reasons for using or not using CAM also change over time spent in the United States.

In addition to differing by immigrant status, predisposing, enabling, and need factors likely also vary by ethnicity and modality. Both for specific modalities and with regard to overall CAM utilization, one could hypothesize that for some ethnic groups, nativity differences will be more pronounced due to the legacy of CAM traditions in their homelands or the pace of their acculturation to U.S. health practices; for others, these differences may be more muted. For example, while an Asian immigrant may not use acupuncture because he/she does not have the "need" (or health need) to use it, and a Hispanic immigrant because he/she has never heard of it, lack of knowledge may be the reason for not using chiropractic care for Asian immigrants, compared to lack of need among Hispanic immigrants.

To summarize, this study builds on existing literature by using the Behavioral Model of health services utilization as a framework to compare immigrant status differentials in use and reasons for nonuse of five CAM modalities. Several important contributions include (1) examining use of CAM as well as reasons for nonuse and comparing these across immigrant statuses, (2) comparing immigrant status differences in reasons for nonuse by race/ethnicity, and (3) examining both overall CAM use and five specific CAM modalities, (4) comparing the dynamics of predisposing, enabling, and need factors, as well as the differing effects of immigrant status on use and reasons for nonuse by modality.

I hypothesize that immigrants, especially recent ones, have lower overall CAM use compared to the U.S.-born. Specifically, I explain nativity differences in CAM use as a combination of lack of knowledge (predisposing), cost (enabling), and need factors. I compare use across five specific CAM practices: acupuncture, herb use, chiropractic/osteopathic, yoga/tai chi/qi gong, and relaxation therapies. The study focuses on these modalities primarily because they are the modalities about which nonusers were asked to give the reasons why they have not used them. Nevertheless, this group of modalities is ideal for this study because (1) it encompasses categories of CAM that immigrants are thought to use most (i.e., herbs), as well as those they use least (i.e., chiropractic), (2) it includes practitioner-based modalities as well as some that may be personal practices, and (3) it spans a wide range of costs. For example, relaxation and yoga/tai chi/qi gong can be practiced on one's own and incur minimal or no cost or can be practiced with a practitioner for a fee, while acupuncture and chiropractic require a practitioner which may incur out-of-pocket expense if the modality is not covered by health insurance. Given the diversity and popularity of this group of modalities, it is particularly appropriate for this study.

Furthermore, I hypothesize that the reasons for nonuse vary by CAM modality. For example, for some modalities the cost may be the deterrent factor, while for other modalities it is the lack of knowledge that prohibits use. Finally, I also expect that ethnicity will moderate the relationship between immigrant status and use (and reasons for nonuse) of specific CAM modalities. I hypothesize that immigrants are more likely than the U.S.-born to cite cost as a reason for not using acupuncture and chiropractic care (since these are provider-based and therefore more costly practices), and they are also more likely to cite knowledge as a reason for not using modalities that are not considered specific to their ethnic group. For example, Asian immigrants will be less likely than U.S.-born Asians to cite lack of knowledge as a reason for not using yoga/tai chi/qi gong, acupuncture or herbs, while at the same time they will be more likely to cite lack of knowledge of chiropractic therapy than White immigrants.

METHODS

Data and Sample

The aim of this study is to explain the nativity gap in CAM use. To this end, I analyze data from the 2007 NHIS Supplement on Complementary and Alternative Medicine, a nationally representative survey of the U.S. civilian, noninstitutionalized population. The survey is conducted by the National Center for Health Statistics and administered through computer-assisted personal interview (CAPI) by U.S. Census Bureau interviewers. In 2007, 23,393 sample adults were administered the CAM Supplement of the NHIS, and the conditional final response rate for sample adults was 78.3% (National Center for Health Statistics, 2008).

The final sample size for this study is 22,748, which excludes missing cases for education and length of residence, as well as those categorized as "Other race." Of the final sample, nearly 78% have used some form of CAM in the year preceding the interview. Approximately 20% of the sample is foreign-born ($N = 4,540$), and the racial composition is as follows: non-Hispanic White (70.5%), non-Hispanic Black (11.7%), Asian (4.6%), and Hispanic (13.2%). The sample design includes stratification, clustering, and multistage sampling. To compensate for the complex sample design, analyses were done in STATA 10.1 utilizing the "svy" suite of commands and included weights based on design, ratio, nonresponse, and poststratification adjustments. This allows the generalization of findings to the national level.

Measures

Dependent Variables

CAM Use. The NHIS includes questions about use of 18 CAM modalities: acupuncture, ayurveda, biofeedback, chelation therapy, chiropractic or osteopathic manipulation (hereafter chiropractic), energy therapy, hypnosis, massage, naturopathy, traditional medicine, movement therapies, vitamin use, homeopathy, diet, herb use, prayer, yoga/tai chi/qi gong (the survey question does not distinguish between them; I refer to them as yoga hereafter), and relaxation therapies (i.e., deep breathing exercises, meditation, guided imagery, progressive relaxation, support group, stress management class). I examine use in the past 12 months of any of the 18 modalities, coding this "Any CAM" variable as 1 if the respondent mentioned trying at least 1 of the 18 modalities in the past year, and 0 otherwise. I also examine use of the top 10 individual CAM modalities (acupuncture, chiropractic, herb use, yoga, relaxation therapies, prayer, diet, vitamin use, homeopathy, or massage) coding each outcome as 1 if the respondent used the modality in the year before the interview and 0 otherwise. These modalities have the highest percentage of respondents who have ever tried each, with the highest percentage having ever tried vitamins and prayer (64% and 60%, respectively) and the lowest percentage having used homeopathy (3.65%). The remaining eight modalities were excluded because less than 3% of the sample had ever tried each one.

Next, I focus on the following five modalities: acupuncture, chiropractic, herbs, yoga, and relaxation. To reiterate, I focus on these modalities because they are the only ones for which questions were asked about why an individual had not used them. Nevertheless, these five modalities are a particularly relevant and important group for this study for the reasons outlined earlier. Again, I create a variable coded 1 if the individual has used any of the five aforementioned CAM modalities in the past 12 months, and 0 otherwise.

Reasons for Not Using CAM. The second set of dependent variables of interest are three reasons (categorized as predisposing, enabling, and need factors) why the respondent has not used each of the five CAM modalities, both ever and in the past 12 months: knowledge, cost, and need. Specifically, the question first asks those who have never tried a modality, "Please tell me the reasons why you have never used [specific modality]." Then, for those who have tried it, but not in the past year, "Please tell me the reasons why you have not used [specific modality] during the past 12 months." Respondents were allowed to offer multiple reasons for not using a modality. I examine the responses, "Never heard of it/Don't know much about it," "It costs too much," and "Didn't need it," as predisposing (i.e., knowledge), enabling or in this case impeding (i.e., cost), and need factors, respectively. Each reason was coded as a dichotomous outcome (1 for mentioned reason and 0 for did not mention reason).

Independent Variables
Immigrant Status and Race/Ethnicity. I use both nativity (U.S.-born versus foreign-born) and length of residence in the United States (recent immigrants with less than 15 years in the United States and established immigrants of 15 years or more) as measures of immigrant status. Together with immigrant status, I examine race and ethnicity. Owing to small cell sizes when analyzing by length of residence and origin, measurement of racial/ethnic differences is limited to the following four groups: non-Hispanic White, Hispanic, non-Hispanic Black, and non-Hispanic Asian.

Other Independent Variables. I control for other factors, predisposing, enabling, and need, associated with CAM use and healthcare utilization. Predisposing factors include age, sex, marital status, and education. A quadratic age term is also included in analyses to capture the curvilinear relationship between reasons for CAM use and age (Grzywacz et al., 2005). Although language of interview (English = 0 or other = 1) may be considered both a predisposing and an enabling factor, I include it as a predisposing factor, as it may be related to immigrants' understanding of the names of the CAM modalities and may also be a measure of acculturation or cultural knowledge of specific modalities. As enabling factors, I include health coverage (coded as 1 if the individual has any health coverage, public or private, and zero otherwise), employment (coded as 1 if the individual was working for pay last week and zero otherwise), and U.S. region of residence (West, South, Northeast, or Midwest). I also use family income as a ratio to the poverty threshold, including a dummy for missing income to maintain sample size, but which is not presented or interpreted here in the interest of space. I consider income, health coverage, and employment as enabling resources related to cost, and region of residence as a measure of access. I explain the importance of this distinction subsequently.

Finally, I measure need through a dichotomous measure of fair or poor subjective health status (fair/poor health = 1, excellent, very good or good health = 0), bodily pain (a continuous measure of areas of the body experiencing pain, ranging from 0 to 5), and a scale of functional limitation (ranging from 0 to 48, where 0 is not limited at all), created by summing responses to questions about how difficult it is to perform 12 specific tasks such as climbing stairs, reaching for objects or stooping.

Analytic Strategy

To analyze the effects of nativity and U.S. length of residence on CAM use, I conduct several logistic regression analyses. The analyses are presented as follows: first, I present the weighted characteristics of the sample, with the results of Pearson chi-square test and Analysis of Variance (ANOVA) to assess significant nativity differences (Table 1). Second, I present logistic regression results estimating odds ratios of use in the past 12 months of "any CAM" and use of the 10 aforementioned modalities, by immigrant status and race, controlling for predisposing, enabling, and need factors (Table 2). Then, I focus on five specific modalities, estimating logistic regressions of use of any of the five modalities in the past 12 months (Table 3), and additively assessing the contributions of predisposing, enabling, and need factors in explaining immigrant status differences in use. (I also examined ethnicity-by-immigrant status interactions in separate analyses, but few differences were significant, therefore I exclude those results.) Next, I examine each of the five modalities separately, analyzing the reasons for nonuse among those who did not use it in the past year: first, the likelihood of not using CAM because of a lack of knowledge of the specified modality (Table 4a), then because CAM is too expensive (Table 4b), and finally because the individual feels he/she has no need for CAM (Table 4c).

Each set of regressions includes distinct controls to avoid including measures of the outcome variable on the right-hand side of the model (e.g., including need measures as covariates in the models measuring need as a reason for nonuse). In the "knowledge" regressions, I include controls for enabling and need factors, as well as demographic and sociostructural factors. Although both knowledge and demographic/structural characteristics are predisposing factors, the Behavioral Model distinguishes between them conceptually and my aim is to assess knowledge net of demographic and structural differences. I also include language as a predisposing factor, although it could also be classified as an enabling factor, because I examine

Table 1. Weighted Characteristics of U.S. Adults by Immigrant Status.

Characteristics (%)	All (n = 22,748)	U.S.-Born (n = 18,405)	Immigrant, <15 Years (n = 1,867)	Immigrant, 15+ Years (n = 2,476)	Significant Immigrant Status Difference[a]
CAM use in the past 12 months					
Any CAM	77.98	78.86	67.91	77.48	***
Acupuncture	1.41	1.34	1.11	2.32	***
Chiropractic/osteopath	8.44	9.28	2.27	5.32	***
Herb use	17.46	18.63	6.79	14.79	***
Yoga/tai chi/qi gong	6.49	6.58	5.7	6.18	
Relaxation	16.27	17.23	10.14	12.05	***
Reasons for not using CAM[b]					
Never heard of	19.96	19.21	28.1	20.76	***
Costs too much	5.4	5.57	4.11	4.8	*
Did not need it	47.56	47.87	44.61	47.01	
Predisposing					
Race and ethnicity					
White	70.53	80.07	15.08	23.50	***
Hispanic	13.24	6.24	54.53	47.28	***
Black	11.66	12.39	7.99	7.61	***
Asian	4.56	1.29	22.41	21.61	***
Language of interview, English only	94.23	99.23	59.76	74.00	***
Mean age (in years)	45.79	46.38	34.54	49.39	***
Female	51.72	52.02	48.32	51.32	*
Education					
Less than high school	15.51	12.44	33.60	30.49	***
High school graduate	57.36	60.37	40.02	42.40	***
Bachelor's degree or higher	27.13	27.19	26.38	27.11	
Married	55.94	54.67	59.12	65.48	***
Enabling					
U.S. region of residence					
West	21.88	19.30	32.52	37.86	***
Midwest	24.35	26.53	13.23	12.44	***
Northeast	17.23	16.40	20.94	22.15	***
South	36.55	37.77	33.31	27.54	***
Employed last week	61.3	60.54	68.09	63.20	***
No health coverage	16.63	13.47	45.26	21.26	***
Family income below poverty line	10.23	9.24	21.13	11.10	***

Table 1. (*Continued*)

Characteristics (%)	All (n = 22,748)	U.S.-Born (n = 18,405)	Immigrant, <15 Years (n = 1,867)	Immigrant, 15+ Years (n = 2,476)	Significant Immigrant Status Difference[a]
Need					
Fair/poor self-reported health	13.29	13.63	6.25	16.10	***
Activity limitation scale	3.09	3.35	0.74	2.61	***
Bodily pain scale	0.63	0.66	0.38	0.58	***

Source: NHIS 2007.
*$p<0.05$; **$p<0.01$; ***$p<0.001$, two-tailed test.
[a]Chi-square or ANOVA tests used to assess immigrant status differences.
[b]Reported reason for at least one of the five modalities.

Table 2. Logistic Regression Results: Adjusted Odds Ratios[a] of CAM Use in Past Year.

	Immigrant Status			Race/Ethnicity			
	U.S.-born	Immigrant, <15 years	Immigrant, 15+ years	Non-Hispanic White	Hispanic	Black	Asian
Any CAM	Ref.	1.002	1.064	Ref.	1.015	1.367***	0.875
Acupuncture	Ref.	1.058	1.485*	Ref.	0.952	0.477*	1.856*
Chiropractic	Ref.	0.558*	0.873	Ref.	0.547***	0.337***	0.523**
Herbs	Ref.	0.582***	0.987	Ref.	0.675***	0.570***	0.780
Yoga/tai chi/qi gong	Ref.	0.935	1.244	Ref.	0.571***	0.555***	1.183
Relaxation	Ref.	0.841	0.848	Ref.	0.743**	0.858*	0.998
Prayer	Ref.	1.060	1.088	Ref.	1.663***	2.775***	0.887
Diet	Ref.	0.906	0.966	Ref.	0.730	0.895	0.930
Vitamins	Ref.	0.833*	0.917	Ref.	0.823**	0.774***	0.858
Homeopathy	Ref.	0.784	0.549*	Ref.	0.824	0.427**	0.643
Massage	Ref.	0.567**	0.771*	Ref.	0.648**	0.510***	0.820
N	22,748	22,748	22,748	22,748	22,748	22,748	22,748

Source: NHIS 2007.
*$p<0.05$; **$p<0.01$; ***$p<0.001$, two-tailed test.
[a]Models control for language, age, age-squared, gender, education, marital status, region, employment status, health coverage, income, pain, activity limitation, and poor health. Respondents with missing income data are included in regression, but results not reported here.

Table 3. Logistic Regression Results: Odds Ratios of Acupuncture, Chiropractic, Herbs, Yoga, or Relaxation Use in Past Year.

	Baseline (1)	Predisposing (2)	Enabling (3)	Need (4)
Nativity (U.S.-born ref.)				
Immigrant, <15 years	0.410***	0.632***	0.660***	0.724**
Immigrant, 15+ years	0.718***	0.963	0.945	0.972
Predisposing factors				
Race/ethnicity (non-Hispanic White ref.)				
Hispanic		0.684***	0.652***	0.661***
Black		0.500***	0.557***	0.593***
Asian		0.969	0.867	0.922
Other language of interview (English ref.)		0.539***	0.527***	0.543***
Age		1.058***	1.057***	1.042***
Age-squared		0.999***	0.999***	1.000***
Female		1.483***	1.503***	1.401***
Education (less than high school ref.)				
High school or equivalent		1.902***	1.833***	1.918***
College degree or higher		2.964***	2.789***	3.071***
Married (unmarried ref.)		0.858***	0.847***	0.852***
Enabling factors				
U.S. region of residence (Northeast ref.)				
Midwest			1.176**	1.195**
South			0.868*	0.876*
West			1.511***	1.489***
Employed last week (not employed ref.)			0.891**	0.950
No health coverage (covered ref.)			1.076	1.058
Family poverty ratio (below poverty line ref.)				
1–1.99 times poverty line			1.019	1.052
2+ times poverty line			1.190**	1.324***
Need factors				
Pain				1.491***
Activity limitation				0.999
Fair/poor health (excellent/very good/good)				0.820**
N	22,748	22,748	22,748	22,748

Source: NHIS 2007.
Notes: Reference groups in parentheses. Respondents with missing income information are included in regression, but results not reported here.
*$p<0.05$; **$p<0.01$; ***$p<0.001$, two-tailed test.

Table 4a. Reason for Not Using CAM: Knowledge – Logistic Regression Odds Ratios of Not Using CAM Modality Because Never Heard of it.

	Acupuncture	Chiropractic	Herbs	Yoga/Tai Chi/Qi Gong	Relaxation
Nativity (U.S.-born ref.)					
Immigrant, <15 years	1.354*	1.403**	0.982	1.146	1.551**
Immigrant, 15+ years	1.026	1.032	0.920	1.012	1.122
Predisposing factors					
Race/ethnicity (non-Hispanic White ref.)					
Hispanic	1.437**	1.173	1.187	1.257	1.065
Black	1.441***	1.306**	1.232*	1.460***	1.283**
Asian	1.112	1.251	1.025	0.870	0.747
Other language of interview (English ref.)	0.941	1.090	0.923	1.119	1.021
Age	0.962***	0.968**	0.985	0.974*	0.981
Age-squared	1.000***	1.000**	1.000	1.000***	1.000*
Female	1.019	1.067	0.967	0.941	1.002
Education (less than high school ref.)					
High school or equivalent	0.575***	0.670***	0.618***	0.611***	0.635***
College degree or higher	0.376***	0.430***	0.487***	0.448***	0.424***
Married (unmarried ref.)	1.139*	1.170*	1.064	1.169*	1.028
Enabling factors					
U.S. region of residence (Northeast ref.)					
Midwest	1.070	0.722*	0.823	1.057	0.937
South	1.211	0.989	0.987	1.289	1.177
West	0.779	0.607***	0.697*	0.873	0.931
Employed last week (not employed ref.)	0.954	0.940	0.978	0.935	0.868
No health coverage (covered ref.)	1.160*	1.090	1.173	1.145	1.293**
Family poverty ratio (below poverty line ref.)					
1–1.99 times poverty line	0.936	0.935	0.906	0.903	0.953
2+ times poverty line	0.610***	0.617***	0.743*	0.645***	0.755*
Need factors					
Pain	0.959	1.000	1.007	0.988	1.032
Activity limitation	1.007	1.004	1.012*	1.006	1.009
Fair/poor health (excellent/very good/good)	1.123	1.030	0.955	1.044	1.052
N	20,563	17,041	16,519	19,779	19,197

Source: NHIS 2007.
Notes: Reference groups in parentheses. Respondents with missing income information are included in regression, but results not reported here.
*$p<0.05$; **$p<0.01$; ***$p<0.001$, two-tailed test.

Table 4b. Reason for not Using CAM: Cost – Logistic Regression Odds Ratios of Not Using CAM Modality Because it was too Expensive.

	Acupuncture	Chiropractic	Herbs	Yoga/Tai Chi/Qi Gong	Relaxation
Nativity (U.S.-born ref.)					
Immigrant, <15 years	0.87	0.860	0.937	1.674	1.300
Immigrant, 15+ years	1.127	0.807	0.932	1.292	1.223
Predisposing factors					
Race/ethnicity (non-Hispanic White ref.)					
Hispanic	0.941	0.764	1.012	1.749*	1.683
Black	0.449***	0.461***	0.594*	0.693	1.373
Asian	0.621	0.549	0.529	0.727	1.788
Other language of interview (English ref.)	0.816	0.819	0.750	0.455	0.830
Age	1.088***	1.077***	1.114***	1.037	1.087
Age-squared	0.999***	0.999***	0.999***	0.999	0.999*
Female	1.887***	1.745***	1.434*	2.998***	1.151
Education (less than high school ref.)					
High school or equivalent	1.272	0.881	1.281	0.996	0.875
College degree or higher	1.282	0.557**	0.920	1.205	0.605
Married (unmarried ref.)	0.583***	0.526***	0.591***	0.534***	0.874
Enabling factors					
U.S. region of residence (Northeast ref.)					
Midwest	1.082	1.612**	1.718*	1.646	1.702
South	0.938	1.308	1.304	1.815*	1.321
West	1.917***	2.056***	2.820***	2.045*	1.544
Employed last week (not employed ref.)	–	–	–	–	–
No health coverage (covered ref.)	–	–	–	–	–
Family poverty ratio (below poverty line ref.)					
1–1.99 times poverty line	–	–	–	–	–
2+ times poverty line	–	–	–	–	–
Need factors					
Pain	1.473***	1.564***	1.299***	1.429***	1.289*
Activity limitation	1.026***	1.011	1.035***	1.003	1.036
Fair/poor health (excellent/very good/good)	1.077	1.213	1.230	0.870	0.792
N	21,733	20,249	18,095	20,649	19,805

Source: NHIS 2007.
Notes: Reference groups in parentheses. Respondents with missing income information are included in regression, but results not reported here.
*p<0.05; **p<0.01; ***p<0.001, two-tailed test.

Table 4c. Reason for Not Using CAM: Need – Logistic Regression Odds Ratios of Not Using CAM Modality Because Did Not Need it.

	Acupuncture	Chiropractic	Herbs	Yoga/Tai Chi/Qi Gong	Relaxation
Nativity (U.S.-born ref.)					
Immigrant, <15 years	1.093	0.849	1.147	1.197	1.126
Immigrant, 15+ years	1.056	0.967	1.134	1.300**	1.034
Predisposing factors					
Race/ethnicity (non-Hispanic White ref.)					
Hispanic	1.210**	1.230**	1.312***	1.200	1.272**
Black	0.918	0.978	0.993	1.108	1.019
Asian	1.297**	1.096	1.326*	1.147	0.946
Other language of interview (English ref.)	1.048	0.910	1.177	1.495**	1.209
Age	0.985*	0.984*	0.986	0.980*	0.981*
Age-squared	1.000**	1.000**	1.000	1.000**	1.000**
Female	0.998	0.956	0.911	0.660***	0.760***
Education (less than high school ref.)					
High school or equivalent	1.339***	1.285***	1.207**	1.239**	1.178*
College degree or higher	1.646***	1.470***	1.351***	1.079	1.276**
Married (unmarried ref.)	1.035	0.995	0.974	0.992	1.087
Enabling factors					
U.S. region of residence (Northeast ref.)					
Midwest	1.462***	1.553***	1.550***	1.728***	1.632***
South	1.248**	1.262**	1.431***	1.482***	1.360**
West	1.342***	1.367***	1.541***	1.612***	1.485***
Employed last week (not employed ref.)	1.093	1.088	1.064	1.032	1.150**
No health coverage (covered ref.)	0.916	0.937	0.885	0.894	0.884
Family poverty ratio (below poverty line ref.)					
1–1.99 times poverty line	1.048	1.158*	1.145	0.931	1.001
2+ times poverty line	1.368***	1.426***	1.282**	1.072	1.096
Need factors					
Pain	–	–	–	–	–
Activity limitation	–	–	–	–	–
Fair/poor health (excellent/very good/good)	–	–	–	–	–
N	21,733	20,249	18,095	20,649	19,805

Source: NHIS 2007.
Notes: Reference groups in parentheses. Respondents with missing income information are included in regression, but results not reported here.
*$p<0.05$; **$p<0.01$; ***$p<0.001$, two-tailed test.

it as a possible measure of cultural knowledge rather than a measure of access due to language barriers. In the "cost" regressions, I exclude measures of income, health coverage, and employment, as these are all enabling resources that directly affect the outcome variable – nonuse because CAM is too expensive. For the same reason, because they are measures of the outcome, in the "need" regressions I exclude health conditions – pain, self-rated health, and activity limitation. In analyses not presented here, I also estimated models for each of the three reasons for not using CAM (knowledge, cost, and need) including measures of each of those factors. For example, I estimated a model with cost as the outcome, including income, employment, and health coverage. The effect of including these controls is as would be expected: their main effects are significant, but the effect on the nativity gap is minimal. Thus, I only present the more parsimonious models excluding these redundant controls.

Finally, in Table 5, I present results from interactive models assessing the moderating impact of ethnicity on the relationship between nativity and reasons for not using CAM. To facilitate interpretation of the interactions, I conduct separate regressions for each racial/ethnic group and test for significant race-immigrant status interactions by estimating logistic regression models (not shown here) interacting race with every covariate in the model. This tests whether each racial/ethnic group differs significantly by nativity from non-Hispanic Whites (e.g., whether the odds ratios for Asian recent immigrants differs significantly from White recent immigrants, or whether Hispanic established immigrants differ from White established immigrants). As in the previous regressions, the outcome variables are knowledge, cost, and need for each of the five CAM modalities and, although I present only nativity effects, all models control for the same factors (except language, for which cell sizes were too small for most racial groups).

RESULTS

Immigrant Status and CAM Use

Bivariate results reveal that immigrant status is related to use of all the CAM modalities, except yoga (Table 1). Notably, immigrants have lower usage than the U.S.-born of all five forms of CAM. For example, 18% of the U.S.-born have used herbs in the past year compared to 7% of recent immigrants (less than 15 years in the United States) and 15% of established

Table 5. Adjusted[a] Odds Ratios: Ethnic Differences in Reasons for Not Using CAM by Immigrant Status.

	Acupuncture				Chiropractic				Herbs			
	White	Hispanic[b]	Black[b]	Asian[b]	White	Hispanic[b]	Black[b]	Asian[b]	White	Hispanic[b]	Black[b]	Asian[b]
Knowledge												
U.S.-born	Ref.	Ref.	Ref.	Ref.	Ref.	Ref.	Ref.	Ref.	Ref.	Ref.	Ref.	Ref.
Immigrant, <15 years	1.623	1.230	1.647*	1.469	1.690	1.414	1.165	3.084***	1.167	0.912	1.237	0.692
Immigrant, 15+ years	0.686	1.130	0.685	1.273	0.690	1.237	0.713	2.234[†]	0.709	1.031	0.624	0.524
Cost												
U.S.-born	Ref.	Ref.	Ref.	Ref.	Ref.	Ref.	Ref.	Ref.	Ref.	Ref.	Ref.	Ref.
Immigrant, <15 years	1.059	0.674	0.483	1.948	0.615	0.743	1.920	0.964	0.448	0.754	—[c]	8.430[†]
Immigrant, 15+ years	1.056	1.179	1.849	1.821	1.126	0.386***,[††]	1.291	1.497	0.936	0.816	—[c]	1.848
Need												
U.S.-born	Ref.	Ref.	Ref.	Ref.	Ref.	Ref.	Ref.	Ref.	Ref.	Ref.	Ref.	Ref.
Immigrant, <15 years	1.140	0.952	1.035	1.439	0.779	0.661**	1.250	1.028	0.950	1.094	1.543	0.856
Immigrant, 15+ years	1.251	0.943	0.821	1.307	1.055	0.850	1.035	0.966	1.437*	1.068	1.577	0.691[†]

Table 5. (Continued)

	Yoga/Tai Chi/Qi Gong				Relaxation			
	White	Hispanic[b]	Black[b]	Asian[b]	White	Hispanic[b]	Black[b]	Asian[b]
Knowledge								
U.S.-born	Ref.	Ref.	Ref.	Ref.	Ref.	Ref.	Ref	Ref.
Immigrant, <15 years	1.342	1.482*	1.267	0.810	1.561	1.847***	1.367	1.876
Immigrant, 15+ years	0.691	1.391[†]	0.655	0.654	0.804	1.434*,[†]	0.804	1.317
Cost								
U.S.-born	Ref.	Ref.	Ref.	Ref.	Ref.	Ref.	Ref.	Ref.
Immigrant, <15 years	1.311	1.225	—[c]	7.109	—[c]	0.981	—[c]	—[c]
Immigrant, 15+ years	1.673	0.864	—[c]	2.962	—[c]	0.420	—[c]	—[c]
Need								
U.S.-born	Ref.	Ref.	Ref.	Ref.	Ref.	Ref.	Ref.	Ref.
Immigrant, <15 years	1.119	1.223	1.230	1.189	1.366	1.024	1.182	0.983
Immigrant, 15+ years	1.449*	1.278	1.716*	1.322	1.156	0.978	1.402	0.847

Source: NHIS 2007.

*$p<0.05$; **$p<0.01$; ***$p<0.001$ (two-tailed test). [†]$p<0.05$; [††]$p<0.01$; [†††]$p<0.001$, (two-tailed test for significant difference compared to Whites).

[a] All models adjusted for age, age-squared, gender, education, region, marital status. In addition, knowledge regressions include employment, poverty, health coverage, pain, poor self-rated health and limitation. Cost regressions include pain, poor self-rated health, and limitation. Need regressions include employment, poverty, and health coverage.

[b] Wald test for significant difference compared to Whites.

[c] Results not presented due to small cell counts.

immigrants (15 or more years in the United States). Of the five CAM modalities examined here, herbs and relaxation are the most widely used CAM types among both the U.S.-born and immigrants; however, among the U.S.-born and established immigrants herb use is most prevalent followed by relaxation, while among recent immigrants the pattern is reversed.

Immigrant status is also significantly related to two of the three reasons for not using CAM. Recent immigrants are much more likely to report not knowing about CAM modalities than are more established immigrants and the U.S.-born, while the U.S.-born are slightly more likely to cite cost as a reason for not using CAM. There is no significant nativity difference in reports of the need for CAM. Moreover, established immigrants' patterns of use are distinct from more recently arrived immigrants. For example, established immigrants use all types of CAM more often than more recent immigrants. The largest differences in CAM use between immigrant groups are in herb use and chiropractic, with the percentage users being greater among established immigrants compared to recent immigrants by 7% and 3%, respectively.

Although established immigrants resemble the U.S.-born more than recent immigrants with regard to CAM use, they differ substantially from the U.S.-born in many other ways, notably ethnicity, age, and education. In terms of sociodemographic characteristics, immigrants who have lived in the United States 15 or more years are more likely to be White, married, older, slightly more educated, and have poorer health.

Given the substantial sociodemographic differences by immigrant status, I now turn to logistic regression results estimating odds ratios of use of "Any CAM" (using at least one of 18 CAM modalities) and of using 10 specific modalities in the past 12 months, while controlling for potentially confounding predisposing, enabling, and need factors (Table 2). The results presented are main effects of immigrant status and race/ethnicity, controlling for predisposing, enabling, and need factors. As hypothesized, even when controlling for these differences, immigrants still have lower odds of usage than the U.S.-born of most CAM modalities, but the differences are most significant for recent immigrants. Recent immigrants are significantly less likely than the U.S.-born to use chiropractic manipulation, herbs, vitamins, and massage. Established immigrants are less likely than the U.S.-born to use homeopathy and massage. Not entirely surprising is the finding that established immigrants have odds of acupuncture use that are 50% higher than the U.S.-born (OR = 1.48, $p<0.05$). This may be driven by Asians' use, which may increase over time in the United States as their health decreases. Therefore, in general, immigrant status is related to lower use of many CAM modalities compared to the U.S.-born, independent of the effects of race/ethnicity and other predisposing, enabling, and need factors. Importantly, the effect of immigrant status is not evident when examining "Any CAM" use, reinforcing the importance of examining subgroups of CAM modalities or individual modalities rather than treating CAM as a homogeneous category. Thus, in subsequent analyses, I turn to use (and then reasons for nonuse) of five specific CAM modalities.

Table 3 presents the odds ratios of using, in the last 12 months, at least one of the following: acupuncture, chiropractic, herbs, relaxation, or yoga. In the baseline model, recent immigrants have 60% lower odds of CAM use than the U.S.-born (OR = 0.410, $p<0.001$) while established immigrants' odds are 28% lower (OR = 0.718, $p<0.001$). Including predisposing factors in the model increases recent immigrants' odds of CAM use vis-à-vis the U.S.-born by about 20%, but they remain significantly lower than the U.S.-born, while the difference between the U.S.-born and established immigrants is no longer significant. Taking the NHIS interview in a language other than English is related to nearly 50% lower odds of CAM use compared to respondents interviewed in English. Adding enabling factors has little impact on the odds ratios for immigrants. Finally, when controlling for predisposing, enabling, and need factors (Model 4), recent immigrants have 28% lower odds of CAM use than the U.S.-born, while established immigrants have slightly lower, but not significantly different, odds of any use of these five modalities than the U.S.-born. These results support the hypothesis that immigrants have lower overall odds of CAM use than the U.S.-born. Why are immigrants, net of the factors posited to explain and/or predict health services use, still less likely than the U.S.-born to use CAM? In Table 4, I turn to knowledge, cost, and need as possible explanations for the nativity gap in CAM use.

Explaining the Nativity Gap: Knowledge, Cost, and Need as Reasons for Not Using CAM

Table 4a presents odds ratios of not using a specified CAM modality because one has never heard of it, net of sociodemographic and health differences.

Results show support for the hypothesis that lack of knowledge of CAM modalities appears to be an important reason for the lesser CAM use of recent immigrants. Recent immigrants have higher odds of reporting lack of knowledge of acupuncture, chiropractic, and relaxation than the U.S.-born. Specifically, recent immigrants' odds of not using CAM because they have not heard of it are 35% higher than the U.S.-born for acupuncture, 40% higher for chiropractic, and 55% higher for relaxation therapies. By contrast, immigrants who have lived in the United States for 15 years or more are just as likely as the U.S.-born to not know of these CAM modalities.

Ethnic differences in the knowledge of CAM are also pronounced. Given the research on ethnic-specific CAM use (Hsiao et al., 2006), it is not surprising that while Hispanics and Black Americans are more likely than White Americans to report not knowing about acupuncture, herbs, and yoga/tai chi/qi gong, Asians do not report lack of knowledge as a reason for not using those CAM modalities. That is, Asians are more likely to know about those modalities than other ethnic groups because they are more commonly used in Asian cultures. Similarly, all other racial/ethnic groups have higher odds than non-Hispanic Whites, and Blacks significantly so, of not using chiropractic because they do not know about it. Other factors predicting lack of knowledge of CAM are low education, low income, living outside the western United States, and being married.

Turning to cost as an explanation for immigrant-native differences in CAM use (Table 4b), we can see that there is no evidence of cost being a factor in immigrants' relatively lower rates of CAM use; therefore, the hypothesis that immigrants will be more likely than the U.S.-born to cite cost as a factor in nonuse of acupuncture and chiropractic is unsupported. There is no significant difference between immigrants and the U.S.-born in the likelihood of not using CAM because of cost limitations for any of the five CAM modalities. However, cost does appear to hinder CAM use for the following groups: females, older adults, those living in the Western United States, and those with pain and activity limitations. However, only two of the included covariates are significantly related to nonuse of relaxation due to cost: quadratic age and pain. This is likely because relaxation can be done without a practitioner, training, and thus in most cases does not incur a cost.

Lastly, in Table 4c, I examine the odds of citing lack of need as a reason for not using CAM and find little support for the hypothesis that immigrants do not use CAM because they do not need it. Controlling for predisposing and enabling factors, the only significant immigrant status difference is for yoga. Specifically, established immigrants are more likely than the U.S.-born to report not using yoga because they do not need it (OR = 1.30, $p < 0.01$). In other words immigrants, more so than the U.S.-born, report that they do not do yoga because they do not need it.

The Interactive Effects of Ethnicity and Immigrant Status

Table 5 presents the results of separate regressions by race, controlling for the factors previously mentioned as important in CAM use and healthcare utilization. Comparing recent and established immigrants of each ethnicity to their U.S.-born counterparts, we can see that there are a few significant nativity differences in all the reasons for not using CAM, but particularly for chiropractic and yoga. With regard to chiropractic use, Hispanic immigrants who have lived in the United States for 15 years or more have 62% lower odds than U.S.-born Hispanics of citing cost a reason for not using chiropractic manipulation (OR = 0.38, $p<0.01$). Also, recent Asian immigrants have odds three times those of U.S.-born Asians of not knowing about chiropractic (OR = 3.084, $p<0.001$). Immigrant–native differentials are also evident among Hispanics in knowledge of yoga and relaxation. For both modalities, recent Hispanic immigrants have significantly higher odds (between 48% and 85%) than U.S.-born Hispanics of not knowing about these modalities.

Turning to the interaction between race/ethnicity and immigrant status, we see significant interactions mainly among Hispanics and Asians, for knowledge and cost as explanations for nonuse. That is, for Hispanics and Asians the effect of immigrant status differs from that of non-Hispanic Whites. For example, while established Hispanic immigrants have much lower odds compared to U.S.-born Hispanics of reporting cost a reason for not using chiropractic (OR = 0.386, $p<0.001$), established White immigrants do not differ from U.S.-born Whites in odds of reporting cost as a reason for not using chiropractic (OR = 1.126, $p>0.1$). This interaction is significant at the 0.01 alpha level. In addition, established Hispanic immigrants significantly differ from established White immigrants in reporting lack of knowledge of yoga and relaxation. While among Hispanics, established immigrants are more likely to report not knowing about these two modalities, there is no nativity difference among Whites. The difference between Asians and Whites is for knowledge as a reason for nonuse of chiropractic and cost and need as reasons for nonuse of herbs. For instance, while odds of established White immigrants citing need as a reason for nonuse of herbs are significantly higher than those of U.S.-born Whites, Asian established immigrants have lower odds (but not significantly) than U.S.-born Asians. Therefore, although there is some support for the hypothesis that ethnicity moderates the immigrant status–CAM relationship, there is no support for the idea that there are significant immigrant status differences in reporting lack of knowledge for one's own ethnic-specific CAM practices.

DISCUSSION

This study is the first, to the author's knowledge, to examine immigrant status differences in use of and reasons for not using specific CAM modalities. The results presented here provide support for the idea that a complex combination of predisposing, enabling, and need factors form the basis for an individual's health service use (and nonuse) and that the Behavioral Model of health service utilization can be fruitfully applied to CAM use. First, using nationally-representative data, this study finds that immigrants, in general, use many CAM modalities less than the U.S.-born do. There are at least a couple of explanations for this nativity gap in CAM use. First, recent immigrants underutilize CAM modalities due to a lack of knowledge about them. Second, established immigrants report lack of need as a reason for nonuse more than the U.S.-born. Furthermore, immigrant–native differences remain even when controlling for established predisposing, enabling, and need factors, suggesting that there are other factors that affect immigrants' knowledge of, and need for, CAM.

Immigrant status differences in the reasons for not using CAM vary by both CAM modality and ethnicity. Established immigrants of certain ethnic groups differ from their U.S.-born counterparts in odds of reporting need as a reason for not using CAM. For example, White and Black established immigrants are more likely than their native-born counterparts to report not needing CAM, but only for yoga and herbs. In addition, compared to their U.S.-born counterparts, Hispanic immigrants tend to report knowledge more as a reason for nonuse of relaxation and yoga, while Asian and Black immigrants report lack of knowledge as a reason for not using chiropractic services and acupuncture, respectively.

Although these results point to some significant immigrant status and ethnic differences in reasons for using or not using CAM, there are several limitations to this study. First, because the NHIS only asks about reasons for not using CAM for only the five modalities presented here, there is a possibility that results could differ for the wide range of modalities that could not be included in this study. However, for the reasons mentioned earlier, such as the range of costs of these modalities and the increasing attention to them by researchers, health providers, and the media, the results for these five modalities may be generalizable to some other modalities as well. There may also be other possible reasons why immigrants appear to underutilize CAM, which could not be addressed here, including measurement issues. The NHIS conducts interviews in English, Spanish, or several other languages, and the analyses here control for language of interview.

However, it is possible that some immigrants interviewed in English, but do not know the English names for CAM modalities, and therefore report that they do not use it because they don't know about it.

Despite these shortcomings, this study's findings provide important insight into immigrants' health service utilization. They point to immigrants being disadvantaged in the early years of their U.S. residence in terms of knowledge of healthcare options, an important access issue. Future research assessing immigrants' health outcomes and access to health care should take CAM into account. More work is needed to clarify why qualitative research finds that immigrants are significant CAM users while large-scale surveys find the U.S-born to be more likely CAM users, whether immigrants use CAM for the same reasons as the U.S.-born (treatment versus wellness, and for what conditions or ailments), and how immigrants' CAM use changes over time in the United States. The ideal study design to answer these questions would be using longitudinal data and mixed methods, which would enable researchers to assess the impact of length of residence in the United States without confounding cohort and period effects and would permit a more culturally centered analysis that might address some of the measurement issues posed by survey methods. Such research could provide insight into immigrants' access to CAM and could ultimately play a role in reducing immigrant and racial/ethnic health disparities in the United States.

REFERENCES

Abraído-Lanza, A. F., Chao, M. T., & Flórez, K. R. (2005). Do healthy behaviors decline with greater acculturation?: Implications for the Latino Mortality Paradox. *Social Science and Medicine*, *61*, 1243–1255.

Ahn, A. C., Ngo-Metzger, Q., Legedza, A. T. R., Massagli, M. P., Clarridge, B. R., & Phillips, R. S. (2006). Complementary and alternative medical therapy use among Chinese and Vietnamese Americans: Prevalence, associated factors, and effects of patient-clinician communication. *American Journal of Public Health*, *96*, 647–653.

Andersen, R. M. (1968). *Behavioral model of families' use of health services*. Research Series. Chicago: University of Chicago.

Andersen, R. M. (1995). Revisiting the behavioral model and access to medical care: Does it matter? *Journal of Health and Social Behavior*, *36*, 1–10.

Barnes, P. M., & Bloom, B. (2008). *Complementary and alternative medicine use among adults and children: United States, 2007*. National Health Statistics Reports. Hyattsville, MD: National Center for Health Statistics.

Barnes, P. M., Powell-Griner, E., Mcfann, K., & Nahin, R. L. (2004). Complementary and alternative medicine use among adults: United States, 2002. *Seminars in Integrative Medicine, 2*, 54–71.

Eisenberg, D. M., Davis, R. B., Ettner, S. L., Appel, S., Wilkey, S., Van Rompay, M., & Kessler, R. C. (1998). Trends in alternative medicine use in the United States, 1990–1997: Results of a follow-up national survey. *JAMA, 280*, 1569–1575.

Garcés, I., Scarinci, I., & Harrison, L. (2006). An examination of sociocultural factors associated with health and health care seeking among Latina immigrants. *Journal of Immigrant and Minority Health, 8*, 377–385.

Gortmaker, S. L., & Wise, P. H. (1997). The first injustice: Socioeconomic disparities, health services technology, and infant mortality. *Annual Review of Sociology, 23*, 147–170.

Grzywacz, J. G., Lang, W., Suerken, C., Quandt, S. A., Bell, R. A., & Arcury, T. A. (2005). Age, race, and ethnicity in the use of complementary and alternative medicine for health self-management: Evidence from the 2002 national health interview survey. *Journal of Aging and Health, 17*, 547–572.

Grzywacz, J. G., Suerken, C. K., Neiberg, R. H., Lang, W., Bell, R. A., Quandt, S. A., & Arcury, T. A. (2007). Age, ethnicity, and use of complementary and alternative medicine in health self-management. *Journal of Health and Social Behavior, 48*, 84–98.

Hsiao, A.-F., Wong, M. D., Goldstein, M. S., Yu, H.-J., Andersen, R. M., Brown, E. R., Becerra, L. M., & Wenger, N. S. (2006). Variation in complementary and alternative medicine (CAM). Use across racial/ethnic groups and the development of ethnic-specific measures of CAM use. *The Journal of Alternative and Complementary Medicine, 12*, 281–290.

Hummer, R. A., Powers, D. A., Pullum, S. G., Gossman, G. L., & Frisbie, W. P. (2007). Paradox found (again): Infant mortality among the Mexican-origin population in the United States. *Demography, 44*, 441–457.

Jasso, G., Massey, D. S., Rosenzweig, M. R., & Smith, J. P. (2004). Immigrant health: Selectivity and acculturation. In: N. B. Anderson, R. A. Bulatao & B. Cohen (Eds), *Critical perspectives on racial and ethnic differences in health in late life*. Washington, DC: The National Academies Press.

Keith, V., Kronenfeld, J., Rivers, P., & Liang, S.-Y. (2005). Assessing the effects of race and ethnicity on use of complementary and alternative therapies in the USA. *Ethnicity and Health, 10*, 19–32.

Kronenfeld, J. J., & Ayers, S. L. (2009). Social sources of disparities in use of complementary and alternative medicine. In: J. J. Kronenfeld (Ed.), *Research in the sociology of health care*. Bingley, UK: Emerald Group Publishing.

Kuo, G., Hawley, S., Weiss, L. T., Balkrishnan, R., & Volk, R. (2004). Factors associated with herbal use among urban multiethnic primary care patients: A cross-sectional survey. *BMC Complementary and Alternative Medicine, 4*, 18.

Leclere, F. B., Jensen, L., & Biddlecom, A. E. (1994). Health care utilization, family context, and adaptation among immigrants to the United States. *Journal of Health and Social Behavior, 35*, 370–384.

Markides, K. S., & Coreil, J. (1986). The health of Hispanics in the Southwestern United States: An epidemiologic paradox. *Public Health Reports, 101*, 253.

Najm, W., Reinsch, S., Hoehler, F., & Tobis, J. (2003). Use of complementary and alternative medicine among the ethnic elderly. *Alternative Therapies in Health and Medicine, 9*, 50–57.

National Center for Health Statistics. (2008). *Data file documentation, national health interview survey, 2007.* Hyattsville, MD: National Center for Health Statistics, Centers for Disease Control and Prevention.

Poss, J., & Jezewski, M. A. (2002). The role and meaning of susto in Mexican Americans' explanatory model of type 2 diabetes. *Medical Anthropology Quarterly, 16,* 360–377.

Sirois, F. M., & Gick, M. L. (2002). An investigation of the health beliefs and motivations of complementary medicine clients. *Social Science and Medicine, 55,* 1025–1037.

Su, D., Li, L., & Pagán, J. A. (2008). Acculturation and the use of complementary and alternative medicine. *Social Science and Medicine, 66,* 439–453.

Upchurch, D. M., Burke, A., Dye, C., Chyu, L., Kusunoki, Y., & Greendale, G. A. (2008). A sociobehavioral model of acupuncture use, patterns, and satisfaction among women in the United States, 2002. *Women's Health Issues, 18,* 62–71.

Xu, J., & Yang, Y. (2009). Traditional Chinese medicine in the Chinese health care system. *Health Policy, 90,* 133–139.

Zolla, C. (2009). Medicina Tradicional Mesoamericana en el Contexto de la Migración. Presented at Curso Internacional Sobre Migracion y Salud. July 3, 2009, Puebla, Mexico.

CLASS AND RACE HEALTH DISPARITIES AND HEALTH INFORMATION SEEKING BEHAVIORS: THE ROLE OF SOCIAL CAPITAL

Cirila Estela Vasquez Guzman, Gilbert Mireles, Neal Christopherson and Michelle Janning

ABSTRACT

Researchers have spent considerable time studying how racial-ethnic minorities experience poorer health than whites [Townsend, P., & Davidson, N. (Eds). (1990). Inequalities in health: The black report. England: Penguin Press; Platt, L. (2006). Assessing the impact of illness, caring and ethnicity on social activity. STICERD Research Paper No. CASE108 London England), and how low socioeconomic status (SES) can negatively influence health status (Lynch, J., & Kaplan, G. (2000). Socioeconomic position. In: L. F. Berkman & I. Kawachi (Eds), Social epidemiology (pp. 13–55). New York: Oxford University Press]. This research investigates the relationship between class and race and perceived health status among patients with chronic conditions. More specifically, we apply the concept of social capital to assess whether the quantity of health information seeking behaviors (HISB) via social networks mediates the relationship between race and health status, and between SES and health status. Regression, t-test and ANOVA analyses of 305 surveys completed at a chronic illness management clinic in a Northwest research hospital reveal three important findings: first, that social class affects perceived health status more strongly than race; second, that frequency and amount of HISB do not play a significant role in perceived health status, regardless of race or SES; and third, that an interaction effect between frequency and amount of HISB suggests that the way that patients seek health information, and the quality of that information, may be more useful indicators of the role of social capital in HISB than our study can provide.

There is a growing population of patients suffering from one or multiple chronic conditions in the United States (Hoffman, Rice, & Sung, 1996). Multiple studies have found that chronic conditions disproportionately affect minority populations (Laditka & Laditka, 2006) and individuals with low socioeconomic status (Dalstra et al., 2005). This chapter investigates the relationship between class and racial-ethnic identity and perceived health status among patients with chronic conditions. More specifically, we apply the concept of social capital to assess whether the quantity of health information seeking behaviors (HISB) via social networks mediates the relationship between race and perceived health status, and between class and perceived health status.

SOCIOECONOMIC AND RACIAL HEALTH DISPARITIES AND CHRONIC CONDITIONS

In 1987, there were 90 million Americans living with chronic conditions and 39 million with more than one chronic condition (Hoffman et al., 1996). As of 2005, there were more than 130 million Americans suffering from chronic conditions and about half were diagnosed with multiple chronic conditions. These numbers are projected to keep increasing. By 2025, it is estimated that nearly half (49%) of our population will be affected by one or more chronic conditions (Wu & Green, 2000). Chronic condition is a long lasting health condition that lasts for three or more months that requires ongoing medical attention and affects a person's daily life. Any of the following is considered to be a chronic condition: asthma, hypertension, diabetes, arthritis, and cancer (MedicineNet.com, 2010).

The rise in the number of individuals coping with chronic conditions disproportionately occurs among minorities and lower class populations. Racial and social class health disparities are well documented in the literature (Oliver, 2008; Issacs & Schroeder, 2004; Wilkinson & Pickett, 2005; Kawachi, Daniels, & Robinson, 2005). Health disparities are defined as "a difference in which disadvantaged social groups such as the poor, racial/ethnic minorities, women and other groups who have persistently experienced social disadvantage or discrimination systematically experience worse health or greater health risks than most advantaged social groups" (Braveman, 2006, pp. 180–181). In terms of race and chronic conditions, heart disease and cancer are both leading causes of death for American Indians and Alaska Natives (Office of Minority Health and Health Disparities, 2008). Diabetes is the condition most prevalent among older Hispanics (20–30%) and African Americans are twice as likely to suffer from a stroke compared to whites (4.6% v 2. 4%) ("Beyond 50.09 ..." 2009). Also, minority populations are more likely to suffer from chronic illness-related complications such as diabetes. For example, end state renal disease (ESRD) is more likely to develop in African Americans than in whites for type 2 diabetes (Perneger, Brancatie, Wheltonn, & Klag, 1994).

Socioeconomic status (SES), like race, is also a widely recognized sociodemographic factor contributing to the gap in health status and well-being. In a progressive pattern those from lower classes die earlier compared to those from higher classes (McDounough, Duncan, Williams, & House, 1997). One study found a correlation between income and health status in 27 OECD countries, and includes a recommendation to increase individuals' per capita real income to positively change self-rated health status (Murthy, 2007). Among patients with chronic conditions, the link between class and health are less clear, but some studies find a significant correlation. Glover, Hetzel, and Tennant (2004) specifically found individuals with low SES had a greater prevalence of chronic conditions. Another study reported income and wealth are significant predictors of having one or more chronic conditions (Kington & Smith, 1997). Approximately 25% of low-income populations are burdened by chronic conditions (Newacheck, Butlet, Harper, Dyan, & Franks, 1980). There is also more frequent prevalence of avoidable hospitalization and/or complications among lower income individuals with chronic conditions. Pappas, Hadden, Kozak, & Fisher (1997) found avoidable hospitalization is most prevalent among middle and lower income groups with chronic conditions compared to higher income groups. In addition, working class individuals with chronic conditions face barriers such as the lack of insurance coverage and/or the inability to cover insurance costs (Hogue, Hargraves, & Collins, 2000; Alegria et al., 2006), which makes it more likely for them to have worse health status, especially when access to needed resources or support dealing with complex chronic condition(s) are absent.

Racial and economic health disparities are well documented and present in our current healthcare system. Patients with chronic conditions reflect similar trends of larger sectors – minority groups and lower income groups with chronic conditions disproportionately have worse health status. Further investigating and understanding of the effects of race and class on health status among patients with chronic conditions is still needed.

COST INCREASES AND CHANGING DEMOGRAPHICS

The United States faces the challenge of increasing healthcare costs. In 2007, according to the National Health Expenditures reports from the Office of Actuary in the Centers for Medicare and Medicaid Services, the U.S. spent $2.26 trillion on health care, or $7,439 per person (2008). Although numerous factors have contributed to increase costs, the literature demonstrates a strong consensus that cost burdens are largely attributed to the increasing population of older patients and patients with chronic conditions (Schneider & Guralnik, 1990; Druss et al., 2001). Expenditures from patients with chronic conditions account for a significant portion of our healthcare costs. Rising healthcare costs are attributed to the rapidly growing populations suffering from one or more chronic conditions. This population sector now accounts for 75% of total healthcare costs (Wolff, Starfield, & Andersen, 2002). Three of every four dollars spent on health care cover the costs of chronic conditions; this is nearly $7,900 for every American with a chronic disease (Center for Disease Control, 2007). The significant health disparities among minorities and lower class groups with chronic conditions further contribute to these already staggering healthcare costs.

The U.S. population is becoming more racially and ethnically diverse. A recent study (Hanchate, Kronman, Young-Xu, Ash, & Emanuel, 2009) found that costs associated with minorities diagnosed with chronic conditions are higher than those associated with whites with chronic conditions. The expenditures are as follows: $20,166 for whites vs. $26,704 for blacks vs. $31,702 for Hispanics during the 6-month period immediately preceding their data collection. End of life costs are greater for Hispanics than other groups because they are more likely to suffer from multiple chronic conditions that lead to greater expenses at life's end. Hispanics. Asian Americans, American Indians, Alaska Natives, and African Americans are less likely to have health insurance, have more difficulty getting healthcare services, and have fewer choices available to them when compared to Whites. They are also more likely to be treated in the emergency room and less likely to have a primary care provider (Collins. Hall, & Neuhaus, 1999). Because of rising healthcare costs and demographic changes, it is imperative to engage in a dialogue and research investigating the means to ameliorate the racial health disparities among patients with chronic conditions.

Patients dealing with chronic conditions are very likely to be from lower social class groups, a segment of the population that also substantially contributes to the healthcare costs. Pickett, Kelly, Brunner, Lobstein, and Wilkinson (2005) found that obesity, diabetes, and mortality rates were all positively correlated with low income. In another study, the prevalence of cardiovascular disease, cancer, chronic respiratory diseases, and diabetes in low- and middle-income countries was highest, accounting for 50% of the total health expenditures in those countries. At a societal level, the age of death in higher income countries was 54% higher for men and 86% for women than in lower income countries (Albegunde, Mathers, Adam. Oregon, & Strong, 2007). Hospitalizations are also more frequent among lower income groups. In New York City, areas with more low-income residents had higher rates of hospitalization compared to higher-income areas where more appropriate and less costly outpatients' procedures were in place (Billings et al., 1993). Researchers consistently report that lower income individuals, and countries with high levels of low-income citizens, have higher healthcare expenditures compared to higher income populations.

DEMOGRAPHIC DIFFERENCES IN HEALTH INFORMATION SEEKING BEHAVIORS

As the number of Americans with chronic health conditions increases and access to information technology improves for larger segments of the population, people are expanding their sources of health-related information. No longer are patients relying exclusively on healthcare professionals to gain access to health information. Instead, patients are now accessing a wide variety of sources including radio, television, newspapers, internet, and others (Lewis, Chang, & Friedman, 2005; Hesse et al., 2005). Unlike acute illness care, managing chronic conditions requires continuous and often complex disease management and care coordination over a prolonged period of time (De Monaco & Hippel, 2007). As a result, more and more of the responsibility for better health in today's healthcare structure falls on the patient. Multiple sources of information are used by patients to cope with this increased responsibility.

Over the past 6 years, from 2001 to 2007, health information seeking from any source has increased by about 20% among all individuals from different educational backgrounds (Tu & Cohen, 2008). This remains the same even when controlling for income, age, or race. Patients with chronic conditions are those most likely to seek health information. One study found that chronic and disabled patients are keen seekers; they are more likely to conduct in-depth searches about specific diseases or conditions, search for their own use or benefit, and use the information found for application or behavior change (Fox, 2009). Research supports the notion that necessity drives frequency: those who need health care the most are more likely to search and use health information.

According to Faircloth, Boylstein, Rittman, Young, and Gubrium (2004), individuals experience a significant disruption when diagnosed with a chronic condition. A diagnosis disrupts the "normal" life conditions as the patient faces numerous physical, emotional, and social struggles every day. Regardless of the specific diagnosis, patients coping with chronic conditions often face the same challenges, such as dealing with symptoms, disability, emotional impacts, complex medication regimens, difficult lifestyle adjustments, and the struggles of obtaining helpful medical care (Wagner et al., 2001). During such times a common response to an illness-related uncertainty is to engage in information management (Mishel, 1988, 1990). People with chronic conditions will seek health information related to their condition to learn more about their diagnosis, to make decisions concerning treatment(s), and to predict their prognosis.

Wilson (2000) defines health information seeking behaviors as the purposive seeking of information to satisfy a health-related goal. This kind of health information seeking behavior excludes passive forms of health information acquisition such as watching television or listening to the radio without intending to seek information. The key feature that characterizes HISB is that it is problem driven. For patients with chronic conditions the problem is self evident.

It is important that patients with chronic conditions access health information because it enables them to better self-manage their conditions. Two of the most commonly searched topics by patients are disease/condition information and medication/treatment information. In a survey investigating patients' use of the internet for health information, 78% of the patients reported searching for information related to their diagnosis and 53% indicated searching for medication information (Schwartz et al., 2006). In another study, the top five topics searched were: diseases, medication, nutrition, exercise, and illness prevention. This information has a direct impact on the patient. Two of the five patients with chronic conditions report using health information to diagnose a health problem and one of the three reports they use the information to treat their health problems (Ybarra & Suman, 2006).

Health information seeking behaviors have been investigated among different racial and income groups. However, research to determine the degree to which race affects health information seeking behaviors remains inconclusive. One study found race to have very little significance. Instead, income, education, and employment had a stronger impact on the degree individuals used the internet for health information (Goldner, 2004). Greater gains have been made in the study of social networks and their impact on health seeking behaviors. Scholars have examined the importance of having an extensive network of contacts to gain appropriate health-related information. Effective communication and access to information are especially important for minorities and other disenfranchised groups (Mahon & Fox, 2002; Lin, 2001; Metoyer-Duran, 1993). Courtright (2005) discusses how newcomers such as Latino immigrants are unable to obtain needed health information to make better decisions about their health because institutions have not yet provided the information in a format best accessible to that population. What this and other researchers strongly suggest is that effective social networks are crucial in order for patients with chronic health conditions to access important information related to their conditions.

SOCIAL CAPITAL AND HEALTH

Scholars have drawn on the work of Bourdieu (1986), Coleman (1989), and Putnam (1995, 2000) to explore the relationship between individuals' networks and their life outcomes. Individuals will make use of their connections to others in an effort to access information or seek some kind of benefit. The set of resources available to a person by virtue of his or her membership in a particular network is referred to as social capital. Putnam (1995) described social capital as "features of social organization such as networks, norms and social trust that facilitate coordination and cooperation for mutual benefit" (p. 67). Social capital is a property of the social networks in which individuals participate. Social capital will include elements of trust and reciprocity. The lack of these will weaken a social network, thereby reducing the degree of social support exchange. Conversely, a greater amount of trust and reciprocity will signal a stronger network and thus more social support.

Research shows that social networks affect a wide range of behaviors such as education, employment opportunities, and criminality (Granovetter, 1973; McCarthy & Hagan, 2001; Portes, 1998). What these studies demonstrate is that the quality and extent of an individual's relationships will variably impact his or her quality of life. With respect to health, those individuals who are better able to exploit the social capital found in their networks are healthier than those who cannot. In *Bowling Alone* Putnam (2000) offers four possible reasons for this. First, he suggests that social networks can provide material support which will in turn reduce stress. Second, social networks will reinforce healthy behaviors. Third, an individual can use his or her networks to lobby for more medical services. Finally, Putnam (2000) suggests that social interaction may help stimulate the body's immune system. Although some of these formulations may rest on empirically dubious ground, other researchers have confirmed the link between health and social networks. House, Landis, and Umberson (1988) found that social capital integration is critical for better health status. Hendryx, Ahern, Lovrich, and McCurdy (2002) found that well-connected individuals were more informed and also better able to influence and access local health services.

Clearly, relationships matter when it comes to health, but how? Drawing on previous research, Kawachi, Kennedy, and Glass (1999) and Kawachi and Berkman (2000) present three primary ways in which health is influenced by social behaviors. First, through norms and attitudes that affect health-related behaviors; second, as a psychological mechanism that influences emotions, confidence, and control; and third, by increasing access to health care and resources. Our study is primarily concerned with this third function. Although it is clear that social capital will influence health information seeking behaviors, what is not clear is how this functions for patients with chronic conditions. Further research regarding the frequency and type of contact are needed.

THE CURRENT STUDY

We investigate the relationship between race and perceived health status and between SES and perceived health status to see how our data fits into past researchers' findings. We complicate this initial analysis by investigating the relationship between both SES and race and amount of health information seeking behaviors. Finally, we uncover whether amount of HISB mediates any effects that race and SES may have on perceived health status.

Based on the aforementioned research findings, several hypotheses emerge:

H1. Racial-ethnic minorities will have lower perceived health status than whites.

H2. Racial-ethnic minorities will have lower levels of health information seeking behaviors (HISB) than whites.

H3. Individuals with lower socioeconomic status will have lower perceived health status than individuals with higher socioeconomic status.

H4. Individuals with lower socioeconomic status will have lower levels of health information seeking behaviors (HISB) than individuals with higher socioeconomic status.

H5. Controlling for HISB will lessen race effects on perceived health status.

H6. Controlling for HISB will lessen socioeconomic status effects on perceived health status.

METHODOLOGY

Participants

A Health Information Seeking Behaviors Survey was sent via mail to patients from a chronic condition clinic at a Northwest Research Hospital in 2009. This survey is available upon request from the authors. This study is part of a larger research project that includes survey questions from the Health Information National Trends Survey (HINTS) and from the Center for Disease Control (CDC) Health Related Quality of Life Survey. In order to solicit survey participants, the researchers contacted all 21 of the providers in the clinic, who gave permission to mail a survey to their eligible patients. From these 21 providers we began with a total of 2,918 potential patients. Of these, 1,855 were excluded because they did not meet criteria of having a diagnosis of one or more chronic conditions, which left us with 1,053 potential participants. An additional 180 were excluded because they had notified the clinic that they do not want to be contacted in regard to any study. We therefore sent out a total of 872 surveys on July 23 and 27, 2009. Eight of these were undeliverable either because we had a wrong address or because patients had passed away. An incentive was provided for patients to return their surveys promptly. Participants who submitted their completed surveys before late August 2009 were entered into a drawing for one of the three $100 grocery-shopping certificates. A total of 305 surveys were completed, which translates into a 34% response rate.

Measures

The survey contained five sections, noted as follows: Section A: Seeking Health Information; Section B: Health Information Needs; Section C: Information Preferences; Section D: Health Status & Health Services; and Section E: About You. The individual variables used in our hypotheses were measured as follows:

Race: Survey respondents were asked "Are you Hispanic or Latino?" and "Which one or more of the following would you say is your race?" Hispanics were included in the minority racial group in our analysis.
Socioeconomic status: Two survey questions were used to assess respondents' socioeconomic status: income and education level. Income categories were measured ordinally with eight income ranges, and education levels were collapsed into four categories: high school or below, vocational or some college, college degree, and postgraduate.
Health Information Seeking Behavior (HISB): Quantity of HISB was assessed using two survey items: first, a question asking respondents to state how many of the listed sources they utilize in seeking health information and second, the frequency with which they seek health information.

The first survey question captures both media and nonmedia or social forms of information channels. We are interested in exploring the role of social capital and therefore the first question is divided into two parts: amount of media-based resources used to retrieve health information and amount of social relationships used to retrieve health information.

Media-based resources measure the number of sources used from the following: books, brochures/pamphlets, internet, magazines, newspapers, telephone information numbers, and television. Social relationships capture the number of resources used from the following: organization, family, friend/co-worker, library, complementary/alternative/unconventional practitioner, and health insurance provider. The second survey item, frequency, is captured with the question "How often do you look for health information about health topics?" Responses were coded at the ordinal level.

Perceived health status: Respondents were asked the question "Overall, how would you rate the quality of health care you received in the past 12 months?"

Data Analysis

In order to test the first four hypotheses, t-tests and ANOVAs were computed to assess mean differences in perceived health status for racial groups and for income and education level groups. T-tests and ANOVAs were also computed to assess mean differences in amount and frequency of HISB for all independent variables. In order to test H5 and H6, two regression analyses were conducted that included the respective independent variables, the amount and frequency of HISB, and perceived health status. Finally, other demographic variables such as age and gender were included in the analyses, as was a test of whether the frequency and amount of HISB were interacting in the regression.

Limitations

With a response rate of 34% and a limited number of racial-ethnic minorities in the sample, it is important to use caution when interpreting the results. This study's design and data collection period occurred within a narrow time frame of 2 months. As a result of the small number of racial-ethnic minorities, we were unable to understand health information seeking behaviors among different racial ethnic groups. Combining all racial groups into two categories ignores features of any single minority racial group. In addition, our SES measures exclude occupational prestige. The median age of the sample is nearly 65 years old and all survey respondents had health insurance when they filled out a survey, both of which lessen the generalizability of the results. Because racial-ethnic disparities are very stark among populations who lack health insurance, this proves to be an important limitation. The data also do not allow for the researchers to assess the quality of the networks consulted in seeking health information, only the quantity and frequency.

RESULTS

The racial groups represented in the sample ($N = 294$; missing $= 11$) are as follows: 88.4% White, 4.1% Asian-American, 2.4% Black/African-American, 0.7% American Indian/Alaska Native, 0.3% Native Hawaiian/Other Pacific, and 4.1% Other. Nearly 95% of respondents ($N = 298$; missing $= 8$) are not Hispanic/Latino. For annual income ($N = 282$; missing $= 22$), 29.2% made less than $35,000, 29.8% made between $35,000 and $75,000, and 33.8% indicated making more than $75,000. Our respondents reported the following levels of education ($N = 305$: missing $= 2$): 12.8% have a HS diploma or less, 29.8% have either vocational or some college education, 24.3% are college graduates, and 32.5% indicated postgraduate schooling. Respondents' ages ranged from 22 to 97, with a median age of 65. Men made up 45% of the sample. Just over 70% reported seeing a health professional 4 or more times in the past 12 months.

Table 1 shows mean differences between whites and nonwhites. Whites were found to have significantly higher levels of income and education, but there were no significant differences on *Perceived Health Status* or the HISB measures *Frequency of Seeking*, *Social Relationships*, and *Media-Based*

Table 1. Mean Differences between Whites and Nonwhites.

	White	Nonwhite	T-Test Significance
Perceived health status	3.08	2.85	
Income	5.59	3.90	**
Education	5.64	4.88	*
Age	66.55	58.30	**
Female	0.54	0.60	
Frequency of seeking	2.38	2.63	
Social relationships	1.38	1.22	
Media-based resources	1.64	1.46	

Notes: ***$p<.1$, *$p<.05$, **$p<.01$.

Table 2. Relationship between Income and Perceived Health Status.

	Perceived Health Status
Income	
<$35,000	2.51
$35,000–$75,000	3.01
Above $75,000	3.54
ANOVA	$p < .001$
Education	
HS or less	2.62
Vocational or some college	3.03
College graduate	3.13
Postgraduate degree	3.23
ANOVA	$p = .035$

Resources. In fact, on the *Frequency of Seeking* measure, nonwhites had a higher mean ($p = .098$). Thus, H1 and H2 are not supported, as we cannot conclude that racial-ethnic minorities have a lower perceived health status, or that they have lower levels of health information seeking behaviors.

To test the relationship between socioeconomic status and *Perceived Health Status* (H3), our income and education measures were first collapsed into fewer categories. Table 2 shows mean differences across these categories.

Both *Income* and *Education* are significantly related to *Perceived Health Status*. Supporting H3, those with higher income levels and higher education levels score higher, on average, on *Perceived Health Status*. The relationship appears to be stronger for *Income*, with those earning over $75,000 per year scoring, on average, nearly one point higher on *Perceived Health Status* than those earning less than $35,000 per year.

Table 3 shows the results of ANOVAs used to test H4 – the relationship between socioeconomic status and HISB measures. Income is not statistically significantly associated with either frequency of seeking or with the number of sources for social relationships. There is a slightly significant relationship with media-based resources ($p < .05$), although the relationship is not linear. The only other significant relationship is between *Education* and *Frequency of Seeking*, due to the difference between the "High School or Less" group and the "Postgraduate Degree" group. Arguably, this partially supports H4, but looking at the means for the other groups, we see again that the relationship is not linear. We conclude that H4 is not supported.

H5 (Controlling for HISB will lessen race effects on perceived health status) and H6 (Controlling for HISB will lessen socioeconomic status

Table 3. Relationship between Socioeconomic Status and HISB Quantity Measures.

	Frequency of Seeking	Number of Social Relationship Resources	Number of Media-Based Resources
Income			
< $35,000	2.41	1.47	1.63
$35,000 to $75,000	2.44	1.35	1.34
> $75,000	2.42	1.26	1.84
ANOVA	$p = .987$	$p = .479$	$p = .027$
Education			
HS or less	2.11	1.08	1.44
Vocational or some college	2.39	1.53	1.70
College graduate	2.29	1.15	1.50
Postgraduate degree	2.63	1.40	1.71
ANOVA	$p = .005$	$p = .097$	$p = .517$

Table 4. Regression Analysis Predicting Perceived Health Status and HISB Quantity.

Race (White)	Model 1	Model 2	Model 3	Model 4	Model 5	Model 6	Model 7
Age	0.246	0.134			−0.1	−0.142	−0.175
Female	−0.003	−0.003			0.002	0.002	0.002
Income	−0.295**	−0.279***			−0.116	−0.104	−0.093
Education			0.178***	0.178***	0.169***	0.173***	0.175***
Frequency			0.003	−0.038	0.015	−0.033	−0.033
Social relationships		0.032		0.016		0.030	0.257*
Media-based sources		−0.092		−0.032		−0.025	−0.022
Frequency* media		0.027		0.004		−0.006	−0.389**
R^2							.158**
	0.024	0.027	0.151	0.138	0.148	0.133	0.163

Notes: *$p<.1$, **$p<.05$, ***$p<.001$.

effects on perceived health status) were tested using multiple regression analysis. Results are shown in Table 4.

Models 1 and 2 test H5. Both are weak models, explaining less than 3% of the variance of perceived health status. Although the effect of race decreases once we control for HISB, race is not significant in either model. Thus, the data fails to support H5.

Models 3 and 4 test H6. The effect of *Education* disappears when we control for *Income*. While these variables are highly correlated ($R = .542$), multicollinearity does not appear to be a problem. The effect of *Income* stays constant when HISB measures are added in Model 4; thus the data does not support H6. Because of some missing data on the *Frequency* variable, an interesting quirk in this analysis is that the model – R^2 value decreases when this variable is added.

Models 5 and 6 include all demographic variables in the same model, and provide further confirmation that the data does not support H5 and H6. The effect of *Income* and *Race* stay consistent when HISB measures are added. Indeed, the only variable in Model 6 that has any effect on *Perceived Health Status* is *Income*. Overall these models are not strong, predicting only about 15% of the variance in *Perceived Health Status*.

To further explore the relationship between HISB and *Perceived Health Status*, an interaction term between *Frequency of Seeking* and *Media Based Relationships* was included in Model 7. Although income remains the most significant predictor, the interaction term and *Frequency* were also significant as well as *Media Based Resources*, indicating that the relationship between *Number of Media Based Resources* and *Perceived Health Status* is dependent on the *Frequency of Seeking*. Table 5 shows predicted scores

Table 5. Interaction between Frequency of Seeking, Number of Media Resources, and Perceived Health Status.

Frequency of Seeking	Number of Media Resources	Predicted Perceived Health Status
Rarely	1	3.72
Rarely	3	3.26
Rarely	5	2.79
Rarely	7	2.33
Sometimes	1	4.13
Sometimes	3	3.99
Sometimes	5	3.84
Sometimes	7	3.69
Often	1	4.55
Often	3	4.72
Often	5	4.89
Often	7	5.06
All the time	1	4.96
All the time	3	5.45
All the time	5	5.93
All the time	7	6.42

(generated from the regression equation in Model 7) for *Perceived Health Status* at different levels of *Number of Media Based Resources* and *Frequency of Seeking*. For these predicted values, *Age, Income, Education,* and *Social Relationships* are held constant at their median values, and race and gender are held constant at the majority values of white and female.

Interestingly, for those who seek information "Rarely," the number of media-based resources used has a negative effect on perceived health status. For those who seek information "All the Time" the number of media-based resources has a positive effect on perceived health status.

Discussion

We investigated the role of health information seeking behaviors as a means to measure social capital in terms of amount of media-based and social resources and frequency in usage of resources for health information among patients with chronic conditions. Among the growing population of patients with chronic conditions the ability to effectively access social relationships is of critical importance. Social capital is necessary to cope with the everyday difficulty of managing a condition that brings many physical and emotional adjustments. It has been shown that a lack of knowledge and an insufficient social support network will function as barriers to higher quality of life perceptions among patients with chronic conditions (Bayliss, Steiner, Fernald, Crane, & Main, 2003; Jerant, Friederichs-Fitzwater, & Moore, 2005). It is thus imperative for these individuals to be socially well integrated to access valuable information concerning health issues.

Our original study design was to assess whether participating in health information seeking behaviors ameliorates any significant relationships between race and income and self-perceived health status. That is, does access to more sources and frequent usage of these sources for health information translate into a better perception of health status, and does this differ by race and class? Contrary to the literature on racial health disparities but consistent with the literature on socioeconomic health disparities, we did not find a significant relationship between racial ethnic minorities and self-perceived health status (H1), but we did find a strong relationship between socioeconomic status and self-perceived health status (H2) for patients with chronic conditions. Our study suggests that income is a better predictor for self-rated health status than race. Although we are unable to conclude that race does not matter because of the small minority population within our sample, it is certain that socioeconomic status is a strong predictor for self-rated health status among patients with chronic conditions. The Gradient of Health and Wealth explains the strong association between income and longevity. Deaton (2002) reported that in the United States, as income rises mortality decreases in equal proportions throughout the income distribution and such relationships persist among other demographics. This conclusion is elaborated by Smith (1999), who found income to be highly correlated with better health status for numerous reasons, including higher income individuals' access to greater resources devoted to health and general better knowledge about health. As far as whether SES is more important than race, however, there is still much debate in this area (see Hayward, Miles, Crimmins, & Yang, 2000).

Our results suggest that the *quantity* of health information that a person seeks via their social networks does not affect self-perceived health status. There were no race or income differences in the degree of health information seeking behaviors in which participants reported engaging (H3 and H4). It is possible, however, that the *quality* of health information seeking behaviors could reveal significant relationships, which future research could investigate. Kawachi, Kennedy, Lochner, and Prothrow-Stith (1991) found that income is associated with degree of social trust. They concluded that quantity and quality of social networks matter. Having access to an extensive social network does not automatically ensure that individuals will make effective use of their social networks to access information. It is necessary to consider the efficacy of the social capital, not simply the expanse of the social network. For example, frequent contact with more effective sources may have a greater influence on the perceived health status of higher SES individuals than a more expansive social network with lower-quality social capital of a person with low SES. Quality may matter as much as, if not more than, quantity when it comes to social capital. This possibility can be justified in our research by the fact that frequency and amount of HISB are interaction variables, as noted in Table 5.

Future research could elaborate on how social capital can vary by type more than we did in this study. Lin (2001), in particular, speaks about how certain social networks have greater weight and therefore are more likely to affect action or behavior changes upon individuals. For example, individuals located in a particular strategic location or position will have valuable social credentials and therefore be able to exercise a greater degree of power. The health information provided by these social networks would have more impact on a patient's decision making. Other scholars (Granovetter, 1973; Wellman & Wortley, 1990) explore the difference between formal and informal social networks, noting the former as more important for achieving social capital, and less accessible for impoverished people. Although research has demonstrated extensively that the number of social networks individuals are part of is important to achieve better health status (Hendryx et al., 2002), our study supports the claim that other researchers have made that we need to further investigate whether certain social networks are better at influencing patients' health more effectively (Lynch, Due, Muntaner, & Smith, 2000; McKenzie, Whitley, & Weich, 2002).

To further understand the relationship between Health Information Seeking Behaviors and Perceived Health Status, we combine the *Number of Media-Based Resources* and *Frequency of Seeking* of health information seeking behaviors. We found that self-perceived health status decreases as the number of media based resources used for health information increases for users who indicated "Rarely" engaging in HISB. However, self-perceived health increases as the number of media-based resources used for health information increases for responders who indicated engaging in HISB "All the time." Quantity of health information seeking behaviors cannot be assumed to be greater in term of higher number of media-based resources *or* frequency of seeking, but instead can be better captured in the interaction *between* these variables. An individual who rarely seeks health information but uses many sources has a more negative perception of their health status than an individual who frequently seeks health information and uses multiple sources. One possible explanation is that some populations have better health information seeking abilities than others such as knowing which key word to insert into the search engine, or being able to frame questions to their health provider in a manner to ensure they receive the specific health information they seek. Of course, one limitation is that media-based information seeking may not capture the ability of patients to utilize social networks, which is the central theoretical focus of our analysis.

Another possible explanation for our results may be that survey respondents receive care from a Northwest clinic that has implemented a model to better meet the needs of older populations and those dealing with chronic conditions. The care model in this clinic uses people and technology to improve care coordination and the quality of care delivered in office based practices. This model specifically implements care managers into practices to facilitate care, motivate behavioral changes, and teach self-management for noncompliant or struggling patients. Under this model, the care team provides the support to help patients make decisions and to take appropriate action(s). This could consist either of providing basic education on their conditions, providing information concerning their condition or treatment, or providing resources to aid patients' ability to manage their conditions. Care managers specifically play an integral role in promoting positive self-management practices among patients.

Although we do not know which patients in our sample currently work with a care manager, all patients do receive care from the clinic where many of the health providers work with care managers. It is possible that health information seeking behavior practices are emphasized and encouraged at this facility with greater frequency than in the overall population. Our study therefore suggests further investigation on the impact of the care models represented here on patients' degree of health information seeking behaviors. Patient participation in such models would exemplify highly effective social capital even if the patient's social network was limited. We hypothesize that minority populations may be receptive to care models that diminish the relationship between racial ethnic minority and self-rated health status. However, more extensive research is needed before this claim can be definitively proven.

ACKNOWLEDGMENTS

The authors would like to thank David Dorr for important help with the facilitation of the survey that formed the basis for this analysis, and to the National Library of Medicine for funding.

REFERENCES

Albegunde, D. O., Mathers, C. D., Adam, T., Oregon, M., & Strong, K. (2007). The burden and costs of chronic diseases in low-income and middle-income countries. *The Lancet*, *370*, 1929–1938.

Alegria, M., Cao, Z., McGuire, T. G., Ojeda, V. D., Scribney, B., Woo, M., & Takeuchi, D. (2006). Health insurance coverage for vulnerable populations: Contrasting Asian Americans and Latinos in the United States. *NIH Public Access*, *43*(3), 231–254.

Bayliss, E. A., Steiner, J. F., Fernald, D. H., Crane, L. A., & Main, D. S. (2003). Descriptions of barriers to self-care by persons with comorbid chronic diseases. *Annals of Family Medicine*, *1*, 15–21.

Beyond 50.09: Chronic Care: A Call to Action for Health Reform. (2009). Washington, DC: AARP Public Policy Institute.

Billings, J., Seitel, L., Lukomnik, J., Carey, T. S., Blank, A. E., & Newman, L. (1993). Impact of socioeconomic status on hospital use in New York City. *Health Affairs*, *12*(1), 162–173.

Bourdieu, P. (1986). The forms of capital. In: J. G. Richardson (Ed.), *Handbook for the theory and research for the sociology of education* (pp. 241–258). New York: Greenwood Press.

Braveman, P. (2006). Health disparities and health equity: Concepts and measurement. *Annual Review Public Health, 27,* 167–194.

Center for Disease Control and Prevention. (2007). Chronic disease overview: Costs of chronic disease. Available at http://www.cdc.gov/inccdphp/overview.htm. Accessed on January 29, 2010.

Coleman, J. (1989). Social capital in the creation of human capital. *American Journal of Sociology, 94,* 95–120.

Collins, K. S., Hall, A., & Neuhaus, C. (1999). U.S. minority health: A chartbook. *The Commonwealth Fund,* 1–160.

Courtright, C. (2005). Health information-seeking among Latino newcomers: An exploratory study. *Information Research, 10*(2), 224.

Dalstra, J. A., Kunst, A. E., Borrell, C., Breeze, E., Cambios Costa, G., Geurts, J. M., Lahemla, E., Van, O. H., Rasmussen, N. K., Regidor, E., Spadea, T., & Mackenbach, J. P. (2005). Socioeconomic differences in the prevalence of common chronic diseases: An overview of eight European countries. *International Journal of Epidemiology, 34*(2), 316–326.

Deaton, A. (2002). Policy implications of the gradient of health and wealth. *Health Affairs, 21*(2), 13–30.

De Monaco, H. J., & Hippel, E. Von. (2007). Reducing medical costs and improving quality via self-management tools. *PLoS Medicine, 4*(4), 609–611.

Druss, B. G., Marcus, S. C., Olfson, M., Tanielian, T., Elinson, L., & Pincus, H. A. (2001). Comparing the national economic burden of five chronic conditions. *Health Affairs, 20*(6), 233–241.

Faircloth, C. A., Boylstein, C., Rittman, M., Young, M. E., & Gubrium, J. (2004). Sudden illness and biographical flow in narratives of stroke recovery. *Sociology of Health and Illness, 26*(2), 242–261.

Fox, S. (2009). The social life of health information. *Pew Internet and American Life Project,* 1–72.

Glover, J. D., Hetzel, D. M. S., & Tennant, S. K. (2004). The socioeconomic gradient and chronic illness and associated risk factors in Australia. *Australia and New Zealand Health Policy, 1*(8), 1–8.

Goldner, M. (2004). Health-related information on the internet: The impact of race, class, and gender. Paper presented at the Annual Meeting of the American Sociological Association, San Francisco, CA.

Granovetter, M. (1973). The strength of weak ties. *American Journal of Sociology, 78,* 1360–1380.

Hanchate, A., Kronman, A. C., Young-Xu, Y., Ash, A. S., & Emanuel, E. (2009). Racial and ethnic differences in end of life costs: Why do minorities cost more than whites? *Archives of Internal Medicine, 9*(169), 493–501.

Hayward, M. D., Miles, T. P., Crimmins, E. M., & Yang, Y. (2000). The significance of socioeconomic status in explaining the racial gap in chronic conditions. *American Sociological Review, 65*(6), 910–930.

Hendryx, M. X., Ahern, M. M., Lovrich, N. P., & McCurdy, A. H. (2002). Access to health care and community social capital. *Health Services Research, 37,* 87–103.

Hesse, B. W., Nelson, D. E., Kreps, G. L., Croyle, R. T., Arora, N. L., Rimer, B. K., & Viswanath, K. (2005). Trust and source of health information: The impact of the internet

and its implications for health care providers: findings from the first health information national trends survey. *Archives of Internal Medicine, 165,* 2618–2624.
Hoffman, C., Rice, D., & Sung, H. Y. (1996). Persons with chronic conditions. *Journal of American Medical Association, 276*(18), 1473–1479.
Hogue, C. J. R., Hargraves, M. A., & Collins, K. S. (2000). Minority health in America: Findings and policy implications from the commonwealth fund minority health survey. *New England Journal of Medicine, 343*(9), 669.
House, J. S., Landis, K. R., & Umberson, D. (1988). Social relationships and health. *American Association for the Advancement of Science, 241*(4865), 540–545.
Issacs, S. L., & Schroeder, S. A. (2004). Class – The ignored determinant of the nation's health. *New England Journal of Medicine, 351*(11), 1137–1142.
Jerant, A. F., Friederichs-Fitzwater, M. M., & Moore, M. (2005). Patients' perceived barriers to active self-management of chronic conditions. *Patient Education and Counseling, 57,* 300–307.
Kawachi, I., & Berkman, L. F. (2000). *Social epidemiology.* New York: Oxford University Press.
Kawachi, I., Daniels, N., & Robinson, D. E. (2005). Health disparities by race and class: Why both matter. *Health Affairs, 24*(2), 343–352.
Kawachi, I., Kennedy, B. P., & Glass, R. (1999). Social capital and self-related health: A contextual analysis. *American Journal of Public Health, 89*(8), 1187–1193.
Kawachi, I., Kennedy, B. P., Lochner, K., & Prothrow-Stith, D. (1991). Social capital, income inequality, and mortality. *American Journal of Public Health, 87*(9), 1491–1498.
Kington, R. S., & Smith, J. P. (1997). Socioeconomic status and racial and ethnic differences in functional status associated with chronic diseases. *American Journal of Public Health, 87*(5), 805–810.
Laditka, J. N., & Laditka, S. B. (2006). Race, ethnicity and hospitalization for six chronic ambulatory care sensitive conditions in the USA. *Ethnicity & Health, 11*(3), 247–263.
Lewis, D., Chang, B. L., & Friedman, C. P. (2005). Consumer health informatics: Informing consumers and improving health care. In: D. Lewis, G. Eysenbach & R. Kukafka (Eds), *Health informatics* (pp. 1–7). New York: Springer Press.
Lin, N. (2001). *Social capital. A theory of social structure and action.* Cambridge: Cambridge University Press.
Lynch, J., Due, P., Muntaner, C., & Smith, G. (2000). Social capital-is it a good investment strategy for public health? *Journal of Epidemiology and Community Health, 54*(6), 404–408.
Mahon, M., & Fox, B. (2002). Minority Americans lag behind whites on nearly every measure of health care quality: Many have communication and financial barriers to care, and lack trust in doctors. *The Commonwealth Fund.*
McCarthy, B., & Hagan, J. (2001). When crime pays: Capital, competence, and criminal success. *Social Forces, 79,* 1035–1060.
McDounough, P., Duncan, G. J., Williams, D., & House, J. (1997). Income dynamics and adult mortality in the United States, 1972 though 1989. *American Journal of Public Health, 87,* 1476–1483.
McKenzie, K., Whitley, R., & Weich, S. (2002). Social capital and mental health. *British Journal of Psychiatry, 181,* 280–283.
MedicineNet.com. (2010). Definition of chronic disease. Available at http://www.medterms.com/script/main/art.asp?articlekey=33490. Retrieved on August 13, 2010.

Metoyer-Duran, C. A. (1993). Information gatekeepers. In: M. E. Williams (Ed.), *Annual review of information science and technology* (Vol. 28, pp. 111–150). Medford, NJ: Learned Information.

Mishel, M. H. (1988). Uncertainty in illness. *Image Journal of Nursing Scholarship*, *20*, 225–232.

Mishel, M. H. (1990). Reconceptulization of the uncertainty in illness theory. *Image Journal of Nursing Scholarship*, *22*, 256–262.

Murthy, V. (2007). Income distribution and health status: econometric evidence from OECD countries. *American Journal of Applied Sciences*, *4*(4), 192–196.

Newacheck, P. W., Butlet, L. H., Harper, A. D., Dyan, L., & Franks, P. E. (1980). Income and illness. *Original Articles*, *18*(12), 1165–1176.

Office of Minority Health and Health Disparities. (2008). *American Indian & Alaska Native (AI/AN) populations* (Available at http://www.cdc.gov/omhd/Populations/AIAN/AIAN.htm#Ten. Retrieved on January 27, 2010.). Office of Minority Health and Health Disparities.

Oliver, M. N. (2008). Racial health inequalities in the USA: The role of social class. *Public Health*, *122*(12), 1440–1442.

Pappas, G., Hadden, W. C., Kozak, L. J., & Fisher, G. F. (1997). Potentially avoidable hospitalizations: Inequalities in rates between US socioeconomic groups. *American Journal of Public Health*, *87*(5), 811–816.

Perneger, T. V., Brancatie, F. L., Wheltonn, P. K., & Klag, M. (1994). End-state renal disease attributable to diabetes mellitus. *Annals of Internal Medicine*, *121*, 912–918.

Pickett, K. E., Kelly, S., Brunner, E., Lobstein, T., & Wilkinson, R. G. (2005). Wider income gaps, wider waistbands? An ecological study of obesity and income inequality. *Journal of Epidemiology and Community Health*, *59*, 670–674.

Portes, A. (1998). Social capital: Its origins and applications in modern sociology. *Annual Review of Sociology*, *24*, 1–24.

Putnam, R. (1995). Bowling alone: America's declining social capital. *Journal of Democracy*, *6*, 65–78.

Putnam, R. (2000). *Bowling alone: The collapse and revival of American community*. New York: Simon and Schuster.

Schneider, E. L., & Guralnik, J. M. (1990). The aging of America. *Journal of the American Medical Association*, *263*(17), 2335–2340.

Schwartz, K., Roe, T., Northrup, J., Meza, J., Seifeldin, R., & Neale, A. V. (2006). Family medicine patients' use of the internet for health information: A metronetstudy. *Journal of the American Board of Family Medicine*, *19*, 39–45.

Smith, J. P. (1999). Healthy bodies and the thick wallets: The dual relation between health and economic status. *Journal of Economic Perspectives*, *13*(2), 145–166.

Tu, H. T., & Cohen, G. R. (2008). *Striking jump in consumers seeking health care information*. Tracking Report no. 20. Center for Studying Health System Change, Washington, DC.

Wagner, E. H., Austin, B. T., David, C., Hidmarsh, M., Schaefer, J., & Bonomi, A. (2001). Improving chronic illness care: Translating evidence into action. *Health Affairs*, *20*(6), 1–7.

Wellman, B., & Wortley, S. (1990). Different strokes from different folks: Community ties and social support. *American Journal of Sociology*, *96*(3), 558–588.

Wilson, T. D. (2000). Human information behavior. *Informing Science*, *3*(2), 49–56.

Wilkinson, R. G., & Pickett, K. E. (2005). Income inequality and population health: A review and explanation of the evidence. *Social Science & Medicine, 62*(7), 1768–1784.

Wolff, J. L., Starfield, B., & Andersen, G. (2002). Prevalence, expenditures, and complications of multiple chronic conditions in the elderly. *Archives of Internal Medicine, 162,* 2269–2276.

Wu, S-Yi., & Green, A. (2000). *Projection of chronic illness prevalence and cost inflation.* Santa Monica, CA: RAND Corporation.

Ybarra, M. L., & Suman, M. (2006). Help seeking behaviors and the Internet: A national survey. *Journal of Medical Informatics, 75,* 29–41.

RACIAL DISPARITIES IN STILLBIRTHS

Vicki Dryfhout

ABSTRACT

Blacks are more likely than white, in the United States, to experience a stillbirth. In this study, I use a structural perspective of race to create a heuristic model that combines medical and social epidemiological explanations to understand the racial disparity in stillbirths. Using data from the National Maternal and Infant Health Survey 1988 (NMIHS), I examine whether racial disparities in stillbirths can be explained by medical and social epidemiological variables. My findings show that medical and social epidemiological explanations do little to reduce the racial disparity. However, many medical model variables were important predictors of stillbirths including multiple gestations, being overweight, obesity, vaginal bleeding, advanced maternal age, and parity.

INTRODUCTION

Scholars have been concerned with the substantial gap in rates of morbidity and mortality between racial groups (Geronimus, 1992; Hummer et al., 1999; Williams & Collins, 2001). Vast inequalities exist in pregnancy outcomes; however, very little research has been conducted investigating the social factors that may account for these differences (Gennaro, 2005). Although a significant amount of research has been conducted on the relationship between social processes and racial inequalities in infant mortality, similar research on racial inequalities in rates of stillbirths is lacking (Hummer et al., 1999; Forbes, Frisbie, Hummer, Pullum, & Echevarria, 2000; Frisbie, Song, Powers, & Street, 2004). A stillbirth has been defined as a fetal loss in pregnancy beyond 20 weeks of gestation (World Health Organization, 1995). This gap in the research is significant, because stillbirths account for the largest share of perinatal losses (Fretts, 2005).

Despite the fact that stillbirths do not have extensive economic costs (compared to, say, preterm births with ongoing medical complications), there are significant emotional costs to parents as well as clinicians (Hughes, Turton & Evans, 1999; Gold, Kuznia, & Hayward, 2008). Parents may suffer from a number of psychological issues including posttraumatic stress disorder and depression and anxiety in future pregnancies (Hughes et al., 1999). A survey of obstetricians found the majority feel stillbirths take a large emotional toll on them personally and they blame themselves or feel guilty (Gold, Kuznia, & Hayward, 2008).

Stillbirth rates tend to be highest for blacks and lowest for whites, whereas Hispanics, Asians, and American Indian/Alaska Natives share rates similar to whites (Martin et al., 2006; MacDorman, Munson & Kirmeyer, 2007). Although the overall stillbirth rate has decreased since 1990, stillbirth rates are still 2.3 times higher for black women versus white women. Specifically, the rate of stillbirths was 4.98 per 1,000 live births plus fetal deaths for white women, but 11.25 per 1,000 live births plus fetal deaths for black women in 2004 (MacDorman et al., 2007). Two major bodies of literature, referred to here as "medical" and "social epidemiological," have addressed the issue of racial disparities in pregnancy outcomes; however, neither has thoroughly explored the multiple mechanisms for the disparity. Within the medical literature, there is disagreement as to whether racial disparities in birth outcomes are simply genetic or whether other factors such as social class, access to treatment, residential segregation, lifestyle behaviors, social networks, or stress explain the racial disparity in stillbirths. Moreover, perinatal researchers often control for race despite the fact that little is known about how race might be linked to pregnancy outcomes.

The social epidemiological model is not an alternative to, but rather an expansion of the medical model. Whereas the medical model focuses solely on medical risks, behavioral risks, and genetics, the social epidemiological model also considers social factors including socioeconomic resources, residential segregation, and healthcare access, quality, and quantity.

Essentially, the social epidemiological model hypothesizes where inequalities in medical and behavioral risks and ultimately pregnancy outcomes originate. By elaborating upon the medical model, the social epidemiological approach, described here, seeks to address the inequities that underlie the medical risks considered in the medical model. Few social epidemiological studies have empirically examined racial disparities in stillbirth, despite the abundance of research on infant mortality (Hummer, 1993; Frisbie, 1994; Frisbie, Forbes, & Pullum, 1996; Hummer et al., 1999; Forbes et al., 2000; Hummer, Powers, Pullum, Gossman, & Frisbie, 2007). A consensus does not exist regarding explanations for racial disparities in pregnancy outcomes within either body of literature. Previous studies have not synthesized these explanations or explored the extent to which they may explain disparities in pregnancy outcomes and, instead, suggest that multiple factors contribute to inequities in stillbirth.

In this chapter, I argue that understanding the ways in which social and economic resources are allocated across racial groups is vital for understanding racial inequality in stillbirth. Although there is some evidence in the medical literature regarding genetic abnormalities and stillbirths, I argue that a much more persuasive explanation for racial inequality in rates of stillbirths lies in social processes that have historically disadvantaged black women relative to their white counterparts.

The meaning of race has changed over time because race is not a biological but rather a socially constructed concept (Bonilla-Silva, 2006). Despite the socially constructed nature of the race concept, it has real effects on the lives of individuals who are defined as black or white because a racialized social system developed conterminously with the concept of race. In this social system, race is used as a stratifying mechanism, systematically awarding privileges and access to goods and resources to those who were white or nonwhite (Bonilla-Silva, 2006). Racial structure is defined as the "totality of social relations and practices that reinforce white privilege (Bonilla-Silva, 2006, p. 9)." For example, some argue that racism resulted in residential segregation and is a principal cause of racial differences in socioeconomic status, which has resulted in racial disparities in health (Williams & Collins, 2001). Understanding the racial structure, how privilege is conferred and maintained among whites versus nonwhites, provides a starting point for examining racial inequalities in health, specifically, racial disparities in stillbirths.

Here, I suggest that racial disparities in birth outcomes are due to several distal and proximate factors. Because there are inequalities in medical risk factors such as preeclampsia, obesity, and diabetes, and therefore, medical risks may be a proximate factor in explaining disparities in stillbirths (Samadi et al., 1996; Rosenberg, Garbers, Lipkind, & Chiasson, 2005). Instead of suggesting several separate explanations for the disparities in stillbirths, I suggest that the medical and social epidemiological explanations work together as a process to explain disparities in medical risks and ultimately stillbirths.

In this chapter, I use a nationally representative sample of live births, fetal deaths, and infant deaths to explore explanations for the racial gap in stillbirths. My goal is to use a sociologically informed comprehensive heuristic model to explain how race is related to stillbirths and test a more comprehensive model of the social antecedents of behavioral and medical risks factors, more fully accounting for racial gaps in stillbirths In the past, researchers have controlled for some factors but not others (e.g., medical risks but not behavioral risk factors, stress but not social and economic risk factors). I use the heuristic model to guide theses analyses and empirically test several of these explanations.

PERSPECTIVES ON INEQUALITY IN STILLBIRTH

Medical Model

Medical Risks
Although researchers do not completely understand the etiology of stillbirths, several medical conditions have been identified as risk factors for a stillbirth, including birth defects, placental and umbilical cord complications, obesity, maternal diabetes, maternal hypertension, infections, postdate pregnancy and multiple gestations, parity, and advanced maternal age (Fretts, 2005; Silver et al., 2007). Obesity and preeclampsia are more common among black women than white women although rates of gestational diabetes are similar (Brown, Chireau, Jallah, & Howard, 2007; Rosenberg, Garbers, Chavkin, & Chiasson, 2003). Women in their first pregnancy are at higher risk for stillbirths than women who had been pregnant before (Raymond, Cnattingius, & Kiely, 2005). Advanced maternal age (≥ 35 years of age) is an important predictor of stillbirths (Fretts, 2005).

Behavioral Risks
Nutrition, prenatal care, tobacco use, alcohol use, and drug use are lifestyle factors that have also been identified to cause stillbirths (Silver et al., 2007). Blacks are less likely than whites to take multivitamin supplements,

67% and 84%, respectively (Yu, Keppel, Singh, & Kessel, 1996). Black and white women are equally likely to smoke during pregnancy (Andreski & Breslau, 1995; Perreira & Cortes, 2006). As education level increases, the probability of smoking decreases for blacks and whites, but the effect is stronger among whites (Andreski & Breslau, 1995). A study investigating barriers to physical activity found neighborhoods with largely black populations and low-socioeconomic status had fewer outdoor public physical activity settings and fewer pay-for-use facilities (Powell, Slater, Chaloupka, & Harper, 2006). Blacks may be less likely than whites to engage in protective behaviors such as taking multivitamins and vigorous leisure activity, which could adversely affect birth outcomes.

Stress
Stress can be classified as acute, related to specific life events, or chronic, an ongoing state. Very little attention has been paid to the role of stress and stillbirth, but a significant body of research has discussed the function of stress in preterm births (Dole et al., 2004; Lu & Chen, 2004; Hogue & Bremner, 2005). There is a significant difference in experiencing stressful life events before and during pregnancy, but they contribute only slightly to the racial disparity in preterm birth (Lu & Chen, 2004). One study found that black women reported a greater number of negative life events and higher levels of depression than white women and were less likely to live with a partner than white women; despite this, they were not at increased risk of preterm birth (Dole et al., 2004). They also found that the association between anxiety and pregnancy outcome weakened after controlling for medical complications, suggesting that stress may act through medical complications. Other researchers argue that chronic stress from racism and discrimination is a prominent part of the lives of black women, which may cause poor pregnancy outcomes (Collins, David, Handler, Wall, & Andes, 2004). Findings from other studies suggest that chronic stress due to discrimination, instead of acute stress, may lead to racial disparities in adverse pregnancy outcomes.

Genetics
Researchers have found that genetic abnormalities cause a proportion of stillbirths. Karyotypic abnormalities including monosomy X, trisomy 21, trisomy 18, and trisomy 14 cause approximately 6–12% of stillbirths. (Wapner & Lewis, 2002; Christiaens, Vissers, Poddighe, & de Pater, 2000). Although it is important to acknowledge the contribution of genetic factors to stillbirth outcomes, a shortcoming of a broader genetic explanation is

that it implies a genetic underpinning of the race concept. Data used in this investigation are insufficient to test genetic factors, and, to my knowledge, no genetic link between stillbirth and race has been demonstrated in the literature.

Social Epidemiological Model

Socioeconomic Resources
Researchers have shown the impact social and economic resources play in rates of mortality and morbidity (Singh & Yu, 1996; Singh & Kogan, 2007; Cockerham, 2005; Link & Phelan, 1995; Phelan, Link, Diez-Roux, Karachi, & Levin, 2004). Resources can be classified into four types including economic capital, human capital, cultural capital, and social capital. Economic capital refers to income or health insurance, which can be used to purchase healthcare services. Social class gradients are evident across numerous diseases. Health insurance and lack of health insurance are associated with better and worse health, respectively. Singh and Kogan (2007) found higher rates of neonatal, postneonatal, and infant mortality among the lowest socioeconomic status groups.

A second form of capital is human capital and refers to an individual's skills or education level and is associated with quality of health. One study found college graduates reported better health than people without a high school degree, although the largest health disparities were reported among the elderly (Goesling, 2007). Cultural capital is a third form of capital, which can be defined as knowledge, relationships, and behaviors that an individual can enact to facilitate a benefit in a social situation. Malat (2006) suggests racial disparities in health care may be a result of differences in cultural capital. Cultural capital may play an important part in the health care and health behaviors individuals engage in. Blacks or low-income individuals may not have the social networks or behaviors to facilitate advantage in the healthcare system, thereby potentially resulting in adverse health outcomes.

Finally, social capital refers to social networks and supports that may also explain the disparity in adverse birth outcomes. Race and social class may affect kin, social ties, and segregation, which may play into the availability of healthcare information patients have access to. Having personal ties to families, neighborhoods, friendship, work groups, and healthcare professionals could result in differing levels of health (Malat, 2006). Researchers do not understand why this association between health and social ties exists, but, they propose that being married may contain a greater amount of social support and less stress. Wilson (1996) argues that poor economic conditions, largely due to residential segregation, have weakened support for husband–wife families and increased out-of-wedlock births. Blacks are less likely to marry than whites putting them at higher risk of a stillbirth. Key predictors of health outcomes include social and economic resources such as economic, human, cultural, and social capital, which are important predictors of health outcomes. Overall, blacks may more likely to suffer poor birth outcomes because they are less likely than whites to have access to these different forms of capital, which can be used to obtain advantages in the healthcare system.

Health Care
Health care is an important factor of the racial disparity in stillbirths and is composed of three components that include access to health care, quality of health care, and physician bias. Access to medical treatment includes both monetary and physical access. Monetary access includes having insurance and quality of insurance, whereas physical access refers to the place of patient's residence in relation to healthcare facilities. Blacks are less likely than whites to receive prenatal care, and lack of care is associated with an increased risk of adverse pregnancy outcomes (Greenberg, 1982). Infections, maternal disease, umbilical cord accidents, and intrauterine growth restriction, which are causes of stillbirths, could potentially be prevented or monitored with regular prenatal care (Echevarria & Frisbie, 2001). However, researchers have found that after controlling for adequate prenatal care, black women were still more likely than white women to be at risk for a stillbirth (Vintzileos, Ananth, Smulian, Scorza, & Knuppel, 2002). Residential segregation can effect income and ability to purchase goods and services that support good health and may explain, in part, black and white differences in prenatal care and health outcomes (Williams & Collins, 2001).

Inequalities in access to health care can also create variation in quality of health care. Studies have shown that black patients tend to be treated by physicians who have lower quality clinical training and these physicians have a more difficult time accessing high-quality subspecialists, diagnostic imaging and nonemergency admission to the hospital (Bach, Pham, Schrag, Tate, & Hargraves, 2004). Research suggests that, apart from access to and quality of health care, the racial disparity in health can be partially explained by physician bias where healthcare providers recommend different courses of treatment to blacks and whites (Epstein et al., 2000; Peterson, Wright, Daley, & Thibault, 1994; Schulman et al., 1999; Van Ryn, Burgess, Malat, & Griffin, 2006). For example, studies have found blacks with end-stage renal disease were less likely than whites to be told about transplantation, referred for renal transplantation, referred for cardiac catheterization, or to have received a recommendation for coronary artery bypass graft surgery (Epstein et al., 2000; Peterson et al., 1994; Van et al., 2006). With respect to stillbirths, physician bias may influence the counseling or treatment options provided by physicians to black and white patients.

Residential Segregation
Neighborhood context and residential segregation have a strong impact on health and racial disparities in health (Williams & Collins, 2001; Collins & Williams, 1999; Grady, 2006; Massey, Condran, & Denton, 1987; Morenoff, 2003; Morenoff et al., 2007; Robert, 1998; Robert, 1999; Robert & Reither, 2004; Weden, Carpiano, & Robert, 2008). Health may be negatively affected by social and physical risks in residential environments created by residential segregation (Williams & Collins, 2001). Educational and employment opportunities, housing quality, health behaviors, and access to and quality of health care may be limited by residential segregation. Limited employment opportunities may result in unemployment or lower levels of income. Residential segregation and exposure to adverse neighborhood conditions are related to racial disparities in birth outcomes, specifically, preterm birth, low birthweight, and infant mortality (Culhane & Elo, 2005).

Comprehensive Heuristic Model

Despite the importance of the variables discussed in the literature earlier, there is little understanding of how they may operate together. In this study, I use a structural interpretation of race to examine how privilege is conferred and maintained among whites versus blacks. This perspective provides a starting point for understanding how medical and social epidemiological variables act together and, ultimately, racial disparities in pregnancy outcomes such as stillbirths. On the basis of this literature, I have developed a heuristic model to explain racial disparities in pregnancy outcomes shown in Fig. 1. In Fig. 1, shaded boxes indicate a primary causal relationship indicated by the medical model, whereas the nonshaded boxes indicate the relationship indicated by the social epidemiological model. On the basis of my interpretation of the medical literature, all of the elements in the model are funneled through medical risks. Black women may experience medical risks such as preeclampsia, hypertension, and gestational diabetes more than white women, which affect the probability of stillbirth (Fretts, 2005).

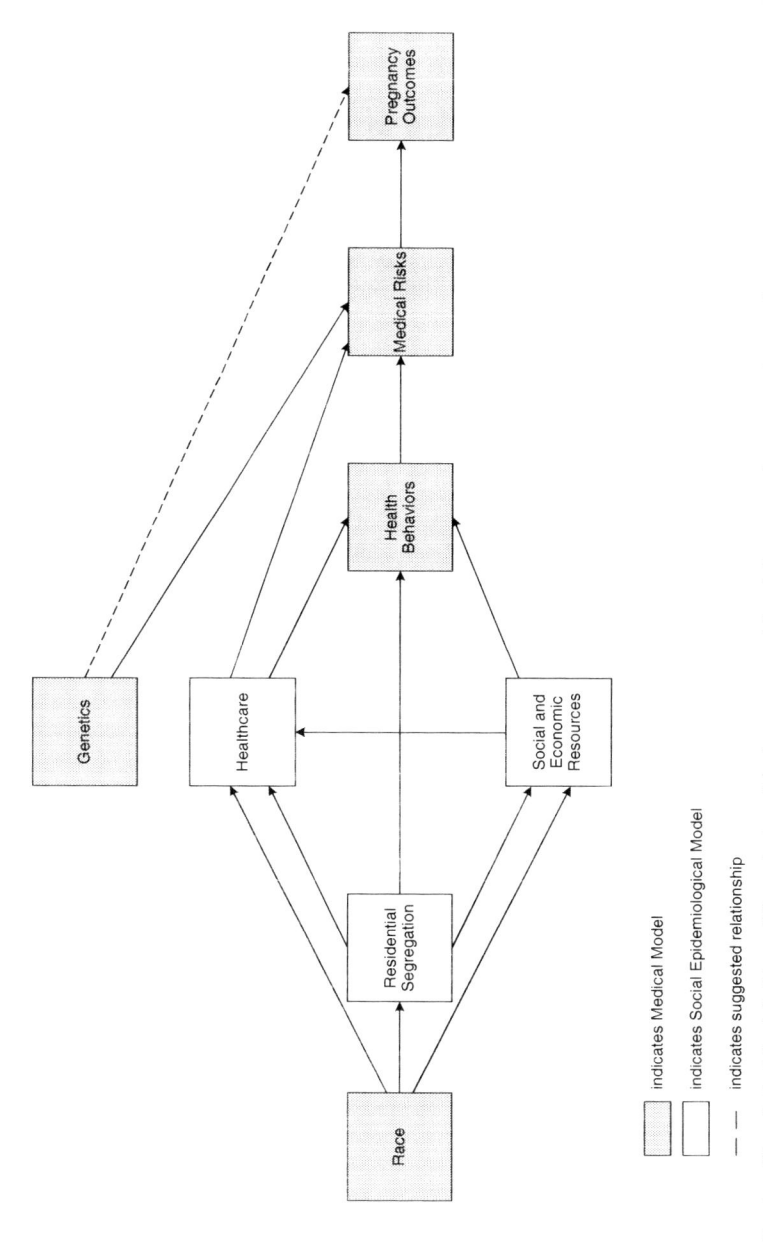

Fig. 1. Heuristic Model. *Note:* The relationship between residential segregation, genetics, and pregnancy outcome cannot be assessed with the available data. Health care refers to health system, provider, and patient variables.

I argue that inequalities between black and white women may be due to differences in health behaviors. For example, poor diet and tobacco use may lead to medical conditions such as preeclampsia, obesity, and gestational diabetes, which are risk factors for stillbirths. Inequalities in health behaviors may be a direct result of differences in social economic resources and health care, indicated by the nonshaded boxes in Fig. 1. These factors are not assumed to act alone but operate through medical risks. Lack of prenatal care could result in an increased number of or severity of negative medical conditions and ultimately negative pregnancy outcomes. Provider bias may result in differing prenatal care recommendations and clinical care for black women versus white women. Inequalities in social and economic resources and health care may be a result of residential segregation, which is largely explained by race. Race is hypothesized to affect residential segregation, social and economic resources, and health care. Residential segregation may affect access to healthcare facilities and access to public transportation impacting access to health care. Residential segregation may also result in number and quality of jobs, poorer quality schools, available recreational facilities, and even the quality of grocery stores and nutritious foods available.

Empirical Goals

Because many scholars interested in birth outcomes control for race, several pathways through which race may operate have not been evaluated. The data that I propose to use in this chapter are subject to these limitations rendering some aspects of the comprehensive heuristic model, shown in Fig. 1, untestable. Proxies and other indirect measures will be used in the analysis whenever possible. While it would be ideal to test the entire model, laid out earlier, the data do not provide information to test the relationship between residential segregation, genetics, and only access to health care can be tested within the healthcare explanation, but, I will discuss the way race operates through residential segregation.

DATA

Data for this study come from the National Maternal and Infant Health Survey 1988 (NMIHS), sponsored by the United States Department of Health and Human Services, National Center for Health Statistics, designed and conducted by the Gallup Organization. The NMIH is a nationally representative sample of live births, fetal deaths, and infant deaths and combines a questionnaire with vital records information.

A stratified systematic random sample of live birth, late fetal death, and infant death vital records were drawn from the 48 states, District of Columbia, and New York City in 1988. Of the 26,355 live birth, late fetal death, and infant death records sampled, interviews were completed with 18,594 individuals, a 71% response rate. Hispanics ($n = 1{,}269$), all cases missing on parity ($n = 197$) and gestational age ($n = 1{,}153$), were excluded resulting in a final sample size of 15,975. There are two reasons Hispanics are excluded from the analyses: (1) the largest gap in stillbirths is between blacks and whites and (2) Hispanics tend to have better health than expected based on socioeconomic factors, which has been termed the "epidemiologic paradox" (Markides & Coreil, 1986). Data from the NMIH are 20 years old, but it is the most recent data set including information on insurance coverage (e.g., private, public, or self-pay) and barriers obtaining medical care (e.g., transportation, childcare, distance, and cost).

MEASURES

Dependent Variable

Stillbirth is a dichotomous variable computed using the self-reported gestational age variable. Stillbirth is coded 0 for full-term live birth (a live birth at ≥ 37 weeks gestation), and 1 for stillbirth (a fetal loss at 20 or more weeks gestation). Preterm births (live birth at less than 37 weeks gestation) are omitted from this analysis because I am interested in focusing on the comparison between stillbirths and live births.

Independent Variable

I expect independent variables measuring the medical and social epidemiological models to be related to the racial disparity in stillbirth, each are described below.

Baseline Model

The only variable included in the baseline model is race, a binary variable coded 1 for blacks and 0 for whites.

Medical Model

Behavioral Risks
Smoking during pregnancy and exercising during pregnancy are behavioral risks, each are dichotomous variables coded 1 for yes and 0 for no.

Medical Risks
Medical risks include multiple gestations, underweight, overweight, obesity, abdominal cramps, vaginal bleeding, advanced maternal age, and parity. Multiple gestation is a dichotomous variable coded 1 for multiple gestations such as twins, triplets, or quadruplets and 0 for singletons. Underweight is coded 1 for body mass index (BMI) below 18.5 (kg/m^2) and 0 for other. Overweight is coded 1 for a BMI of 25.0–29.9 and 0 for other. Obesity is coded 1 for BMI 30.0 and above and 0 for other. Abdominal cramps and vaginal bleeding are dummy variables coded 1 for yes and 0 for no. Advanced maternal age is a dichotomous variable coded 1 for 35 years or older (e.g., advanced maternal age) and 0 for less than 35 years of age. Parity is defined as the number of times a woman has given birth including the focal birth. Parity is a dichotomous variable with primiparous (giving birth once) coded 1 and multiparous (given birth more than once) coded 0.

Social Epidemiological Model

Social and Economic Resources
Marital status, household income, education level, occupation, and health insurance are social and economic resource variables included in the model. Marital status is a dichotomous variable coded 1 for married and 0 for not married. Household income is a series of seven dummy variables including: $0–$9,999 versus other, $10,000–$19,999 versus other, $20,000–$29,999 versus other, $30,000–$39,999 versus other, $40,000–$49,999 versus other, $50,000–$59,999 versus other, and $60,000 and over versus other. The reference category for household income is $0–$9,999 and is omitted from the analyses. Education is a dichotomous variable coded 1 for 12 years or more and 0 for less than 12 years. Occupation is composed of four exclusive dichotomous variables. Nonmanual occupation refers to managerial, professional, technical, sales, and administrative positions and is coded 1 for nonmanual and 0 for all other. Manual occupation refers to service occupations, farming, forestry, fishing, precision, craft repair, fabricator, laborer, and operators and is coded 1 for manual and 0 for all other.

Armed forces is a dichotomous variable coded 1 for armed forces and 0 for all other. Unemployed is coded 1 for yes and 0 for no is the reference category and excluded from analyses. Insurance status is a dichotomous variable with having insurance coded 1 and no insurance coded 0.

Health Care
Healthcare variables in the model include prenatal care provider type; prenatal care, parsed into care received during the first, second, and third trimesters, respectively; and number of healthcare visits. Provider type is a dichotomous variable with private physician coded 1 and clinic or other physician coded 0 derived from a question where respondents were asked "what type of place they went for their prenatal care?" Other physician includes county or city health department, community health center, health maintenance organization, clinic at work or school, clinic at hospital, emergency room in hospital, and other. Three exclusive dichotomous variables were created to indicate if prenatal care was initiated in the first trimester, second trimester, or third trimester and coded 1 for yes and 0 for no. Respondents were asked, "How many weeks pregnant were you on your first prenatal visit?", which was recoded into trimester of initiation. Number of healthcare visits is a continuous variable ranging from 0 to 26 and coded 0 for no prenatal visits and 1 for one prenatal visit through 26 for 26 prenatal visits.

METHODS

Statistical analyses were performed using Stata version 9.0 (StataCorp, 2005), and the following commands were employed: (1) svy and robust commands for adjusting standard errors in complex survey designs; (2) the pweight command was used with the finwgt or final weight provided by the NMIH; and (3) logit command for logistic regression and prtab for predicted probabilities. In the next section, I describe the measurement of the variables used in the analysis.

Analytic Plan

Weighted bivariate distributions of blacks and whites were calculated to show differences and similarities between blacks and whites on variables used in the analysis (Table 1). Next, a series of logistic regression models

Table 1. Percent Distribution for Variables in Analysis (Weighted).

	Entire Sample (%)	Black (%)	White (%)	x^2/df
Dependent variable				
Outcome***				470.994/1
Stillbirth	0.3	0.5	0.3	
Full-term	99.7	99.5	99.7	
Independent variables				
Race				
Black	16.7	*	*	
White	83.3	*	*	
Health behaviors				
Smoking***				4293.813/1
Yes	22.9	19.7	23.6	
No	77.1	80.3	76.4	
Exercise***				322.396/1
Yes	42.7	43.7	42.5	
No	57.3	56.3	57.5	
Medical risks				
Multiples***				2081.720
Multiple gestation (twins, triplets, and quads)	2.1	2.9	2.0	
Singleton gestation	97.9	97.1	98.0	
Underweight***				809.935/1
Yes	14.9	13.8	15.2	
No	85.1	86.2	84.8	
Overweight***				3337.694/1
Yes	14.9	17.2	14.4	
No	85.1	86.8	85.6	
Obese***				8058.156/1
Yes	7.2	9.9	6.6	
No	92.8	90.1	93.4	
Abdominal cramps***				7502.060/1
Yes	23.5	27.8	22.7	
No	76.5	72.2	77.3	
Vaginal bleeding***				317.466/1
Yes	14.7	13.9	14.8	
No	85.3	86.1	85.2	
Advanced maternal age***				6144.984/1
Yes	7.6	5.2	8.1	
No	92.4	94.8	91.9	
Parity***				
Primaparous	35.0	29.9	36.1	8428.673/1
Multiparous	65.0	70.1	63.9	

Table 1. (Continued)

	Entire Sample (%)	Black (%)	White (%)	x^2/df
Social and economic resources				
Martial status***				590194.30/1
Married	72.8	32.9	80.8	
Not married	27.2	67.1	19.2	
Household income***				
$0–$9.999				274000.75/1
Yes	22.5	47.9	17.3	
No	77.5	52.1	82.7	
$10,000–$19,999***				3446.229/1
Yes	21.3	24.1	20.7	
No	78.7	75.9	79.3	
$20,000–$29,999***				29632.866/1
Yes	18.4	10.6	20.0	
No	81.6	89.4	80.0	
$30,000–$39,999***				23169.785/1
Yes	14.9	8.6	16.1	
No	85.1	91.4	83.9	
$40,000–$49,999				21997.096/1
Yes	9.4	4.4	10.5	
No	90.6	95.6	89.5	
$50,000–$59,999***				14934.848/1
Yes	5.4	2.2	6.1	
No	94.6	97.8	93.9	
>$ 60,000***				34282.488/1
Yes	8.2	2.3	9.4	
No	91.8	97.7	90.6	
Education***				80195.609/1
12 years or more	86.3	74.9	88.6	
<12 years	13.7	25.1	11.4	
Occupation				
Nonmanual***				57910.182/1
Yes	57.0	43.1	59.8	
No	43.0	56.9	40.2	
Manual***				23528.779/1
Yes	28.7	36.8	27.1	
No	71.3	63.2	72.9	
Armed forces				.940/1
Yes	0.4	0.4	0.4	
No	99.6	99.6	99.6	
Unemployed***				20725.951/1
Yes	13.9	19.7	12.7	
No	86.1	80.3	87.3	

Table 1. (*Continued*)

	Entire Sample (%)	Black (%)	White (%)	x^2/df
Health insurance***				
Yes	67.8	51.3	71.2	92585.582/1
No	32.2	48.7	28.8	
Health care				
Prenatal care Provider***				199440.15/1
Private physician	63.5	38.5	68.6	
Other	36.5	61.5	31.4	
Prenatal care initiated During first trimester***				98221.400/1
Yes	78.0	62.9	81.1	
No	22.0	37.1	18.9	
Prenatal care initiated during second trimester***				59671.991/1
Yes	17.3	28.1	15.2	
No	82.7	71.9	84.8	
Prenatal care initiated during third trimester***				16747.675/1
Yes	3.5	6.2	2.9	
No	96.5	99.8	97.1	
Number of visits***	12.7 ± 5.9	10.8 ± 5.9	13.1 ± 5.9	

***$p<.001$; **$p<.01$; *$p<.05$ based on chi-square test of association for categorical variables and *t*-tests for continuous variables.

were estimated, in which the response categories stillbirth is contrasted with the reference category full term. To examine the utility of the medical and social epidemiological explanations for racial differences in stillbirth, three regression models are nested. The baseline model is race and variables representing the medical model and social epidemiological model are entered in subsequent models. By nesting the regression models, I can see the extent to which controlling for the mechanisms linking race to stillbirth results in attenuation of the racial gap.

RESULTS

Bivariate Analyses

Descriptive statistics, in Table 1, report that there are statistically significant differences between blacks and whites on all variables. Approximately

.3% of the total sample had a stillbirth. Whites were less likely than blacks to have a stillbirth (.3% versus .5%) versus full-term live birth.

Blacks and whites differed substantially on healthcare-related variables and social and economic resources variables. Similar percentages for blacks and whites were found on all health behavior and medical risk variables. Having health insurance varied tremendously between blacks (51.3%) and whites (71.2%), and seeing a private physician was much less likely for blacks (38.5%) than whites (68.6%). Blacks were less likely than whites to initiate prenatal care in the first trimester (62.9% versus 81.1%) but more likely than whites to initiate prenatal care in the second trimester (28.1% versus 15.2%) and third trimester (6.2% versus 2.9%). In comparison to blacks, whites had a greater number of prenatal care visits (13.1 ± 5.9 versus 10.8 ± 5.9).

To a large extent, blacks had less access to social and economic resources than whites. Specifically, blacks were less likely to be married (32.9%) than whites (80.8%), approximately half of all blacks had a household income ranging from $0 to $9,999 compared to 17.3% of whites, blacks were less likely than whites to be in nonmanual (43.1% versus 59.8%), and blacks were less likely to have 12 or more years of education (74.9% versus 88.6%).

Multivariable Analyses

To assess racial differences in stillbirth, I use logistic regression to predict a two-category dependent variable called *stillbirth*, which enables comparisons between stillbirth and full-term birth. Coefficients presented in Table 2 indicate how each variable is related to the log odds of having a stillbirth versus full-term birth.

Stillbirth versus Full-Term Birth

Model 1 shows that blacks were more likely than whites to have a stillbirth versus full-term birth. The odds of blacks having a stillbirth were 1.79 times greater than whites ($e^{.581} = 1.79$). In this model, the predicted probability of blacks having a stillbirth is .49% versus .31% for whites.

In model 2, medical variables are added to the baseline model; the association between race and stillbirth remains unchanged. In this model, the predicted probability of blacks having a stillbirth is .51% versus .33% for whites when all other variables in the model are held at the mean. Smoking, multiples, overweight, obesity, and vaginal bleeding are positively

Table 2. Coefficients for Logistic Regression Comparing Stillbirth to Full-Term Birth.

	Stillbirth versus Full-Term		
	Model 1	Model 2	Model 3
Race (1 = black)	0.581***	0.586***	0.526***
Health behaviors	–		
Smoking (1 = yes)	–	0.158**	0.180**
Physical activity (1 = yes)	–	−0.248***	−0.276
Medical risks	–		
Multiples (1 = yes)	–	1.745***	1.909***
Underweight (1 = yes)	–	−0.024	−0.020
Overweight (1 = yes)	–	0.256***	0.329***
Obese (1 = yes)	–	0.551***	0.635***
Abdominal cramps (1 = yes)	–	0.054	0.033
Vaginal bleeding (1 = yes)	–	0.177*	0.260**
Advanced maternal age (1 = yes)	–	−0.450***	0.423***
Parity (1 = primiparous)	–	0.146**	0.189**
Social and economic resources	–	–	
Marital status (1 = married)	–	–	0.419***
Income $10,000–$19,999			0.093
Income $20,000–$29,999			−0.064
Income $30,000–$39,999			−0.128
Income $40,000–$49,999			−0.127
Income $50,000–$59,999			−0.089
Income > $60,000			−0.058
Education (1 = 12 years or more)	–	–	0.258**
Occupation (1 = nonmanual)	–	–	−0.085
Occupation (1 = manual)			0.075
Occupation (1 = armed forces)			0.392
Health insurance (1 = yes)	–	–	0.114
Healthcare			
Prenatal care provider (1 = private physician)	–	–	0.022
Prenatal care initiated first trimester (1 = yes)	–	–	−0.192
Prenatal care initiated second trimester (1 = yes)	–	–	−0.290
Prenatal care initiated third trimester (1 = yes)	–	–	−0.421
Number of prenatal visits (0–26)	–	–	−0.133***
df	2	22	60
R^2	0.028	0.064*	0.107*

*$p < .05$; **$p < .01$; $p < .001$ for two-tailed z-test of parameter estimate.

associated with the probability of a stillbirth. In contrast, exercising is negatively associated with the probability of a stillbirth.

In model 3, social epidemiological variables are added and the racial gap in stillbirths remains nearly unchanged. The odds of blacks having a stillbirth drops to 1.69 times greater than whites ($e^{.526} = 1.69$). With the inclusion of social epidemiological variables, the racial gap in stillbirths increases by 9.4% ([.581−.526]/.581 = .094). In this model, the predicted probability of blacks having a stillbirth is .51% versus .34% for whites when all other variables in the model are held at the mean. Marital status and education are positively associated with stillbirth. Number of prenatal visits is negatively associated with stillbirth. Analyses (not shown) show trimesters of prenatal care initiation are significant predictors of stillbirths when number of prenatal care visits is not controlled. Controlling for number of prenatal care visits eliminates the effect of prenatal care initiation.

DISCUSSION

The goal of this study was to explain the racial gap in stillbirths; however, neither the medical nor the social epidemiological model mediates this relationship. Very little of the racial gap in stillbirths is explained by the medical or the social epidemiological model, and one reason for this may be that overall researchers have very little understanding of the causes of stillbirths. Lack of uniform protocols for evaluating and classifying stillbirths in the United States and the decreasing number of autopsies performed on stillborn fetuses make it too difficult to identify causes of stillbirths (American College of Obstetricians and Gynecologists, 2009).

Recently, the American College of Obstetricians and Gynecologists (ACOG) released a practice bulletin recommending guidelines for clinicians managing a stillbirth, which could aid in improving understanding of factors causing stillbirths and, more specifically, the racial gap in stillbirths. ACOG called for general examination of stillborn fetuses; examination of the placenta, cord, and membranes; karyotype evaluation; and maternal evaluation (American College of Obstetricians and Gynecologists, 2009). The recommended maternal evaluation including information on family, maternal, and obstetric history along with information on the current pregnancy may be most helpful in identifying causes for racial disparities in stillbirths. Assessing explanations for the racial gap in stillbirths remains difficult with such little understanding on the underlying mechanisms of stillbirths. As more information is gathered on causes of stillbirths, further understanding of the racial gap in stillbirths may be developed.

Although the racial gap in stillbirths was not explained in this study, results from this study are consistent with previous studies showing that blacks are more likely than whites to have a stillbirth

(MacDorman et al., 2007). The probability of black women having a stillbirth was still greater than white women for women who were average on all medical and social epidemiological variables. Findings from this study are concurrent with other studies showing that health behaviors and medical risks are significant predictors of stillbirths (Fretts, 2005; Silver et al., 2007). Factors such as smoking, multiple gestations, being overweight, and obesity increase the probability of stillbirth, whereas engaging in physical activity during pregnancy decreases the probability of stillbirth. Blacks, in this study, were less likely to smoke and more likely to exercise than whites. However, blacks were more likely to be overweight and obese and had slightly higher rates of multiple gestations than whites. Other studies suggested that blacks have a higher rate of stillbirths because of factors such as hypertensive disorders and diabetes, and while these could not be directly measured in this study, they are indirectly measured by strong correlates overweight and obesity (Fretts, 2005). Findings from this study reiterate the importance of medical risks and health behaviors in the probability of a stillbirth, but future research should further examine racial disparities in these factors.

The racial gap in stillbirths is slightly reduced when the social epidemiological variables are added to the model, but, again, the racial gap is not fully explained with the inclusion of social economic resources and healthcare variables. Other studies have also found that after controlling for prenatal care, blacks are still more likely than whites to experience a stillbirth (Vintzileos et al., 2002). In this study, blacks were still more likely than whites to have a stillbirth, after controlling for number of prenatal care visits. However, while controlling for healthcare variables, including number of prenatal care visits, does not eliminate the racial gap, it does reduce the racial gap. Fretts (2005) argues that access to prenatal care and identifying high-risk patients based on medical and socioeconomic factors is an important component with respect to reducing the racial gap in stillbirths. Residential segregation reduces access to and quality of health care, and bivariate findings from this study show that blacks are less likely than whites to initiate health care in the first trimester and have fewer prenatal care visits overall.

While the racial gap in rates of stillbirths is slightly reduced with the introduction of social epidemiological variables, explanations for the remaining racial disparity may be due to chronic stress from discrimination, which could not be measured in this study due to the nature of the survey data. As mentioned earlier, chronic stress from discrimination has been found to be a predictor of poor pregnancy outcomes (Collins et al., 2004).

Another possible explanation for the persistent racial gap in rates of stillbirths may be physician bias, which could result in different treatment plans or recommendations for black versus white patients.

Data for this study relied on self-reports of behaviors during pregnancy; pregnancy of interest ranged from one to two years before the interview, which is subject to recall bias and produces lower quality data than if respondent's behavior was directly observed during pregnancy (Kogan, Alexander, Kotelchuck, Nagey, & Jack, 1994). This study could not capture residential segregation, physician bias or chronic stress, and discrimination explanation, which may play an important role in poor pregnancy outcomes. Future researchers should focus attention on explaining the racial gap in rates of stillbirth and examine explanations of residential segregation, physician bias, chronic stress, and discrimination explanations. Use of qualitative interviews, focus groups, or ethnographies could highlight important variables future quantitative studies should seek to measure. The racial disparity in rates of stillbirth may be a multifaceted problem, and increasing access to and consistency of prenatal care may be one avenue to reduce the racial gap in rates of stillbirths.

REFERENCES

American College of Obstetricians and Gynecologists. (2009). Management of stillbirth. ACOG practice bulletin #102. *Obstetrics and Gynecology, 113*(3), 748–761.

Andreski, P., & Breslau, N. (1995). Maternal smoking among blacks and whites. *Social Science Medicine, 41*(2), 227–233.

Bach, P. B., Pham, H. H., Schrag, D., Tate, R. C., & Hargraves, J. L. (2004). Primary care physicians who treat blacks and whites. *New England Journal of Medicine, 351*(6), 575–584.

Bonilla-Silva, E. (2006). *Racism without racists.* Lanham, MD: Rowman and Littlefield Publishers, Inc.

Brown, H. L., Chireau, M. V., Jallah, Y., & Howard, D. (2007). The "Hispanic paradox": An investigation of racial disparity in pregnancy outcomes at a tertiary care medical center. *American Journal of Obstetrics and Gynecology, 197*(2), 197.e1–197.e2.

Christiaens, G. C., Vissers, J., Poddighe, P. J., & de Pater, J. M. (2000). Comparative genomic hybridization for cytogenetic evaluation of stillbirth. *Obstetrics and Gynecology, 96*(2), 281–286.

Cockerham, W. C. (2005). Health lifestyle theory and the convergence of agency and structure. *Journal of Health and Social Behavior, 46*(1), 51–67.

Collins, C. A., & Williams, D. R. (1999). Segregation and mortality: The deadly effects of racism? *Sociological Forum, 14*(3), 495–523.

Collins, J. W., Jr., David, R. J., Handler, A., Wall, S., & Andes, S. (2004). Very low birthweight in African American infants: The role of maternal exposure to interpersonal discrimination. *American Journal of Public Health, 94*(12), 2132–2138.

Culhane, J. F., & Elo, I. T. (2005). Neighborhood context and reproductive health. *American Journal of Obstetrics and Gynecology, 192*(5 Suppl.), S22–S29.

Dole, N., Savitz, D. A., Siega-Riz, A. M., Hertz-Picciotto, I., McMahon, M. J., & Buekens, P. (2004). Psychosocial factors and preterm birth among African American and white women in central North Carolina. *American Journal of Public Health, 94*(8), 1358–1365.

Echevarria, S., & Frisbie, W. P. (2001). Race/ethnic-specific variation in adequacy of prenatal care utilization. *Social Forces, 80*(2), 633–655.

Epstein, A. M., Ayanian, J. Z., Keogh, J. H., Noonan, S. J., Armistead, N., Cleary, P. D., Weissman, J. S., David-Kasdan, J. A., Carlson, D., Fuller, J., Marsh, D., & Conti, R. M. (2000). Racial disparities in access to renal transplantation. *The New England Journal of Medicine, 343*(21), 1537–1545.

Forbes, D., Frisbie, W. P., Hummer, R. A., Pullum, S. G., & Echevarria, S. (2000). A comparison of Hispanic and Anglo compromised birth outcomes and cause-specific infant mortality in the United States 1989–1991. *Social Science Quarterly, 81*(1), 439–458.

Fretts, R. C. (2005). Etiology and prevention of stillbirth. *American Journal of Obstetrics and Gynecology, 193*(6), 1923–1935.

Frisbie, W. P. (1994). Birth weight and infant mortality in the Mexican origin and Anglo populations. *Social Science Quarterly, 74*(4), 881–895.

Frisbie, W. P., Forbes, D., & Pullum, S. G. (1996). Compromised birth outcomes and infant mortality among racial and ethnic groups. *Demography, 33*(4), 469–481.

Frisbie, W. P., Song, S.-E., Powers, D. A., & Street, J. A. (2004). The increasing racial disparity in infant mortality: Respiratory distress syndrome and other causes. *Demography, 41*(4), 773–800.

Gennaro, S. (2005). Overview of current state of research on pregnancy outcomes in minority populations. *American Journal of Obstetrics and Gynecology, 192*, S3–S10.

Geronimus, A. T. (1992). The weathering hypothesis and the health of African-American women and infants: Evidence and speculation. *Ethnicity and Disease, 2*(3), 207–221.

Gold, K. J., Kuznia, A. L., & Hayward, R. A. (2008). How physicians cope with stillbirth or neonatal death: A national survey of obstetricians. *Obstetrics and Gynecology, 112*, 29–34.

Goesling, B. (2007). The rising significance of health. *Social Forces, 85*(4), 1621–1644.

Grady, S. C. (2006). Racial disparities in low birthweight and the contribution of residential segregation: A multilevel analysis. *Social Science and Medicine, 63*, 3013–3029.

Greenberg, R. S. (1982). The impact of prenatal care in different social groups. *Obstetrics and Gynecology, 145*(7), 197–801.

Hogue, C., & Bremner, D. (2005). Stress model for research into preterm delivery among black women. *American Journal of Obstetrics and Gynecology, 192*(5), S47–S55.

Hughes, P. M., Turton, P., & Evans, C. D. (1999). Stillbirth as a risk factor for depression and anxiety in the subsequent pregnancy: Cohort study. *British Medical Journal, 318*(7200), 1721–1724.

Hummer, R. A. (1993). Racial differentials in infant mortality in the U.S: An examination of social and health determinants. *Social Forces, 72*(2), 529–554.

Hummer, R. A., Biegler, M., De Turk, P. B., Forbes, D., Frisbie, W. P., Hong, Y., & Pullum, S. G. (1999). Race, nativity and infant mortality in the United States. *Social Forces, 77*(3), 1083–1118.

Hummer, R. A., Powers, D. A., Pullum, S. G., Gossman, G. L., & Frisbie, W. P. (2007). Paradox found (again): Infant mortality among the Mexican-origin population in the United States. *Demography, 44*(3), 441–457.

Kogan, M. D., Alexander, G. R., Kotelchuck, M., Nagey, D. A., & Jack, B. W. (1994). Comparing mothers' reports on the content of prenatal care received with recommended national guidelines for care. *Public Health Reports, 109*(5), 637–646.

Link, B. G., & Phelan, J. (1995). Social conditions as fundamental cause of disease. *Journal of Health and Social Behavior, 35*(Extra Issue), 80–94.

Lu, M. C., & Chen, B. (2004). Racial and ethnic disparities in preterm births: The role of stressful life events. *American Journal of Obstetrics and Gynecology, 191*(3), 691–699.

MacDorman, M. F., Munson, M. L., & Kirmeyer, S. (2007). Fetal and perinatal mortality, United States, 2004. *National Vital Statistics Reports, 56*(3), 1–20.

Markides, K. S., & Coreil, J. (1986). The health of Hispanics in the South-western United States: An epidemiologic paradox. *Public Health Reports, 101*, 253–265.

Malat, J. (2006). Expanding research on the racial disparity in medical treatment with ideas from sociology. *Health, 10*(3), 259–282.

Martin, J. A., Hamilton, B. E., Sutton, P. D., Ventura, S. J., Menacker, F., Kirmeyer, S., & Munson, M. L. (2006). Births: Final data for 2005. *National Vital Statistics Report, 56*(6), 1–104.

Massey, D. S., Condran, G. A., & Denton, N. A. (1987). The effects of residential segregation on black social and economic well-being. *Social Forces, 66*(1), 29–56.

Morenoff, J. D. (2003). Neighborhood mechanisms and the spatial dynamics of birth weight. *American Journal of Sociology, 108*(5), 976–1017.

Morenoff, J. D., House, J. S., Hansen, B. B., Williams, D. R., Kaplan, G. A., & Hunte, H. E. (2007). Understanding social disparities in hypertension prevalence, awareness, treatment, and control: The role of neighborhood context. *Social Science and Medicine, 65*, 1853–1866.

Perreira, K. M., & Cortes, K. E. (2006). Race/ethnicity and nativity differences in alcohol and tobacco use during pregnancy. *American Journal of Public Health, 96*(9), 1629–1636.

Peterson, E. D., Wright, S. M., Daley, J., & Thibault, G. E. (1994). Racial variation in cardiac procedure use and survival following acute myocardial infarction in the department of veterans affairs. *The Journal of the American Medical Association, 271*(15), 1175–1180.

Phelan, J. C., Link, B. G., Diez-Roux, A., Karachi, I., & Levin, B. (2004). Fundamental causes of social inequalities in mortality: A test of the theory. *Journal of Social Behavior, 45*(3), 265–285.

Powell, L. M., Slater, S., Chaloupka, F. J., & Harper, D. (2006). Availability of physical activity-related facilities and neighborhood demographic and socioeconomic characteristics: A national study. *American Journal of Public Health, 96*(9), 1676–1680.

Raymond, E. G., Cnattingius, S., & Kiely, J. L. (2005). Effects of maternal age, parity and smoking on the risk of stillbirth. *British Journal of Obstetrics and Gynecology, 101*(4), 301–306.

Robert, S. (1998). Community-level socioeconomic status effects on adult health. *Journal of Health and Social Behavior, 39*, 18–37.

Robert, S. (1999). Socioeconomic position and health: The independent contribution of community socioeconomic context. *Annual Review of Sociology, 25*, 489–516.
Robert, S., & Reither, E. N. (2004). A multilevel analysis of race, community disadvantage, and body mass index among adults in the US. *Social Science and Medicine, 59*, 2421–2434.
Rosenberg, T. J., Garbers, S., Chavkin, W., & Chiasson, M. A. (2003). Prepregnancy weight and adverse perinatal outcomes in an ethnically diverse population. *Obstetrics and Gynecology, 102*(5), 1022–1027.
Rosenberg, T. J., Garbers, S., Lipkind, H., & Chiasson, M. A. (2005). Maternal obesity and diabetes as risk factors for adverse pregnancy outcomes among 4 racial/ethnic groups. *American Journal of Public Health, 95*(9), 1545–1551.
Van Ryn, M., Burgess, D., Malat, J., & Griffin, J. (2006). Physicians' perceptions of patients' social and behavioral characteristics and race disparities in treatment recommendations for men with coronary artery disease. *American Journal of Public Health, 96*(2), 351–357.
Samadi, A., Mayberry, R., Zaidi, A., Pleasant, J., McGhee, N., & Rice, R. (1996). Maternal hypertension and associated pregnancy complications among African-American and other women in the United States. *Obstetrics and Gynecology, 87*(4), 557–563.
Schulman, K. A., Berlin, J. A., Harless, W., Kerner, J. F., Sistrunk, S., Gersh, B. J., Dube, R., Taleghani, C. K., Burke, J. E., Williams, S., Eisenberg, J. M., Escarce, J. J., & Ayers, W. (1999). The effect of race and sex on physicians' recommendations for cardiac catheterization. *The New England Journal of Medicine, 340*(8), 618–626.
Silver, R. M., Varner, M. W., Reddy, U., Goldenberg, R., Pinar, H., Conway, D., Bukowski, R., Carpenter, M., Hogue, C., Willinger, M., Dudley, D., Saade, G., & Stoll, B. (2007). Work-up of stillbirth: A review of the evidence. *American Journal of Obstetrics and Gynecology, 196*(5), 433–444.
Singh, G. K., & Kogan, M. D. (2007). Persistent socioeconomic disparities in infant, neonatal, and postneonatal mortality rates in the United States, 1969–2001. *Pediatrics, 119*(4), e928–e939.
Singh, G. K., & Yu, S. M. (1996). Trends and differentials in adolescent and young adult mortality in the United States, 1950 through 1993. *American Journal of Public Health, 86*(4), 560–564.
StataCorp. (2005). *Stata statistical software: Release 9*. College Station, TX: StataCorp LP.
Vintzileos, A. M., Ananth, C. V., Smulian, J. C., Scorza, W. E., & Knuppel, R. A. (2002). Prenatal care and black-white fetal death disparity in the United States: Heterogeneity by high-risk conditions. *Obstetrics and Gynecology, 99*, 483–489.
Wapner, R. J., & Lewis, D. (2002). Genetics and metabolic causes of stillbirth. *Seminars in Perinatology, 26*(1), 70–74.
Weden, M. W., Carpiano, R. M., & Robert, S. A. (2008). Subjective and objective neighborhood characteristics and adult health. *Social Science and Medicine, 66*(6), 1256–1270.
Williams, D. R., & Collins, C. (2001). Racial residential segregation: A fundamental cause of racial disparities in health. *Public Health Reports, 116*(5), 404–416.
Wilson, W. J. (1996). *When work disappears: The world of the new urban poor*. New York: Random House Publications.
World Health Organization. (1995). *The OBSQUID Project: Quality development in perinatal care, final report*. Publ Eur Serv. WHO Regional Publications European Series.
Yu, S. M., Keppel, K. G., Singh, G. K., & Kessel, W. (1996). Preconceptional and prenatal multivitamin-mineral supplement use in the 1988 National Maternal and Infant Health Survey. *American Journal of Public Health, 86*(2), 240–242.

SECTION III
GEOGRAPHIC AND COMMUNITY FACTORS IN DIFFERENCES IN HEALTH AND HEALTH CARE

HABILITATIVE THERAPY AMONG PRESCHOOL CHILDREN: REGIONAL DISPARITIES IN THE EARLY INTERVENTION POPULATION[☆,☆☆]

Richard Lee Rogers

ABSTRACT

Using data on children under three years of age from the 2003 National Survey of Children's Health (n = 16,953), this study uses logistic regression to identify the presence of disparities in the use of habilitative therapy (physical therapy, occupational therapy, and speech therapy) among all children, strong candidates for therapy due to physical or developmental issues, and children for whom there is a parental concern about speech. Region of residence emerges as a source of disparity: (1) Children in the South exhibit consistently low levels of therapy use,

---

[☆] The National Center for Health Statistics is responsible only for the initial data, and analyses, interpretations, and conclusions are solely the responsibility of the author.
[☆☆] An earlier version of this chapter was presented at the annual meeting of the Southern Sociological Society in Richmond, VA, April 9–12, 2008.

and (2) children with speech concerns in all regions of the country outside the Northeast are less likely to use therapists than children in the Northeast. Other variables gaining significance include age of child, gender, race, presence in a nuclear family, and insurance status, though the influence of these variables is not consistent.

INTRODUCTION

Habilitative therapy is an important component of health care for preschool children with disabilities, disorders, and delays. Addressing these problems early in life has been shown to be highly effective in lessening the degree of disadvantage and more cost efficient than delaying treatment until the child is older (McLean & Cripe, 1997). To guarantee a minimum level of care for all children, Part C of the Individuals with Disabilities Education Act (IDEA) provides federal funding for state-sponsored early intervention programs assisting children under the age of three years whose families lack health insurance or for whom private insurance does not cover habilitative therapy (Danaher, Shackelford, & Harbin, 2004). The 2003 National Survey of Children's Health (NSCH) estimates that 3.4 percent of children under three – almost 377,000 kids – use a therapist, and as of fall of 2007, over 300,000 children received early intervention under Part C of IDEA (U.S. Department of Education, 2008).

However, it is widely believed that participation in pediatric therapy programs should be much higher. For example, Rosenberg, Zhang, and Robinson (2008) estimate that only one in 10 children with developmental delays receive services during the first 24 months. Why are these services underutilized? The answers are surprisingly unclear. Gaps in health care are usually tied to disparities associated with demographic, social, and economic characteristics, but these inequalities are less salient when dealing with therapeutic services in general and barely researched in pediatrics (Smedley, Stith, & Nelson, 2003, p. 66; National Research Council and Institute of Medicine, 2004, pp. 86–87). In assessing this situation among children under the age of three – the age eligible for early intervention – this study uses the 2003 NSCH to introduce into the literature the importance of regional variations in the quality of care. Two populations are analyzed: (1) children who are strong candidates for therapy based on medical evaluations for physical and developmental issues and (2) an additional group of children for whom parents have a concern about speech delays but who are otherwise not regarded as strong candidates for therapy.

BACKGROUND

Health disparities can be described as systematic differences in health associated with social position (Braveman, 2006). The discussion assumes that good health is a basic human right and access to quality health care should be based on need – disparities are seen as obstacles to the acquisition of this right. Socio-economic factors such as income and education are regarded as a form of inequality of considerable importance (Barr, 2008; Haggerty & Johnson, 1996). The reception of quality health care is tied to the ability to pay – low-income populations have fewer financial resources from which to draw and are less likely to have health-insurance coverage (DeNavas-Walt, Proctor, & Smith, 2008). In addition, the well educated are more likely to engage in healthy lifestyles and have access to working conditions and social–psychological resources indirectly associated with good health (Ross & Wu, 1995).

Demographic and cultural factors are also important markers of health disparities because individuals who are not part of dominant groups face barriers in health care not experienced by whites and males. Race and ethnicity capture cultural differences among groups and also identify populations subject to patterns of direct, perceived, and institutional discrimination (Gabard & Cooper, 1998; Smedley et al., 2003; Guevara, Mandell, Rostain, Zhao, & Hadley, 2006; Malat & Hamilton, 2006; Ngui & Flores, 2007; Williams, Neighbors, & Jackson, 2003). Females have more problems accessing quality health care than males (Gorman & Read, 2006). Age is an indirect measure for developmental milestones among children and functional limitations among the elderly (Leung & Kao, 1999; Kelley-Moore, Schumacher, Kahana, & Kahana, 2006).

The existence of disparities among children is regarded as an especially important issue. Poor health when young not only affects present-day quality of life but can undermine the foundations of succeeding stages of development (Case, Lubotsky, & Paxson, 2002; National Research Council and Institute of Medicine, 2004). Many long-term initiatives to improve children's health have been highly successful, such as the minimization of the spread of disease through the use of vaccinations (Roush & Murphy, 2007), the improvement of dental health with water fluoridation (see Milgrom & Reisine, 2000), and the reduction of exposure to lead (Lanphear, Dietrich, & Berger, 2003). At the same time, there remains considerable work to be done: Relative to other industrialized nations, the United States has high rates of low birth weights and infant mortality. Estimates of chronic illness range from 6.5 to 19 percent of children (Newacheck & Halfon, 1998).

Many of the disparities in the society at large are replicated among children. In terms of general health, children have better health and fewer unmet medical needs as parental socioeconomic status increases (Newacheck, Jameson, & Halfon, 1994; Brooks-Gunn & Duncan, 1997; Newacheck, Hughes, Hung, Wong, & Stoddard, 2000; Hughes & Ng, 2003). Poverty decreases access to care, although its effects are minimized by school-based health care and publicly supported insurance programs like Medicaid and State Children's Health Insurance Program (Newacheck et al., 1994; Dick et al., 2004; Dubay & Kenney, 2004; Kenney, 2007). Childhood health disparities are also tied to demographic and social characteristics such as race, age (older children are less likely to have their needs met), gender, absence of both parents, large family size, lack of education, region of residence, and nonmetropolitan status (Newacheck et al., 2000; Hughes & Ng, 2003; Lieu, Newacheck, & McManus, 1993; Bauman, Silver, & Stein, 2006; Guevara et al., 2006; Stevens, Seid, Mistry, & Halfon, 2006; Weinick & Krauss, 2000).

Pediatric habilitative therapy targets a population of vulnerable children with chronic illnesses, special needs, and functional limitations. These children consume a disproportionately large percentage of pediatric health services due to their need for expanded care and/or assistive devices (Smyth-Staruch, Breslau, Wietzman, & Gortmaker, 1984; Newacheck & Kim, 2005). Unlike other forms of children's health care, the existence of disparities in the use of therapy is difficult to establish (Smedley et al., 2003). On the surface, the use of habilitative therapy appears associated with many of the same barriers inhibiting the delivery of quality health care in other populations (Table 1). However, a more careful reading of this literature highlights ambiguities related to socioeconomic status and race. Four of the six most relevant studies highlight a measure of socioeconomic status, such as income, poverty, or efforts to bridge socioeconomic differences through insurance (Smyth-Staruch et al., 1984; Mayer, Skinner, & Slifkin, 2004; Dusing, Skinner, & Mayer, 2004; Benedict, 2006). In these studies, race and ethnicity are not significantly associated with therapy use. In the other two studies, race and ethnicity are significant, but measures of socioeconomic status and insurance availability are not (Rosenberg et al., 2008; Kuhlthau, Hill, Fluet, Meara, & Yucel, 2008).

Why does this inconsistency exist? One possibility is that socioeconomic status and race are confounding factors, but other research suggests that the effects of socioeconomic status on children's health do not disappear when controlling for race (Ashiabi, 2008). Inconsistencies on findings about race in particular are also emerging in studies about the time until diagnosis

Table 1. Summary of Major Studies on Disparities in the Children's Use of Habilitative Therapy.

Dependent Variable (Study)	Data Source	Population	Disparities Established	Disparities Not Established
Use of physical therapy (Smyth-Staruch et al., 1984)	Patients at four specialty clinics in Cleveland, OH	Children aged 3–18 years with chronic congenital conditions	Income (+)	Education Race
Use of specialty care (Mayer, Skinner, & Slifkin, 2004)	National Survey of Children with Special Health Care Needs, 2000–2002	Children aged ≤18 years with special needs	Pediatric subspecialists (+) Metropolitan residence (−) Age (−) Poverty (−) Availability of insurance (+)	General pediatricians Internists per population Maternal education Gender Race/ethnicity Site of care
Use of therapy (Dusing, Skinner, & Mayer, 2004)	National Survey of Children with Special Health Care Needs, 2000–2002	Children aged ≤18 years with special needs	Availability of insurance (+) Metropolitan residence ( )	Maternal education Gender Race/ethnicity Poverty
Use of therapy in all settings (Benedict, 2006)	National Health Interview Survey, Disability Supplement, 1994–1995	Children aged 5–17 years	Household education (+) Family income (+) Public insurance (+) Family size (+) Age (−)	Family structure Race/ethnicity Gender Note: All variables except age if therapy is school based
Use of early intervention (Rosenberg et al., 2008)	Early Childhood Longitudinal Study, 2001 Birth Cohort	Children at 9 and 24 months	Black ( ) Hispanic ( )	Insurance status Poverty
Use of therapy and associated expenditures (Kuhlthau et al., 2008)	Medical Expenditure Panel Survey, 1996–2001	Children aged 0–17 years	Black ( ) Hispanic ( ) Male (+)	Age Maternal education Metropolitan residence Poverty Insurance status

Note: Establishment of disparities based on multivariate analyses. (+) indicates an increase in likelihood of care and (−) indicates decrease.

(Mandell, Listerud, Levy, & Pinto-Martin, 2002; Mann, Crawford, Wilson, & McDermott, 2008). A second explanation suggests that the dynamics of children's health care are changing due to the introduction of public insurance programs like Medicaid and the State Children's Health Insurance Program and the growth of supportive services such as early intervention and school-based therapy. For example, Benedict (2006) finds that disparities disappear with the use of therapy in educational settings.

This chapter is an effort to build on the current research to determine the presence of disparities related to habilitative therapy during the early intervention years – children under three years of age. To date, only one study focuses exclusively on the use of therapeutic services in this population (Rosenberg et al., 2008). The aims of this study are two. The first aim is to establish whether disparities exist in the early intervention population. It is suspected that developmental delays often go untreated because of the inability to describe early suspicions of the onset of some conditions in strictly medical terms – a requirement for participation in early intervention programs – and the misguided belief that children always grow out of these problems naturally (Perry, 2007). This latter point is exacerbated among minority groups where cultural perceptions minimize the need for therapy (Garcia, Perez, & Ortiz, 2000; Kolobe, 2004; Kummerer, Lopez-Reyna & Hughes, 2007).

Second, this study explores the addition of region of residence as an environmental factor in predicting the use of pediatric habilitative therapy. As Table 2 indicates, there are substantial variations in the use of early intervention by region. The Northeast is highest with 4.01 percent of children under three participating in early intervention programs, while the West and South are lowest at 2.30 and 1.95 percent, respectively. The low levels of use in the South are especially surprising – one would

Table 2. Use of Early Intervention Services among Children Aged 0–2 Years by Region.

	All Children (0–2 Years)	Children Using Early Intervention Services	%
Northeast	1,982,373	79,583	4.01
Midwest	2,656,207	71,955	2.71
West	3,127,363	71,806	2.30
South	4,783,706	93,386	1.95
Total United States	12,549,649	316,730	2.52

Source: U.S. Department of Education, Office of Special Education Programs (http://www.ideadata.org).

anticipate that use is *higher* in the South because the region's poverty and high percentage of babies born with low birth weights are factors frequently associated with the delays and disorders that early intervention programs are intended to serve.

METHODOLOGY

Data

Data for this study come from the public-use files of the 2003 NSCH, a tool used to benchmark progress toward *Healthy People 2010* (National Center for Health Statistics, 2005; Blumberg et al., 2005; Van Dyck et al., 2004). The survey, sponsored by the Maternal and Child Health Bureau within the Health Resources and Services Administration, draws on the capabilities of the State and Local Area Integrated Telephone Survey program. The total number of completed interviews is 102,353 and reflects a response rate of 55.3 percent nationally. The subset of data used in this study is children under three years of age, for whom there are 16,953 interviews.

Although research on children's health routinely relies on surveys with problems similar to ones described here (e.g., National Health Interview Survey and National Survey of Children Having Special Health Care Needs), the shortcomings should nevertheless be noted due to the potential for bias or inaccuracy. First, the objective measurement of children's health is problematic. Chronic conditions and acute illnesses are more difficult to recognize because of the rapidity of physical changes during childhood and the methodological problems of locating illnesses within the population (Beal et al., 2004). Second, the survey relies on the interpretations of an adult respondent, usually a parent, regarding the state of the child's health without independent verification from a health professional or health records. Subjective assessments of health cannot always be taken at face value (Angel & Gronfein, 1988), and the ways in which caregiver subjectivity complicates this process have not been fully assessed (Beal et al., 2004).

Dependent Variable

The dependent variable is the use of a habilitative therapist. This is taken directly from survey question S2Q13: "Does [CHILD] need or get special therapy, such as physical, occupational, or speech therapy?" The result is a dichotomous variable (1 = yes and 0 = no), which is referred to as use of a therapist throughout this chapter.

According to the survey, 3.4 percent of children (weighted) use a therapist. However, it should be noted that some of the children "needing" a therapist might not be "using" one given the way in which the question is written, but it is assumed here that the number of children in this position is relatively small.

Independent Variables

Demographic and social characteristics included in this analysis are age, gender, race and ethnicity, and family structure (Table 3). Child's age in years is operationalized as a series of dichotomous variables ranging from 0 to 2 with each year accounting for approximately one-third of the sample. Gender is whether the child is male or female – there are slightly more males than females. Race and ethnicity are mutually exclusive categories for white (57.4 percent of respondents), black (13.4 percent), Hispanic (21.1 percent), and other (8.2 percent). Family structure identifies those in a nuclear family – approximately two-thirds of children – and total children in the household, which has two children as the modal category. Insurance type divides children into mutually exclusive categories of those using public insurance such as Medicaid or State Children's Health Insurance Program (35.4 percent of respondents), other (private) providers (58.8 percent), and no insurance (5.9 percent). Region is classified using U.S. Census Bureau definitions for Northeast (17.0 percent of respondents), Midwest (22.1 percent), South (36.6 percent), and West (24.4 percent).

Controlling for Health Conditions

The severity of health conditions is an important control, which is handled in this analysis by identifying two subsets of children – strong candidates for therapy and speech-only candidates. The designation of a child as a strong candidate for therapy is based on medically evaluated needs and functional limitations. Such controls have been consistently shown to be highly significant in understanding the use of therapy. Medically evaluated needs are identified using questions on health in Section 2 of the NSCH (Blumberg et al., 2005). Children are defined as strong candidates for therapy if they meet one of three conditions: (1) they have a functional limitation,

Table 3. Characteristics of Preschool Population.

Variable	All Children N	All Children %	Strong Candidates N	Strong Candidates %	Speech N	Speech %
Age in years						
Less than 1 year	5,729	33.8	177	27.7	333	16.9
1 year old	6,050	35.7	216	33.8	901	45.6
2 years old	5,175	30.5	246	38.6	742	37.6
Gender						
Male	8,615	50.8	393	61.5	1,129	57.2
Female	8,332	49.2	246	38.5	847	42.9
Race and ethnicity						
White	9,625	57.4	395	62.4	929	47.7
Black	2,247	13.4	90	14.3	378	19.4
Hispanic	3,530	21.1	105	16.6	408	20.9
Other	1,371	8.2	43	6.8	232	12.0
Family structure						
Nuclear	12,883	77.1	414	66.4	1,352	69.7
Other	3,830	22.9	109	33.6	588	30.3
Total children in household						
1	5,274	31.1	180	28.1	644	32.6
2	6,151	36.3	229	35.9	769	38.9
3	3,491	20.6	139	21.8	397	20.1
4 or more	2,036	12.0	91	14.3	168	8.5
Insurance type						
Public	5,988	35.4	315	49.2	745	37.7
Other	9,949	58.8	294	46.1	1,085	54.9
None	998	5.9	30	4.7	145	7.4
Region						
Northeast	2,884	17.0	127	19.8	338	17.1
Midwest	3,737	22.1	168	26.4	416	21.1
South	6,201	36.6	229	35.9	725	36.7
West	4,131	24.4	114	17.9	497	25.2
Strong level of candidacy						
Yes	639	3.8				
No	16,314	96.2				

Note: Results weighted to population. Totals may not equal sum of columns due to rounding.

Table 4. Frequency and Percent Distributions of Medical Condition by Level of Candidacy.

Condition	% of Affected Children Using a Therapist
Strong candidates	
Functional limitation	59.7
Bone, joint, or muscle problem	57.5
Development delay or physical impairment	57.4
All strong candidates	48.3
Moderate candidates	
Behavioral or conduct problems	30.5
Hearing or vision loss	21.5
Asthma	6.4
Food allergy	5.5
Respiratory allergy	4.1
Skin allergy	4.1
All moderate candidates	12.7
Weak candidates	1.5
All children	3.4

Note: Results weighted to population. Individual conditions are not mutually exclusive, and percentages for individual conditions look higher than overall percentages for the associated level of candidacy due to comorbidities.

(2) a doctor or other health professional has expressed concern about bone, joint, or muscle problems, or (3) a doctor or other health professional has expressed concern about developmental delays or physical impairments. Each of these conditions is associated with use of a therapist at least 50 percent of the time (Table 4).

Strong candidates for therapy account for 3.8 percent of the population and 54.1 percent of all children receiving habilitative therapy (Table 5). However, attention must also be given to concerns for speech even when the child is otherwise not a strong candidate. Speech delays do not in themselves trigger eligibility for publicly funded early intervention – the survey itself does not even ask about medical evaluations of speech until children are at least three – but speech concerns must nevertheless be regarded as an important subset of the target population inasmuch as they account for nearly a third (29.8 percent) of all children using a therapist. For this reason, a second subset of children is referred to as speech or speech-only candidates – children who are not strong candidates for therapy but who have a parental concern for speech. This segment accounts for 12.5 percent

Table 5. Use of a Therapist by Condition.

Use of a Therapist	Strong Candidates			Speech-Only Candidates			Other Children			All Children		
	N	Column %	Row %	N	Column %	Row %	N	Column %	Row %	N	Column %	Row %
Yes	309	48.3	54.1	170	8.0	29.8	92	0.7	16.1	571	3.4	100.0
No	330	51.7	2.0	1,950	92.0	11.9	14,102	99.4	86.1	16,382	96.6	100.0
Total	639	100.0	3.8	2,120	100.0	12.5	14,194	100.0	83.7	16,953	100.0	100.0

Note: Results are weighted. Totals may not equal the sum due to rounding error.

of the population, and coupled with strong candidates makes it possible to account for nearly 84 percent of all children using therapy.

Although the focus of this study is disparities related to the use of a therapist, it is important to note that the designation of children as strong or speech-only candidates is tied to disparities as well (Table 3). Designation as a strong candidate increases with age because many types of delays cannot be identified until the child clearly misses a developmental benchmark (Landy, 2002; Leung & Kao, 1999). Boys are also more likely to be strong candidates than girls because some conditions affect boys more than girls and also because boys are more demonstrative in their behaviors when a problem is present (e.g., Wing, 1981; Underwood, 2002). The representation of children from nonnuclear families among strong candidates increases more than 10 percent relative to the population at large. Use of public insurance is also higher than the population among strong candidates.

Similarly, there are also differences between speech-only candidates and the population at large. Speech-only candidates are disproportionately represented among one- and two-year olds. As with strong candidates, the likelihood of a speech concern is higher among boys than girls, while the likelihood decreases among whites.

Analysis

All statistics are calculated using Stata/SE 10.0 and are weighted to the population distribution. Individual analyses may have numbers of observations lower than 16,953 due to missing data in the independent variables, although for any individual variable, the loss of observations due to missing data is less than 2 percent. Table 6 reports the odds ratios (ORs) for block

Table 6. Odds Ratios for Use of a Therapist.

	All Children		Strong Candidates	Speech Candidates
	Block regressions	Multivariate regression	Multivariate regression	Multivariate regression
Age (ref. = less than 1 year)				
1 year old	1.37 (0.91–2.08)	1.42 (0.90–2.22)	1.15 (0.63–2.11)	0.75 (0.28–2.04)
2 years old	2.69 (1.83–3.96)***	2.82 (1.79–4.46)***	1.28 (0.70–2.36)	3.82 (1.55–9.39)**
Male	1.76 (1.32–2.36)***	1.51 (1.08–2.10)*	1.07 (0.66–1.74)	1.01 (0.59–1.75)
Race and ethnicity (ref. = other)				
White	1.49 (0.88–2.52)	1.06 (0.56–2.02)	2.38 (0.98–5.75)****	0.95 (0.39–2.30)
Black	1.98 (1.03–3.79)*	1.68 (0.73–3.86)	5.19 (1.65–16.3)**	0.85 (0.24–2.99)
Hispanic	1.56 (0.84–2.90)	1.57 (0.72–3.41)	2.25 (0.76–6.71)	1.12 (0.37–3.36)
Nuclear family	0.81 (0.58–1.11)	1.73 (1.11–2.69)*	1.27 (0.72–2.26)	2.36 (1.13–4.90)*
Total children in household	1.13 (0.97–1.33)	1.06 (0.88–1.27)	1.22 (0.94–1.57)	1.09 (0.81–1.47)
Insurance (ref. = none)				
Public	2.34 (1.31–4.19)**	2.23 (1.03–4.81)*	2.02 (0.65–6.24)	2.01 (0.61–6.62)
Other	1.26 (0.71–2.24)	1.30 (0.60–2.79)	1.34 (0.43–4.22)	1.28 (0.40–4.11)
Region (ref. = Northeast)				
Midwest	0.81 (0.54–1.20)	0.72 (0.44–1.18)	1.29 (0.60–2.76)	0.40 (0.18–0.86)*
South	0.54 (0.36–0.80)**	0.45 (0.27–0.78)**	0.40 (0.18–0.89)*	0.42 (0.22–0.82)*
West	0.38 (0.24–0.61)***	0.33 (0.19–0.57)***	0.91 (0.40–2.06)	0.10 (0.04–0.23)***
Strong level of candidacy	57.21 (41.0–79.9)***	59.30 (41.7–84.3)***		
Observations		16,752	633	1,947

*$p \leq 0.05$; **$p \leq 0.01$; ***$p \leq 0.001$; ****$p \leq 0.10$

and multivariate logistic regressions for all children under the age of three and the two population subsets. (Blocks of variables are run in lieu of bivariate statistics where an independent factor has two or more responses in addition to the reference category.) Variable blocks are age (age 1 and age 2), race and ethnicity (white, black, Hispanic), insurance type (public and other), and region (Midwest, South, and West). Single-variable blocks (bivariate analyses) are conducted for male, nuclear family, total children in the household, and strong level of candidacy.

In the interest of parsimony, the number of independent and control variables is based on preliminary analyses. These analyses included fully loaded, forward stepwise, and backward stepwise regressions for the predecessors of the final models reported in Table 6 as well as equations to predict strong candidacy. To qualify for inclusion in the final models, a variable or one variable from the related block of variables had to achieve 0.05-level significance in at least one model. Several variables – household education, primary language spoken at home, foreign-born status, poverty, use of a personal doctor or nurse, having an examination or checkup in the previous 12 months – failed to meet the criteria in preliminary analyses and are excluded in the creation of the final models reported in Table 6.

RESULTS

The results clearly demonstrate the importance of the severity of conditions in determining the use of a therapist. In block analysis, children who are strong candidates for therapy are 57 times more likely to see a therapist than other children (OR = 57.21), and this relationship remains strong in multivariate analysis, which has strong candidates as 59 times more likely (OR = 59.30).

Region, the key variable of interest in this study, emerges as a source of disparity in two ways. First, the use of a therapist consistently declines with residence in the South. Among all children, Southern residents are 46 percent less likely (OR = 0.54) than Northeastern residents (the reference group) to use a therapist in block logistic regressions, and in multivariate analysis the gap increases to 55 percent (OR = 0.45). Among strong candidates, there is a 60 percent decline (OR = 0.40), and there is a 58 percent decline among speech-only candidates (OR = 0.42).

Second, among speech-only candidates, there is a decline in the use of a therapist in all regions of the country outside the Northeast. In the West, the decline in the use of a therapist among all children (OR = 0.33) appears to be driven by the decreasing likelihood of using a therapist among speech-only candidates, for whom there is a 90 percent decline (OR = 0.10) relative to the Northeast. The Midwest shows a 60 percent decline (OR = 0.40).

Other variables besides region are seldom of interest. Age and gender emerge as important among all children, but the significance of these variables can be explained in part as indicators of having the initial conditions triggering therapy. The only point where these variables are significant in multivariate analyses is the heightened likelihood of two-year olds to use a therapist, which can be easily explained by the missing of developmental benchmarks rather than disparity. Block regression reveals that black children are almost two times *more* likely to use a therapist than whites (OR = 1.98), but in multivariate analyses, this relationship holds only among strong candidates, where blacks are more than five times more likely to use a therapist (OR = 5.19). In multivariate analyses, presence in a nuclear family increases the likelihood of using a therapist 1.7 times among all children (OR = 1.73), due primarily to the increased likelihood of using a therapist among speech-only candidates (OR = 2.36). Insurance status is significant among all children, but disappears among strong and speech-only candidates largely because these subsets of the population are more likely to have insurance, in part due to public insurance programs.

DISCUSSION

In this analysis, regional variations in the delivery of therapeutic services are introduced as an important consideration in understanding disparities in habilitative therapy. Two aspects of this variation are noticeable. First, residence in the South is consistently associated with an unmet need for services. Second, among speech-only candidates, children in all regions of the country show significant gaps regarding the use of a therapist when compared with the Northeast.

This analysis does not uncover why these geographic disparities exist, but there are two points worth considering as research on this topic continues. First and most obvious is the weakness of the healthcare infrastructure in the West and South (see Fordyce, Chen, Doescher, & Hart, 2007). Second, these two regions are also home to large numbers of blacks and Hispanics, collectively known for their distrust and avoidance of medical professionals (Magilvy, Congdon, Martinez, Davis, & Averill, 2000; Armstrong et al., 2006; Stepanikova, Mollborn, Cook, Thom, & Kramer, 2006; Kennedy, Mathis, & Woods 2007; Musa, Schulz, Harris, Silverman, & Thomas, 2009). This distrust is often difficult to identify directly in survey research.

With regard to other types of social and economic characteristics, the presence of disparities appears less pronounced with children in early intervention ages than one would expect given the salience of disparities in the general population. In conjunction with this, the study does little to resolve the debate over the influence of race. Black children, rather than experiencing a decline in the use of therapists as expected, are found more likely to use early intervention than vulnerable children in other major racial/ethnic groups.

The absence of social and economic disparities should not be celebrated as the successful delivery of habilitative services. Quite the opposite, only about half of strong candidates actually receive therapy (Table 2). One key factor may be the inability to establish the treatment of delays and impairments in early childhood as medically necessary, a standard that usually must be met before early intervention services are offered. As a result, children are not recommended for therapy until after their eligibility for early intervention has passed, which in turn shifts responsibility for treating habilitative disorders to the educational system (Palfrey, Singer, Raphael, & Walker, 1990; Leiter, 2005).

Taken as a whole, the aforementioned patterns suggest that the fastest way to reduce habilitative disparities in the use of early intervention comes through targeting vulnerable populations geographically rather than by demographic, social, or economic characteristics. This is an important consideration as the American healthcare system is modified: Inasmuch as many vulnerable children are already eligible for early intervention, significant improvements in participation in pediatric habilitation may not be associated with universal coverage as much as they are tied to make it easier for families to find the appropriate therapists near their homes. For example, the problems of geographic disadvantage in general health have been overcome in some localities through the use of community centers or mobile clinics staffed with multidisciplinary teams of nurses, university faculty, and student assistants (Sherrill et al., 2005; McDaniel & Strauss, 2006). This structure can be modified to include therapists, therapy assistants, or interns and thus increase the overall level of pediatric habilitation for vulnerable individuals.

ACKNOWLEDGMENTS

I am appreciative to Denise Rogers and Mary Jo Cooley Hidecker for their comments and Chandra Walls for her assistance with the data.

REFERENCES

Angel, R., & Gronfein, W. (1988). The use of subjective information in statistical models. *American Sociological Review, 53*, 464–473.

Armstrong, K., Rose, A., Peters, N., Long, J. A., McMurphy, S., & Shea, J. A. (2006). Distrust of the health care system and self reported health in the United States. *Journal of General Internal Medicine, 21*, 292–297.

Ashiabi, G. S. (2008). African American and non-Hispanic white children's health: Integrating alternative explanations. *Ethnicity & Health, 13*, 375–398.

Barr, D. A. (2008). *Health disparities in the United States: Social class, race, ethnicity, and health.* Baltimore: Johns Hopkins.

Bauman, L. J., Silver, E. J., & Stein, R. E. K. (2006). Cumulative social disadvantage and child health. *Pediatrics, 117*, 1321–1328.

Beal, A. C., Co, J. P. T, Dougherty, D., Jorsling, T., Kam, J., Perrin, J., & Palmer, R. H. (2004). Quality measures for children's health care. *Pediatrics, 113*, 199–209.

Benedict, R. E. (2006). Disparities in use and unmet need for therapeutic and supportive services among school-age children with functional limitations: A comparison across settings. *Health Services Research, 41*, 103–124.

Blumberg, S. J., Olson, L., Frankel, M. R., Osborn, L., Srinath, K. P., & Giambo, P. (2005). Design and operation of the National Survey of Children's Health, 2003. *Vital and Health Statistics, 1*(43). Available at http://www.cdc.gov/nchs/data/series/sr_01/sr01_043.pdf. Retrieved on April 28, 2007.

Braveman, P. (2006). Health disparities and health equity: Concepts and measurement. *Annual Review of Public Health, 27*, 167–194.

Brooks-Dunn, J., & Duncan, G. J. (1997). The effects of poverty on children. *The Future of Children, 7*(2), 55–71.

Case, A., Lubotsky, D., & Paxson, C. (2002). Economic status and health in childhood: The origins of the gradient. *American Economic Review, 92*, 1308–1334.

Danaher, J., Shackelford, J., & Harbin, G. (2004). Revisiting a comparison of eligibility policies for infant/toddler programs and preschool special education programs. *Topics in Early Childhood Special Education, 24*(2), 59–67.

DeNavas-Walt, C., Proctor, B. D., & Smith, J. C. (2008). *Income, poverty, and health insurance coverage in the United States: 2007.* U.S. Census Bureau, Current Population Reports, P60-235. United States Government Printing Office, Washington, DC, USA.

Dick, A. W., Brach, C., Allison, R. A., Shenkman, E., Shone, L. P., Szilagyi, P. G., Klein, J. D., & Lewit, E. M. (2004). SCHIP's impact in three states: How do the most vulnerable children fare? *Health Affairs, 23*(5), 63–75.

Dubay, L., & Kenney, G. (2004). Gains in children's health insurance coverage but additional progress needed. *Pediatrics, 114*, 1338–1340.

Dusing, S. C., Skinner, A. C., & Mayer, M. L. (2004). Unmet need for therapy services, assistive devices, and related services: Data from the National Survey of Children with Special Health Care Needs. *Ambulatory Pediatrics, 4,* 448–454.

Fordyce, M. A., Chen, F. M., Doescher, & Hart, L. G. (2007). *Physician supply and distribution in rural areas of the United States.* Final report no. 116. WWAMI Rural Health Research Center, University of Washington, Seattle, WA, USA.

Gabard, D. L., & Cooper, T. L. (1998). Race: Constructs and dilemmas. *Administration and Society, 30,* 339–356.

Garcia, S. B., Perez, A. M., & Ortiz, A. A. (2000). Mexican American mother's beliefs about distress: Implications for early childhood intervention. *Remedial & Special Education, 21,* 90–101.

Gorman, B. K., & Read, J. G. (2006). Gender disparities in adult health: An examination of three measures of morbidity. *Journal of Health and Social Behavior, 47*(2), 95–110.

Guevara, J. P., Mandell, D. S., Rostain, A. L., Zhao, H., & Hadley, T. R. (2006). Disparities in the reporting and treatment of health conditions in children: An analysis of the Medical Expenditure Panel Survey. *Health Services Research, 41,* 532–549.

Haggerty, M., & Johnson, C. (1996). The social construction of the distribution of income and health. *Journal of Economic Issues, 30,* 525–532.

Hughes, D. C., & Ng, S. (2003). Reducing health disparities among children. *The Future of Children, 13*(1), 153–167.

Kelley-Moore, J. A., Schumacher, J. G., Kahana, E., & Kahana, B. (2006). When do older adults become "disabled"? Social and health antecedents of perceived disability in a panel study of the oldest old. *Journal of Health and Social Behavior, 47*(June), 126–141.

Kennedy, B. R., Mathis, C. C., & Woods, A. K. (2007). African Americans and their distrust of the health care system: Healthcare for diverse populations. *Journal of Cultural Diversity, 14,* 56–60.

Kenney, G. (2007). The impacts of the state children's health insurance program on children who enroll: Findings from ten states. *Health Services Research, 42,* 1520–1543.

Kolobe, T. H. A. (2004). Childrearing practices and developmental expectations for Mexican-American mothers and the development status of their infants. *Physical Therapy, 84,* 439–453.

Kuhlthau, K., Hill, K., Fluet, C., Meara, E., & Yucel, R. M. (2008). Correlates of therapy use and expenditures in children in the United States. *Developmental Neurorehabilitation, 11,* 115–123.

Kummerer, S. E., Lopez-Reyna, N. A., & Hughes, M. T. (2007). Mexican immigrant mothers' perceptions of their children's communication disabilities, emergent literacy development, and speech-language therapy program. *American Journal of Speech-Language Pathology, 16,* 271–282.

Landy, S. (2002). *Pathways to competence: Encouraging healthy social and emotional development in young children.* Baltimore: Paul H. Brookes.

Lanphear, B. P., Dietrich, K. N., & Berger, O. (2003). Prevention of lead toxicity in U.S. Children. *Ambulatory Pediatrics, 3,* 27–36.

Leiter, V. (2005). The division of labor among systems of therapeutic care for children with disabilities. *Journal of Disability Policy Studies, 16,* 147–155.

Leung, A. K. C., & Kao, C. P. (1999). Evaluation and management of the child with speech delay. *American Family Physician, 59,* 3121–3128.

Lieu, T. A., Newacheck, P. W., & McManus, M. A. (1993). Race, ethnicity, and access to ambulatory care among U.S. adolescents. *American Journal of Public Health, 83*, 960–965.

Magilvy, J. K., Congdon, J. G., Martinez, R. J., Davis, R., & Averill, J. (2000). Caring for our own: Health care experiences of rural Hispanic elders. *Journal of Aging Studies, 14*, 171–190.

Malat, J., & Hamilton, M. A. (2006). Preference for same-race health care providers and perceptions of interpersonal discrimination in health care. *Journal of Health and Social Behavior, 47*, 173–187.

Mandell, D. S., Listerud, J., Levy, S. E., & Pinto-Martin, J. A. (2002). Race differences in the age at diagnosis among Medicaid-eligible children with autism. *Journal of the American Academy of Child & Adolescent Psychiatry, 41*, 1447–1453.

Mann, J. R., Crawford, S., Wilson, L., & McDermott, S. (2008). Does race influence age of diagnosis for children with developmental delay? *Disability and Health Journal, 1*(3), 157–162.

Mayer, M. L., Skinner, A. C., & Slifkin, R. T. (2004). Unmet need for routine and specialty care: Data from the National Survey of Children with Special Health Care Needs. *Pediatrics, 113*, 109–115.

McDaniel, J., & Strauss, S. S. (2006). Development of a nurse practice arrangement in rural Appalachia: Trends and challenges. *Nursing Education Perspectives, 27*, 302–307.

McLean, L. K., & Cripe, J. W. (1997). The effectiveness of early intervention for children with communication disorders. In: M. J. Guvalnick (Ed.), *The Effectiveness of Early Intervention* (pp. 349–428). Baltimore: Paul H. Brookes.

Milgrom, P., & Reisine, S. (2000). Oral health in the United States: The post-fluoride generation. *Annual Review of Public Health, 21*, 403–436.

Musa, D., Schulz, R., Harris, R., Silverman, M., & Thomas, S. B. (2009). Trust in the health care system and the use of preventive health solutions by older blacks and white adults. *American Journal of Public Health, 99*, 1293–1298.

National Center for Health Statistics. (2005). *National Survey of Children's Health, 2003.* Public-use data file and documentation. Available at http://www.cdc.gov/nchs/about/major/slaits/nsch.htm. Retrieved on April 28, 2007.

National Research Council and Institute of Medicine. (2004). *Children's health, the nation's wealth: Assessing and improving child health.* Committee on Evaluation of Children's Health. Board of Children, Youth, and Families, Division of Behavioral and Social Science and Education. Washington, DC: The National Academies Press.

Newacheck, P., Jameson, W. J., & Halfon, N. (1994). Health status and income: The impact of poverty on child health. *Journal of School Health, 64*, 229–234.

Newacheck, P. W., & Halfon, N. (1998). Prevalence and impact of disabling chronic conditions in childhood. *American Journal of Public Health, 88*, 610–617.

Newacheck, P. W., Hughes, D. C., Hung, Y.-Y., Wong, S., & Stoddard, J. (2000). The unmet health needs of America's children. *Pediatrics, 105*, 989–997.

Newacheck, P. W., & Kim, S. E. (2005). A national profile of health care utilization and expenditures for children with special health care needs. *Archives of Pediatric and Adolescent Medicine, 159*, 10–17.

Ngui, E. M., & Flores, G. (2007). Unmet needs for specialty, dental, mental, and allied health care among children with special health care needs: Are there racial/ethnic disparities? *Journal of Health Care for the Poor and Underserved, 18*, 931–949.

Palfrey, J. S., Singer, J. D., Raphael, E. S., & Walker, D. K. (1990). Providing therapeutic services to children in special educational placements: An analysis of the related services provisions of Public Law 94-142 in five urban school districts. *Pediatrics, 85*, 518–525.

Perry, D. F. (2007). A missed opportunity: Categorical programs fail to meet the needs of young children and their caregivers. *Journal of Early Intervention, 29*(2), 107–110.

Rosenberg, S. A., Zhang, D., & Robinson, C. C. (2008). Prevalence in developmental delays and participation in early intervention services for young children. *Pediatrics, 121*, 1503–1509.

Ross, C. E., & Wu, C.-l. (1995). The links between education and health. *American Sociological Review, 60*, 719–745.

Roush, S. W., & Murphy, T. V. (2007). Historical comparisons of morbidity and mortality for vaccine-preventable diseases in the United States. *Journal of the American Medical Association, 298*, 2155–2163.

U.S. Department of Education, Office of Special Education Programs. (2008). *IDEAdata.org.* Available at http://www.ideadata.org. Retrieved on October 4, 2008.

Sherrill, W. W., Crew, L., Mayo, R. M., Mayo, W. F., Rogers, B. L., & Haynes, D. F. (2005). Educational and health services innovation to improve care for rural Hispanic communities in the U.S. *Education for Health, 18*, 356–367.

Smedley, B. D., Stith, A. Y., & Nelson, A. R. (Eds). (2003). *Unequal treatment: Confronting racial and ethnic disparities in health care.* Washington, DC: National Academies Press.

Smyth-Staruch, K., Breslau, N., Wietzman, M., & Gortmaker, S. (1984). Use of health services by chronically ill and disabled children. *Medical Care, 22*, 310–328.

Stepanikova, I., Mollborn, S., Cook, K. S., Thom, D. H., & Kramer, R. M. (2006). Patients' race, ethnicity, language, and trust in a physician. *Journal of Health & Social Behavior, 47*, 390–405.

Stevens, G. D., Seid, M., Mistry, R., & Halfon, N. (2006). Disparities in primary care for vulnerable children: The influence of multiple risk factors. *Health Services Research, 41*, 507–528.

Underwood, M. K. (2002). Sticks and stones and social exclusion: Aggression among girls and boys. In: P. K. Smith & C. H. Hart (Eds), *Blackwell handbook of childhood social development.* Oxford, UK: Blackwell Publisherschap. 27.

Van Dyck, P., Kogan, M. D., Heppel, D., Blumberg, S. J., Cynamon, M. L., & Newacheck, P. W. (2004). The national survey of children's health: A new data resource. *Maternal and Child Health Journal, 8*, 183–188.

Weinick, R. M., & Krauss, N. A. (2000). Racial/ethnic differences in children's access to care. *American Journal of Public Health, 90*, 1771–1774.

Williams, D. R., Neighbors, H. W., & Jackson, J. S. (2003). Racial/ethnic discrimination and health: Findings from community studies. *American Journal of Public Health, 93*, 200–208.

Wing, L. (1981). Sex ratios in early childhood autism and related conditions. *Psychiatry Research, 5*, 129–137.

CONSUMER-DIRECTED HEALTH INSURANCE VS. MANAGED CARE: ANALYSIS OF HEALTHCARE UTILIZATION AND EXPENDITURES INCURRED BY EMPLOYEES IN A RURAL AREA[*]

Cecilia M. Watkins, John White, David F. Duncan, David K. Wyant, Thomas Nicholson, Jagdish Khubchandani and Lakshminarayana Chekuri

ABSTRACT

Consumer-Directed Health Plans (CDHPs) are proposed as an option to control healthcare costs. No research has addressed their applicability in rural settings. This study analyzes three years (2003–2005) of healthcare

[*] No external support was received for the study. The authors have no proprietary interest in any product or service mentioned in the report. This study was exempt from IRB review.

expenditure and utilization incurred by two employers and a national carrier providing data from a rural state, Kentucky. The study included two measures of expenditures (health care and prescription drugs) and three measures of utilization (physician visits, hospital admissions, and hospital inpatient days). In general, the CDHP successfully controlled the growth of medical costs. These findings suggest that CDHPs may be a viable alternative benefit structure for rural employers.

INTRODUCTION

Healthcare expenditures in the United States continue to increase rapidly. It is projected that by 2014, total healthcare spending in the United States will constitute 18.7% of the gross domestic product (Heffler et al., 2005). Multiple factors have led to these increases in healthcare expenditures including population growth, medical inflation, and general inflation, as well as income, education level, and the demand for health insurance (McBride, 2005). As costs rise and the demand for health insurance increases, employers are expected to provide a stable or even lower share of insurance premiums. These problems are particularly great in rural populations, which are often underserved and must apply more of their income to healthcare costs with less coverage for preventive services, dental care, or drugs (Bailey, 2004).

Eberhardt and Pamuk (2004) found that rural residents have higher rates of premature mortality (before age 75), higher rates of death due to unintentional injuries, chronic obstructive pulmonary disease and suicide when compared to suburban residents. Both the most urban and the most rural areas have higher infant mortality rates and lower rates of health insurance coverage. Socioeconomic and cultural factors must be taken into account as these populations are studied. The most significant differences occurred between rural and suburban areas reflecting the need to include suburban as a separate category from urban for health research. Kronenfeld (2005) points out that low SES, racial and ethnic disparities and overall poor health outcomes can be linked to those that are underinsured and would be less likely to use preventive services. As noted by Meng et al. (2009) rural Americans are more likely to practice poor health behaviors, such as physical inactivity and smoking which can lead to higher rates of obesity, lung cancer, and other chronic diseases.

Rural minorities are at a greater disadvantage than rural residents in general, especially concerning quality of care, access to health insurance and utilization of dental services (Agency for Healthcare Research and Quality [AHRQ], 2005). Rural elderly are more often classified as "poor" and are more likely to be dependent on Medicare and Medicaid than urban elderly. Rural children experience fatal injuries at a rate of 44% higher than urban children (Wilhide, 2002). Rural women are less likely to have mammogram screenings or pap smears than urban women (Hard Times in the Heartland, 2009). A study conducted by Haas et al. (2004) suggests that for blacks, Latinos and whites, the racial and ethnic demographics of one's county of residence is associated with an individual's access to care, due to the social norms within the area that could influence expectations for health care. Residential segregation may also provide fewer economic opportunities, poorer built environments, fewer public resources, lack of adequate housing, more violence, and higher levels of pollution.

The cultural factors in remote rural areas have a significant influence on the health status of their residents. For example, Appalachia experiences dramatically poor health status compared with the rest of the country. Cultural factors that contribute to that status include reliance on informal communication channels (friends, family, and neighbors) instead of health professionals, a historical economic dependence on tobacco, religion as an "external locus of control" used for decision making, and geographical isolation. As a result of the economic and industrial isolation of America's rural areas many individuals/communities may be reluctant to challenge industrial pollution out of fears of the economic consequences (Behringer & Friedell, 2006).

Rural residents make up 20% of the U.S. population, but only 9% of the nation's physicians practice in rural areas (van Dis, 2002). Access to quality health services was ranked in *Rural Healthy People 2010* as the highest priority focus area for rural populations. These priorities were selected by state and local rural health leaders (Gamm & Hutchison, 2004). The general public also views access to care as important, especially when there is a fear of losing their own health insurance due to employers dropping coverage or raising the employees' contribution to premiums (Kronenfeld, 2007). The majority of adults, the working-age population, have no government programs to act as a safety net and protect them against the loss of healthcare coverage. Good jobs that provide healthcare benefits are critical for adequate healthcare access, especially in the current economic downturn (Kronenfeld, 2009).

A study conducted by Brems, Johnson, Warner, and Roberts (2006) revealed that healthcare providers in rural communities faced more challenges in providing care than providers in urban communities.

These challenges included limited resources, confidentiality concerns, overlapping roles, provider travel, training constraints, lack of access to services, language differences, and patient avoidance of care.

Rural areas are not only medically underserved, but also suffer from inadequate access to health insurance coverage, having large numbers of uninsured, and underinsured persons. For a variety of social, economic, and systemic reasons rural areas suffer high levels of health problems (Beck, Jijon, & Edwards, 1996; Johnson, Murdock, Hoque, & McGehee, 2003; van Dis, 2002) which are only worsened by poor access to health care and lack of health insurance (Gamm, Hutchison, Dabney, & Dorsey, 2003). Furthermore, while even those rural residents who have health insurance tend to have lesser benefits (Hartley, Quam, & Lurie, 1994), the cost of providing health care in rural areas has been found to be greater (Asthana, Gibson, Moon, & Brigham, 2003; Asthana & Halliday, 2004). These realities have resulted in the identification of increasing access to health insurance in rural areas as a national public health priority (Gamm et al., 2003).

The business sector of rural communities has not generally contributed much toward the amelioration of these problems (Morton, 2001). The contribution of employer-sponsored health insurance is limited by the fact that in rural areas residents rely more on small employers and these are the very businesses that are most likely to experience higher than average insurance premium increases (Scorsone, 2002).

The current economic downturn has resulted in rural jobs being lost at a faster rate than the national average, which in turn results in the loss of healthcare benefits. Since the beginning of the 2008–2009 recession, manufacturing in rural areas, which typically offer the best benefits, have loss nearly 5% of their jobs (Hard Times in the Heartland, 2009). Kronenfeld (2008) reveals that many health experts conclude that part of the cause of disparities in health and health care use in America are the vast amounts of economic inequality and poverty found in this country. Kronenfeld (2008) also notes that market ideology is the most important barrier to healthcare equity due to the market theory which supports that distribution will follow economic demand rather than need.

Health benefit programs have been attempting to offset some of the expenditure growth and a consumer-directed health plan (CDHP) is one possible strategy for doing so. CDHPs combine high deductible insurance for major expenses with a tax-advantaged savings account – such as an individual Health Reimbursement Account (HRA) or a Health Savings Account (HSA) – to cover routine medical expenses (RAND Health, 2007). A major goal of the CDHP is to reduce over-utilization of healthcare services, which in turn would lower healthcare costs. Research suggests that when consumers are faced with higher cost sharing, they will respond to financial incentives and consume fewer services in order to control their costs (RAND Health, 2007; Beeuwkes-Buntin et al., 2006). Also, it is assumed that this plan design will transform enrollees into better consumers of health care, aiding in an overall decline in healthcare costs (Agrawal, Ehrbeck, Mango, & Packard, 2005). Overall, the CDHP is based on the idea that if members are better healthcare consumers, they will use fewer health services and reduce total healthcare expenditures. Motivation for behavior change – reducing healthcare utilization – is encouraged by the employee's ownership of the initial funds of healthcare dollars contributed by the employer (Bandura, 1986).

CDHPs have received praise as well as criticism since they have been available as a health plan option. Researchers have looked into their effect on the quality of health care that individuals receive as well as the financial benefits CDHPs provide to employers and their employees in comparison to the traditional health plans that are provided today. A study conducted by Parente, Feldman, and Christianson (2004) measured the impact of a CDHP on an employer with more than 20,000 employees grouped into one of the three cohorts: HMO, PPO, or CDHP. They found that over the period from 2000 to 2002 the CDHP enrollees had lower total expenditures than the PPO enrollees, but higher expenditures than enrollees in the HMO after 2 years. Of particular note, however hospital admissions and expenditures did increase relatively dramatically for the CDHP cohort. The authors concluded that the CDHP was a "viable alternative" to traditional health plans (Parente et al., 2004). In a national survey, it was found that because of higher out-of-pocket costs, individuals in CDHPs were less satisfied than members of more comprehensive plans (Fronstin & Collins, 2005).

A major problem arises from decision-support tools that do not provide enrollees with adequate information concerning the quality of health care or cost of healthcare services. Paul Keckley, of the Deloitte Center for Health Solutions (2008) notes, "The trend seems clear: Most Americans will be paying a larger role in purchasing health services, either directly through individual health insurance policies and high deductible plans, or indirectly by using tools to make comparisons among doctors, hospitals, treatment options and insurance products." In addition, some argue that CDHPs favor risk-segmentation, resulting in a stronger preference for CDHPs in healthier people than in less healthy individuals (Tollen, Ross, & Poor, 2004). This could influence the average healthcare costs incurred by a subscriber of a CDHP. When employers offer a CDHP as one of the two or more options, enrollment in the CDHP is generally lower than in traditional plans. According to a 2005 national employer benefit survey, only 1% of U.S. employers offered an exclusive CDHP option, without any other traditional plans in conjunction with it (United States Governmental Accountability Office, 2006).

Despite mixed opinions, enrollment in CDHPs is on the rise. In January 2005, 3 million people were enrolled in these plans. By April 2006, the number increased to approximately 5 million (United States Governmental Accountability Office, 2006). In a March 2004 study nearly 75% of employers said they are very or somewhat likely to offer their employees a high-deductible health plan with a HSA by 2006 (Mercer Human Resource Consulting, 2004).

CDHPs have been under scrutiny, but research has not examined their effects in the rural setting. Both rural and urban families experienced similar increases in health spending from 2001 to 2002 (McBride, 2005). Dealing with these increased costs, however, presents particular challenges for rural communities. The rural economy consists largely of smaller employers and the self-employed. Rural residents are often more likely to have fewer health insurance choices, higher premium rates, or be uninsured (Bailey, 2004). For some smaller employers, implementing a CDHP may be the difference between offering employee health benefits or not.

This study analyzes the healthcare expenditures and utilization incurred by two employers in South Central Kentucky and regional data for Kentucky for one health insurer. One employer offered the CDHP only, the other employer offered a traditional managed care plan. An additional comparison used regional data from a national carrier in Kentucky for the years 2003, 2004 and 2005. Aggregate claims and enrollment data were obtained from the employers and reports released by the health insurance carrier. The study included two measures of expenditures (health care and prescription drugs) and four measures of utilization (physician visits, hospital admissions, hospital length of stay, and emergency room visits).

MATERIAL AND METHODS

The study population includes employees and their dependents enrolled in the healthcare plans offered by two employers during the calendar years 2003, 2004, and 2005. The two employers; Company A (a manufacturing industry) and Company B (a university), are located in South Central Kentucky. The South Central area of Kentucky is considered rural.

Company A's location is strictly rural, Company B is located in a smaller metropolitan area, whereas the regional data is a combination of mostly rural and small towns, with some metropolitan and urban areas. Both employers offered exclusively one type of self-funded health insurance plan to their respective employees. Company A offered a CDHP and Company B offered the traditional managed care plan. The regional data, from a national carrier, was comprised of mostly PPO data, although a minimal amount of consumer-driven and HMO data was also included.

The data for this study came from three distinctive sources; the CDHP data were collected from the manufacturer's health insurance service provider; the managed care data came from the university's human resource department; and the regional data came from a national carrier. Healthcare expenditures and utilization incurred by the respective members were analyzed by comparing claims and enrollment data. Claims data consisted of the total healthcare costs incurred per calendar year, in 2003, 2004, and 2005, including the deductible, co-pay, and co-insurance. Prescription drug expenditures incurred by the members were also analyzed. Similarly, an analysis of the total number of physician office visits, hospital admissions, and hospital inpatient days incurred by members was also carried out. For companies A and B, data were collected in the month of March, after the claims audit was done for the prior year. These helped to reduce errors such as duplication of entries and loss of claims data. Enrollment data were obtained from the records provided by the respective employers. This data included the total number of subscribers in each of the years, their mean age, and the ratio of males to females. For each year, gross healthcare expenditures were obtained by combining the total net pay medical, co-insurance, co–pay, and the deductible. This amount was divided by the total number of members to get an average per capita healthcare expenditure, which was compared among the employers for each of the years and from one year to the next for each of the employers.

The Kentucky regional data were obtained from a report provided by a national carrier located in Kentucky. Before the national carrier adopting a new data-reporting platform in mid-2004, all Kentucky businesses were grouped into three areas. Their new platform allowed them to break their data into five more refined areas, however, this did not happen immediately. Beginning in June 2004, as groups came up for renewal, they were rolled into the new platform. Consequentially, the data revealed gradual growth from June 2004 to June 2005 in the three new areas and a gradual decline in two. This was not real growth and decline, but rather limitations in the data.

Bearing in mind the issue of risk-segmentation, in an attempt to eliminate possible selection bias in this study, we chose employers who offered only one type of health plan to their employees. However, differences in prior health status of the enrolled groups could potentially influence healthcare costs and utilization. The data from the Kentucky regional area came mainly from private sector PPOs, with no Medicare or Medicaid data included.

Company A

Company A's healthcare plan had a 3-year average membership of 2,953, with a mean age of 31. The 3-year average gender mix for Company A was male, 51% and female, 49%.

This manufacturing company offered an exclusive CDHP to all of their employees. The members of this plan included the employees, their dependents, retirees, and the long-term disability recipients. The company switched to the CDHP due to the rising healthcare costs as well as to encourage their employees along with their dependents to become more involved in healthcare decisions. As a part of this plan structure, the employer established a health fund for each eligible employee.

When CDHPs first began, plans offered one account option: the HRA, but employers now have added three options that include health savings accounts (HSA), retiree reimbursement accounts (RRA), and a flexible spending account (FSA). An HRA is a source of funding that the employer establishes and solely sponsors, in which employees can use to pay for qualified medical expenses. Account balances can be carried over at the end of the year. However, it is company specific, whereas, if the employee leaves the company, the account does not travel with them.

The health savings account is a tax-advantaged account created to pay for medical care expenses. With this account, the employer, employees, and their family members (or any combination) may make contributions to the account. Employees can contribute to the HSA on a pre-tax basis. HSA funds can be invested for tax-free growth and withdrawals for qualified medical expenses are also tax-free. In addition, leftover HSA funds automatically roll over from year to year. Unlike an HRA, the money in an HSA is not company specific and is portable. Retiree reimbursement accounts are like the original HRAs, except they reimburse medical costs only after a worker retires. Employers create RRAs for active employees, and then only the employer credits the accounts. A flexible spending account allows an employer, an employee, or both to make regular deposits to an account through salary deduction. For employees, this money avoids both income tax and Social Security tax. Money in the FSA can only reimburse qualified medical expenses. However, unlike HRAs, HSAs, and RRAs, the balances in an FSA cannot carry forward.

In 2003 and 2004, the company offered one plan, an HRA with the option to elect an FSA. However in 2005, the company added a second plan option, an HSA. The amounts in the funds varied depending on the employee's family size. Aetna was chosen to be the third party administrator for this fund. As long as money was available in this account, it could be used to pay for 100% of healthcare expenses. Expenses above the deductible were paid by the employer for all in-network services. In addition to CDHP, Company A also made substantial changes to their wellness programs, which included providing financial incentives to their employees for filling out health risk appraisals (Tables 1 and 2). As is the case with many CDHPs, Company A offers a PPO network for enrollees in its health plan.

Company B

Company B's healthcare plan had a 3-year average membership of 2,835, with an average age of 35. The 3-year average gender mix for Company B was male, 48% and female, 52%.

This employer offered a traditional managed care (PPO) plan to all of their employees. There were three plan designs from which to choose when selecting from their health insurance option: Blue Access High, Blue Access Low, and Blue Access Economy. All three plans utilized the same network.

Table 1. An Overview of Company A's Plan 2003 and 2004.

	Employee	Employee+1	Employee+2 or More
Annual employer's allocation to an employee's deductible (this allocation is the first dollar coverage used)	$400[a]	$600[a]	$800[a]
Employee's out of-pocket expense (deductible)	$600	$900	$1,200

Notes: Employer pays for PPO coverage above the deductible at 100% with no contributions by employee and no co-insurance.
Above is the plan for the Health Reimbursement Account (HRA) with the option to elect a Flexible Savings Account (FSA) to fund employee's out-of-pocket expense.
[a]Includes $200 bonus for completion of Health Risk Appraisal.

Table 2. An Overview of Company A's Plan 2005.

	Employee	Employee+1	Employee+2 or More
Annual employer's allocation to an employee's deductible (this allocation is the first dollar coverage used)	$450[a]/$500[b]	$675[a]/$800[b]	$900[a]/$1,100[b]
Employee's out-of-pocket expense (deductible)	$650/$800[b]	$975/$1,300[b]	$1300/$1,800[b]

Notes: Employer pays for PPO coverage above the deductible at 100% with no contributions by employee and no co-insurance.
Above is the plan for the Health Reimbursement Account (HRA) with the option to elect a Flexible Savings Account (FSA) or a Health Savings Account (HSA) to fund employee's out-of-pocket expense.
In 2005, Pharmacy became integrated into the plan.
[a]Includes $200 bonus for completion of Health Risk Appraisal.
[b]HSA option.

The differences in the plans are the deductibles, co-pays, co-insurances, number of visits for certain services and out of pocket maximums, with Blue Access High being the highest coverage plan. This employer also offers an FSA as an additional option (Table 3). The PPO network for Company B is somewhat larger than that of Company A, but includes the providers in the Company A network.

Kentucky Regional Data

A national insurance carrier with a multiline of businesses in Kentucky supplied the regional data. The Kentucky regional healthcare plan had a 3-year average membership of 355,368, with an average age of 33. The 3-year average gender mix for the region was male, 48% and female, 52%. This insurance carrier offered a mix of HMO, PPO, and consumer-directed healthcare plans. There was a very small percentage of HMO and consumer-directed business, with the majority of the data coming from PPO.

RESULTS

Descriptive statistics for the three groups are shown in Table 4. The numbers of members were consistent throughout the 3-year period for

Table 3. An Overview of Company B Plan 2003/2004[a]/2005[b].

Plan Name (Blue Access)	Total Premium/ Month ($)	Employer Monthly Share ($)	Employee Monthly Share ($)	Deductible ($)	Co-Pay ($)	Co-Insurance (%)
High						
Self only	341.00 381.00[a] 390.00[b]	341.00 381.00[a] 390.00[b]	0.00	400.00	15.00	10
Self and spouse	593.00 638.00[a] 707.00[b]	341.00 381.00[a] 390.00[b]	252.00 257.00[a] 317.00[a]	800.00[c]	15.00	10
Self and children	503.00 546.00[a] 555.00[b]	341.00 381.00[a] 390.00[b]	162.00 165.00[a] 165.00[b]	800.00[c]	15.00	10
Self, spouse, and children	722.00 872.00[a] 881.00[b]	341.00 381.00[a] 390.00[b]	481.00 491.00[a] 491.00[b]	800.00[c]	15.00	10
Low						
Self only	341.00 381.00[a] N/A[b]	341.00 381.00[a] N/A[b]	0.00	750.00	25.00	20
Self and spouse	526.00 580.00[a] 690.00[b]	341.00 381.00[a] 390.00[b]	185.00 189.00[a] 219.00[b]	1,500.00	25.00	20
Self and children	445.00 487.00[a] 496.00[b]	341.00 381.00[a] 390.00[b]	104.00 106.00[a] 106.00[b]	1,500.00	25.00	20
Self, spouse, and children	721.00 769.00[a] 778.00[b]	341.00 381.00[a] 390.00[b]	380.00 388.00[a] 388.00[b]	1,500.00	25.00	20
Economy						
Self only	341.00 381.00[a] N/A[b]	341.00 381.00[a] N/A[b]	0.00	1,000.00	30.00	30
Self and spouse	464.00 506.00[a] 530.00[b]	341.00 381.00[a] 390.00[b]	123.00 125.00[a] 140.00[b]	2,000.00	30.00	30
Self and children	393.00 434.00[a] 443.00[b]	341.00 381.00[a] 390.00[b]	52.00 53.00[a] 53.00[b]	2,000.00	30.00	30
Self, spouse, and children	627.00 673.00[a] 682.00[b]	341.00 381.00[a] 390.00[b]	286.00 292.00[a] 292.00[b]	2,000.00	30.00	30

High, Low, and Economy are the three types of plans.
[a]Indicates 2004 adjustments.
[b]Indicates 2005 adjustments.
[c]$800 is a collective maximum deductible amount when covering more than just the employee.

Table 4. Member Characteristics and Outcomes.

	2003	2004	+/−	2005	+/−
Company A	2,994	2,945	−1.6%	2,920	−0.85%
Company B	2,702	2,790	3.3%	3,014	8.03%
KY regional	267,328	414,413	55.0%	384,362	−7.25%
Mean age					
Company A	30	31	0.7	31.5	0.9
Company B	35	35	0.0	35	0.0
KY regional	33	34	1.0	33	−1.0
Percentage of female					
Company A	48.9	49	0.2%	48.7	−0.61%
Company B	52.7	54.6	3.6%	49.9	−8.61%
KY regional	52	53	1.9%	52	−1.89%
Admissions per 1,000 members					
Company A	71	72	1.4%	81	12.50%
Company B	145	175	20.7%	152	−13.14%
KY regional	79	85	7.6%	80	−5.88%
Inpatient days per 1,000 members					
Company A	162	208	28.4%	223	7.21%
Company B	883	670	−24.1%	418	−37.61%
KY regional	342	366	7.0%	348	−4.92%
Physician office visits per 1,000 members					
Company A	3,393	3,420	0.8%	3,559	4.06%
Company B	11,739	13,125	11.8%	12,960	−1.26%
KY regional	3,120	3,295	5.6%	3,230	−1.97%
Drug costs per member					
Company A	$398.20	$402.42	1.1%	$475.09	18.06%
Company B	$371.28	$425.71	14.7%	$512.86	20.47%
KY regional	$280.49	$329.99	17.6%	$430.14	30.35%
Total medical costs per member					
Company A	$2,003.11	$2,131.00	6.4%	$2,378.53	11.62%
Company B	$2,058.53	$1,595.17	−22.5%	$2,142.38	34.30%
KY regional	$1,809.97	$2,129.38	17.6%	$2,413.28	13.33%

companies A and B. For the regional plan data, the number of members in the region for the national carrier increased significantly from 2003 to 2004 due to the change in the national insurance company's territorial reporting structure. A significant number of members were added in 2004, only to lose them in 2005. Owing to the structure change and the significant shift in members, the national insurance company's confidence for the regional numbers from 2003 is not as high as for 2004 and 2005 (Table 4). The average age and gender ratio of members is similar across the 3-year period for each of the three groups.

The data in Table 4 demonstrates similar patterns for the CDHP and regional data, particularly for the years 2004 and 2005, during which medical costs increased 11.62% for CDHP and 13.33% for the regional data. Thus, the cost increase was slower for the CDHP than for the regional carrier. This contrasts with previously reported studies which showed decreased utilization patterns among members of CDHP (Beeuwkes-Buntin et al., 2006). Given the strength of the similarities, it appears that the experience of the CDHP largely mirrored the experience of the traditional plan in the region. If this trend continued over a significant period of time, CDHP could be a major factor in cost containment.

The measures for utilization (admissions, hospital inpatient days and office visits) are shown in Table 4. For admissions and office visits the experiences of the CDHP plan of Company A were similar to the regional plan data. However, the strong year to year variation for Plan B contrasts with both the CDHP and the regional data. Speculation of the reasons for this variation cannot be supported by reliable data and will not be presented in this study.

Table 4 also shows total medical costs per member and total drug costs per member. The year to year variation in Plan B continues to be evident. Costs for Company A are rising slower than for either Company B or the region.

DISCUSSION

This study has several limitations. One is the short-time frame of the study. Three years of data, especially involving a new program, may not accurately reflect a long-term trend. Another is the small number of companies participating in the study. Although CDHPs are increasing in number, relatively few companies in Kentucky appear to have implemented consumer-directed health insurance plans and even fewer make their aggregate data available for research. The fact that the data available for this study were aggregate data means that it was not possible to partial out the influence of a number of potentially confounding variables that might have been of interest. This is an important limitation because racial and class disparities must both be considered to get a true picture of the challenges in equal access to quality health care (Kronenfeld, 2005).

Generalization from this study is further limited, not only by the fact that we are looking at two companies and one regional provider, but also by changes that occurred in the plans over the course of the study. Changes in the geographic region covered by the national carrier data and in services covered under the company health plans occurred during the course of the study. These are inherent problems in conducting research in real world, applied settings. As plans are adjusted, the data may change accordingly.

This study compares a rural employer offering a CDHP plan, another offering a traditional health plan, and regional health plan data. The rural CDHP experience was similar to the regional health plan data. The traditional health plan had significant variation during the period, which made it very different from both the CDHP and regional data.

As was the case in a previous study of a large scale CDHP (Parente et al., 2004), this study has also found evidence that for rural employers a CDHP is "a viable alternative." The present study is not offered as a definitive evaluation of the efficacy of these plans but rather as a first examination of their potential in rural health care. Many factors, including implementation methods, demographics of the employee population and consumer information could influence the success of a CDHP. This study should be viewed as one data point, as different designs of the CDHP are likely to yield different results.

Over time, as employees become more familiar with the CDHP, and as consumers receive better information which allows better choices, cost savings are likely to improve. In short, if, as Beeuwkes-Buntin et al. (2006) suggest, CDHP makes consumers more "prudent managers of their own health and health care" we should see slower cost increases as members make smarter choices with their healthcare dollars.

Taking into consideration the concern that efficient operation of a CDHP requires informed consumers, it is noteworthy that this plan involved a small rural company with factory workers. This contrasts with the population studied by Parente et al. (2004). To some extent, the present study, with a different design and population, supports their conclusion regarding the viability of CDHPs.

Future research on rural health insurance needs to address the realities of consumer choice in rural settings. The entire issue of consumer choice in the healthcare system has been underexamined in economic analyses of healthcare financing (Ryan, 2006). The difficulties consumers encounter in making wise choices among providers of health care and ancillary services may be even greater in the rural setting. Sources of consumer-accessible data may be fewer and the choices of services themselves may be far more restricted than in urban settings. Rural patients, for instance, cannot choose ambulatory surgery over inpatient surgery if there is no ambulatory surgery center in their area. Given the constraints of the local market, the fact cost savings were still evident in the CDHP is encouraging.

Our report is an attempt to open a professional dialogue on CDHPs for rural health. Our results suggest that they have potential in rural as well as urban settings. Problems with implementation and management of CDHPs will determine how successful they can be in any setting but may present special challenges in rural health. However, these findings suggest that CDHP plans may be a viable alternative benefit structure for rural employers concerned about the costs of providing more traditional PPO or HMO insurance plans.

Population health studies have determined that social status, income, education, occupation, and place of residence have more significance in life expectancy and health than the healthcare system does. Hartley (2004) points out that rural health in particular, when immersed in "traditional" cultures may have a health-enhancing effect, whereas cultural transition results in increases in stress related illnesses such as mental illness and poor cardiovascular health. He warns, however, that we should not reify culture into a "tacit assumption that rural culture is based on standard societal roles that have evolved out of an agrarian history."

CDHP represents only one of the number of potential ways to address issues of healthcare access for the rural population. Research on rural health needs to examine both individual influences such as education and attitudes and ecological influences such as the environment, culture, and health services (Eberhardt & Pamuk, 2004; Hartley, 2004). No insurance plan alone will provide the answer to the problems of rural health disparities, but a plan such as CDHP may contribute to the solution.

A study conducted by Probst, Moore, Glover, & Samuels (2004) concluded that a future of better health for rural minorities must include better surveillance by improved sampling of rural racial and ethnic minority populations. This would require a cross-sectional approach, which is tailored to local socioeconomic environments, with input from local community members. A broad multidisciplinary and multi-institutional approach must be included in data collection and healthcare research to insure that all population groups are accounted for and considered in policy development and reform.

REFERENCES

Agency for Healthcare Research and Quality. (2005). Health care disparities in rural area. *2004 National Healthcare Disparities Report.* AHRQ Pub No. 05-P022. Available at http://www.ahrq.gov. Retrieved on November 3, 2009.

Agrawal, V., Ehrbeck, T., Mango, P., & Packard, K. O. (2005). Consumer directed health plan report: Early evidence is promising. *McKinsey & Co. North American Payer Provider Practice,* 1–9.

Asthana, S., Gibson, A., Moon, G., & Brigham, P. (2003). Allocating resources for health and social care: The significance of rurality. *Health and Social Care in the Community, 11*(6), 486–493.

Asthana, S., & Halliday, J. (2004). What can rural agencies do to address the additional costs of rural services? A typology of rural service innovation. *Health and Social Care in the Community, 12*(6), 457–465.

Bailey, J. (2004). Health care in rural America. *Center for Rural Affairs Newsletter.* Available at http://www.cfra.org/files/Health_Care_in_Rural_America_0.pdf. Retrieved on September 22, 2008.

Bandura, A. (1986). *Social foundations of thought and action.* Englewood Cliffs, NJ: Prentice-Hall.

Beck, R. W., Jijon, C. R., & Edwards, J. B. (1996). The relationships among gender, perceived financial barriers to care, and health status in a rural population. *Journal of Rural Health, 12*(3), 188–189.

Beeuwkes-Buntin, M., Damberg, C., Haviland, A., Kapur, K., Lurie, N., McDevitt, R., & Marquis, M. S. (2006). Consumer-directed health care: Early evidence about effects on cost and quality. *Health Affairs, 25,* 516–530. Available at http://content.healthaffairs.org/cgi/content/full/25/6/w516. Retrieved on September 23, 2008.

Behringer, B., & Friedell, G. (2006). Appalachia: Where place matters in health. *Preventing Chronic Disease.* Available at http://www.cdc.gov/pcd/issues/2006/oct/06_0067.htm

Brems, C., Johnson, M., Warner, T., & Roberts, L. (2006). Barriers to healthcare as reported by rural and urban interprofessional providers. *Journal of Interprofessional Care, 20*(2), 105–118.

Deloitte Center for Health Solutions. (2008). Consumer-directed health plans: Current trends, emerging opportunities. Available at http://www.deloitte.com/dtt/article/0%2C1002%2Ccid%25253D182545%2C00.html. Retrieved on August 14.

Eberhardt, M., & Pamuk, E. (2004). The importance of place of residence: Examining health in rural and nonrural areas. *American Journal of Public Health, 94*(10).

Fronstin, P., & Collins, S. R. (2005). Early experience with high-deductible and consumer-driven health plans: Findings from the EBRI/Commonwealth fund consumerism in health care survey. *EBRI Issue Brief, 288,* 1–29.

Gamm, L., & Hutchison, L. (2004). Rural healthy people 2010 – Evolving interactive practice. *American Journal of Public Health, 94*(10), 1711–1712.

Gamm, L., Hutchison, L., Dabney, B., & Dorsey, A. (Eds). (2003). *Rural healthy people 2010* (Vol. 1). College Station, TX: Southwest Rural Health Research Center.

Haas, J., Phillips, K., Sonneborn, D., McCulloch, C., Baker, L., Kaplan, C., Perez-Stable, E., & Liang, S. (2004). Variation in access to health care for different racial/ethnic groups by the racial/ethnic composition of an individual's county of residence. *Medical Care, 42*(7), 707–713.

Hard Times in the Heartland: Health Care in Rural America. (2009). Health care and the rural economy. Available at http://www.healthreform.gov/reports/hardtimes. Retrieved on November 3.

Hartley, D. (2004). Rural health disparities, population health and rural culture. *American Journal of Public Health*, *94*, 1675–1678. Available at http://www.ajph.org/cgi/content/full/94/10/1675. Retrieved on November 3, 2009.

Hartley, D., Quam, L., & Lurie, N. (1994). Urban and rural differences in health insurance and access to care. *Journal of Rural Health*, *10*(2), 98–108.

Heffler, S., Smith, S., Keehan, S., Borger, C., Clemens, M. K., & Truffer, C. (2005). Trends: U.S. health spending projections for 2004–2014. *Health Affairs 2005*, *W5*, 74–84. Available at http://content.healthaffairs.org/cgi/reprint/hlthaff.w5.74v1.pdf. Retrieved on February 23.

Johnson, K., Murdock, S. H., Hoque, M. N., & McGehee, M. A. (2003). Racial/ethnic diversification in metropolitan and nonmetropolitan population change in the United States: Implications for health care provision in rural America. *Journal of Rural Health*, *19*(4), 425–432.

Kronenfeld, J. (2005). Health care services, racial and ethnic minorities and underserved populations: Patient and provider perspectives. *Research in the Sociology of Health Care*, *23*, 3–13.

Kronenfeld, J. (2007). Access, quality and satisfaction: Concerns of patients, providers and insurers. *Research in the Sociology of Health Care*, *24*, 3–14.

Kronenfeld, J. (2008). Inequalities and disparities in health care and health: Concerns of patients, providers and insurers. *Research in the Sociology of Health Care*, *25*, 3–14.

Kronenfeld, J. (2009). Social sources of disparities in health and health care and linkages to policy, population concerns and providers of care. *Research in the Sociology of Health Care*, *27*, 3–17.

McBride, T. D. (2005). Why are health care expenditures increasing and is there a rural differential? *Rural Policy Brief*, *10*, 1–8.

Meng, H., Wamsley, B., Liebel, D., Dixon, D., Eggert, G., & Van Nostrand, J. (2009). Urban-rural differences in the effect of a Medicare health promotion and disease self-management program on physical function and health care expenditures. *Gerontologist*, *49*(3), 407–417.

Mercer Human Resource Consulting. (2004). *Survey on health savings account*. New York: Mercer Human Resource Consulting.

Morton, L. W. (2001). The contributions of business and civil society sectors to rural capacity to solve local health issues. *Journal of Rural Health*, *17*(3), 167–178.

Parente, S., Feldman, R., & Christianson, J. (2004). Evaluation of the effect of a consumer-driven health plan on medical care expenditures and utilization. *Health Services Research*, *39*, 1189–1209.

Probst, J., Moore, C., Glover, S., & Samuels, M. (2004). Person and place: The compounding effects of race/ethnicity and rurality on health. *American Journal of Public Health*, *94*(10), 1695–1703.

RAND Health. (2007). Consumer-directed health care: Early evidence shows lower costs, mixed effects on quality of care. *Research Highlights*. Available at http://www.rand.org/pubs/research_briefs/RB9234/index1.html. Retrieved on September 23, 2008.

Ryan, M. (2006). Agency in health care: Lessons for economists from sociologists. *American Journal of Economics and Sociology*, *53*(2), 207–217.

Scorsone, E. W. (2002). The national health care debate impact Kentucky's rural economies? *Kentucky Rural Health Works Program.* Available at http://www.ca.uky.edu/KRHW/pubs/02sep_debate_impact.html. Retrieved on September 18, 2008.

Tollen, L. A., Ross, M. N., & Poor, S. (2004). Risk segmentation related to the offering of a consumer-directed health plan: A case study of Humana Inc. *Health Service Research, 39,* 1167–1188.

United States Governmental Accountability Office. (2006). Consumer directed health plans: Small but growing enrollment fueled by rising cost of health care coverage: Report to the Chairman, Committee on the Budget, House of Representatives (GAO-06-514). Washington: Government Printing Office.

van Dis, J. (2002). Where we live: Health care in rural vs urban America. *JAMA, 287,* 108.

Wilhide, S. (2002). Rural health disparities and access to Care. Presented to the Institute of Medicine Committee for Guidance in Designing a National Health Care Disparities Report. Paper presented at the National Rural Health Association, March 20.

SECTION IV
GENDER DIFFERENCES IN HEALTH AND HEALTH CARE

SOME CONSIDERATIONS REGARDING GENDER WHEN A HEALTHCARE INTERPRETER IS HELPING PROVIDERS AND THEIR LIMITED ENGLISH PROFICIENT PATIENTS

Stergios Roussos, Mary-Rose Mueller, Linda Hill, Nadia Salas, Melbourne Hovell and Veronica Villarreal

ABSTRACT

An estimated 50 million people in the United States do not speak the same language as their healthcare provider, and 23 million are considered limited English proficient (LEP). Federal and state laws mandate language assistance services, such as interpreting, to all LEP patients at all points of medical care. Despite longtime and widespread use of interpreting in healthcare, efforts to assure interpreting access and quality are now slowly emerging. An interpreter may be a family member or friend, a bilingual staff member, or professional interpreter. As with trends in other ancillary staff in medicine, the majority of interpreters are female. Research is not available to clarify how gender may influence the process and outcomes of care during an interpreted medical visit. This chapter draws from the results of a brief qualitative study on medical interpreting and published standards on medical interpreting to critically reflect on the role of gender during an interpreted healthcare visit. Recommendations for research and practice are offered to raise awareness of the interpreting process and how it may be influenced by gender. Attention to the role of gender during interpreted medical visits is important to improving healthcare and health for persons with LEP.

INTRODUCTION

Substantial evidence outlines how the gender of the provider and the patient influences the processes of healthcare delivery in ways that can influence medical outcomes (IOM, 2003; Bird & Rieker, 2008). What is discussed during a medical visit, how it is discussed, and how it is understood and applied directly and indirectly vary with gender. However, what is the role of gender when a third person must directly mediate communication between the patient and their provider? The rising urgency to address racial and ethnic disparities in health and healthcare has opened up a new area of inquiry in healthcare research: the role of interpreters in the care of persons with limited English proficiency (LEP) (Flores, 2005; Karliner, Jacobs, Chen, & Mutha, 2007). This chapter provides an early examination within this emerging area of research by outlining some questions and considerations on the role of gender in interpreted healthcare visits.

Since 1964, federal civil rights legislation has mandated language assistance services free of charge for all LEP patients at all points of healthcare (Chen, Youdelman, & Brooks, 2007). Constitutional amendments to address language access evolved over the past 40 to reflect the diversity in our country. Today, over 300 languages are spoken in the United States (U.S. Census, 2000). In the past five years, the U.S. population that speaks a language other than English has increased by more than 7 million, bringing the total to 52 million, while the LEP population has increased by almost 4 million, now at 23 million (U.S. Census, 2005). LEP patients do not understand English at all or well enough to communicate in English during a medical visit. Language assistance is usually in the form of interpreting, with someone who speaks English and the patient's foreign language.

Empirical studies since the late 1990s have shown that the use of interpreters can improve service delivery and medical outcomes for LEP patients (Flores, 2005; Karliner et al., 2007). Interpreters facilitate and enhance the process of care by improving patient–provider communication, patient comprehension of medical advice, provider prescription of appropriate medication, and patient compliance with treatment. Disparities in medial outcomes across various chronic and acute illnesses have been reduced for LEP patients by providing an interpreter. Despite the use of interpreters as a civil right and evidence-based practice, scarce research has occurred to understand and improve the quality of healthcare interpreting Karliner et al., 2007).

At the current time, anyone can interpret in healthcare without any oversight or accountability for quality by professional or governmental entities (Chen et al., 2007). An interpreter may be a family member or friend (sometimes a child), any bilingual staff within a healthcare facility, or a professionally trained medical interpreter. Most often, physicians, nurses, and other providers rely on bilingual medical assistants to interpret because they are widely and readily available, familiar with the providers and facilities, and inexpensive compared to external, professional interpreters. These bilingual staff interpreters are nearly always female given the longstanding dominance of women employed as medical assistants and related allied health professions (Wooten, 1997).

Given that gender and interpreting influence provider–patient communication, the gender of an interpreter likely is associated with variations in communication between LEP patients and their English-speaking providers. Research has not examined the role of gender in interpreted healthcare visits for LEP patients. This may be important given that the vast majority of bilingual staff who interpret in healthcare is female. Studying the influence of gender may also have value because it may clarify an ongoing debate about interpreter roles within the field of healthcare interpreting.

This debate is based on an assumed continuum of the visibility and interaction of the interpreter. On one end, some believe that the role of the interpreter should be less visible and more mechanical. In this view, interpreters are considered better if they are saying the exact language-equivalent words of the conversation and if they act in ways that they are not noticed (e.g., standing outside of the patient's and provider's view, using the first person "I" rather than "she/he said") (Angelelli, 2004a, 2004b). On the other end, some believe that interpreters should not and cannot only "translate words" but actually negotiate the meaning of provider–patient interactions. In this view, the interpreter is better when their role is more visible and acknowledged during the medical visit. Through their own understanding of the languages and cultures in the interaction, and through their own capacity to speak the languages and convey the cultural aspects of the interaction, interpreters may be creating a different (more accurate, more appropriate) meaning than the original words of the provider and the patient. An examination of the role of gender during interpreted healthcare visits inevitably confronts the tensions in this continuum in a manner that may inform how to assess and improve the effectiveness of interpreters in the elimination of disparities for LEP patients.

METHODS

This analysis of the role of gender in interpreted medical visits is informed by two methods. First, findings from the planning phase of a broader study on the role of interpreters are critiqued for the influence of gender. Given no prior evidence to suspect that gender would play a role in interpreting, this qualitative study was not planned to identify the role of gender. To our surprise, the topic of gender was unavoidable. Second, the focus group findings are examined in light of the National Standards of Practice for Interpreters in Health Care (National Council on Interpreting in Health Care [NCIHC], 2005) for circumstances when gender may influence recommended practices.

Focus Groups to Clarify the Role of Interpreters in Healthcare

Focus groups were conducted as part of the planning phase of a broader study to understand how interpreters may influence "shared decision making" between providers and patients in circumstances when medical evidence was insufficient for a provider to make the decision authoritatively. Shared decision making was examined for interpreted medical visits with Latino LEP patients at risk for prostate cancer. The focus group study occurred in one Federally Qualified Health Center (FQHC) in San Diego. Among the center's 72,000 visits per year, patient demographics include 17% Asian, 8% Black, 15% White, 56% Hispanic, and 4% other. Low income, large families, low educational levels, and heads of households who are often non-English speaking characterized the area population. Nearly all interpreting occurred through dual role, bilingual staff members (e.g., no family, friends, or external interpreters). Forty-five bilingual staff (five males) served as interpreters.

Three focus groups provided this study's data: one with monolingual healthcare providers (four females and two males) who have used an interpreter to communicate for LEP Latino men regarding prostate screening; one with Spanish-speaking Latinos (six males) aged 50–70 with a recent history of prostate-specific antigen (PSA) testing; and one with clinical and front office staff (four females and one male) who also serve as interpreters. Focus group scripts and questions were grounded in and derived from (1) the literature on interpretation, shared decision making, PSA testing, and Latino health; (2) review by "experts" in the field; (3) insights derived from audio-recorded medical visits for LEP Latino patients, one with and one without an interpreter; and (4) insights gleaned from an interview to pilot the focus group questions with a physician with a history of using an interpreter to serve LEP Latino patients. Focus group discussions were organized around three topical areas: interpreting practices, decision making, and prostate cancer screening with PSA tests. The focus group with the LEP Latino men was conducted in Spanish; all other groups were facilitated in English. A trained facilitator led discussion ranging from 90 to 120 min. The focus groups were audio-recorded and later transcribed verbatim in English; handwritten notes taken during the focus group were used to further clarify information from the recordings. All participants were assigned a code; focus group data (transcripts, notes, and surveys) were de-identified. Research activities were approved and overseen by the sponsoring Institutional Review Boards: San Diego State University, University of California San Diego, and University of San Diego.

Focus group transcripts were coded, and categories were developed for themes, relations, and patterns. Initial coding was conducted by one of the authors for all focus groups. Subsequently, three of the authors met to organize themes, generate ideas, and determine focused codes and categories to organize the results. Analytic memos were written to elaborate codes and categories. Analytic ideas were informed by the literature on language access and medical interpretation. In the sections to follow, we report on findings pertaining to interpreting practices and the conditions under which they are deployed in interpreted healthcare visits. We did not set out to explore the influence of gender on the interactional dynamics of interpreted healthcare encounters. Nevertheless, study participants seemed to reflect on gender-related issues during focus group interviews.

Critique of Gender within Standards for Interpreting in Healthcare

The National Standards of Practice for Interpreters in Health Care were developed by the NCIHC in 2005. NCIHC is a nonprofit organization led by and representing interpreters in healthcare within the United States. NCIHC has served to organize research and best practice, to facilitate conferences and educational workshops, and to advocate for the professionalization of the healthcare interpreting field. The NCIHC Standards of Practice guide interpreters and consumers of interpreting services on how to ensure high quality and performance. There are eighteen standards organized into six categories: accuracy, confidentiality, impartiality, respect, cultural awareness, and role boundaries. Each standard is written as a specific action or practice that occurs during an interpreted healthcare visit. The standards were examined given the focus group results to outline considerations for how gender may influence interpreted healthcare visits.

RESULTS

Focus Group with Latino Men

For some patients, the gender of providers and interpreters seemed to inhibit full and open interactional exchanges during interpreted healthcare encounters. One patient voiced being embarrassed when discussing male sensitive issues while in the presence of a female interpreter. He noted, "if it is a male interpreter you will tell everything that's about men. But if it's a female [interpreter], you cannot say things that you can tell to a man." Another patient experienced bashfulness when in the presence of a female interpreter, especially if she "is a pretty young lady." Other patients said that professional attitudes and behavior were more important than gender as barriers and facilitators of healthcare communication. One man recalled the ease of conversing with a care provider about prostate health in the presence of a female interpreter; he attributed his comfort to the fact that the interpreter was "doing a job." Another man shared that although he was initially uneasy during a health visit with a female care provider, he was quickly made comfortable by her professional manner.

Focus Groups with Bilingual Staff Who Interpret

Both male and female bilingual staff interpreters suggested that gender served as an impediment to their communication with male patients. One man commented that female patients occasionally appear discomforted by his presence. A female bilingual staff member recounted instances of embarrassment when called on to interpret during discussions of prostate health and during prostate physical examinations. Interpreters noted, however, that they oftentimes overcome and manage personal discomfort though the use of behavioral strategies. One female staff member said, "you can't make it look like [you are embarrassed]. You have to make it appear like you are in the most comfortable setting ever." When asked how she accomplished this, she said, "I distract myself." Another said, "We have to get the patient to trust us. We can tell them 'I'm here to translate. If you need anything, I'm here."

Focus Group with Healthcare Providers

Healthcare providers seemed to hold disparate views on the relationship between gender and healthcare communication. One provider noted that, from his experience, "women [patients] are more forthcoming than men" in discussing health issues. Another provider disagreed with this statement, asserting that it was the patient's "character," and not his or her "gender" or "culture," that determines how easy or challenging it is to communicate. On the influence of gender communication dynamics during interpreted encounters, providers seemed to suggest that gender had variable effects, as is evident in this provider's reflection: "It depends on the interpreter. Some female interpreters are just fine talking about [male specific health issues] and some are a little uncomfortable."

Considerations and Limitations of the Results

The findings and inferences in this study are drawn from a secondary examination of results from another study not explicitly designed to examine the role of gender. Thus, gender-related comments from the focus groups may be limited compared to studies focused on the role of gender. In our study setting, women comprised the majority of both the bilingual staff who served as medical interpreters and the professionals (physicians, nurse practitioners, and physician assistants) who provided healthcare services to patients. Interpretations may be limited to similar settings. The topic of the broader study, shared decision making for PSA test with LEP Latino men, had implications on male sexual organs and practices, which may have predisposed the conversations of the focus groups on gender issues.

DISCUSSION

This analysis of the role of gender in interpreted healthcare visits is intended to raise awareness of the issue of gender within a context that may not be readily recognizable. The role of the interpreter in healthcare is a relatively new area of research emerging from the need to eliminate disparities in health and healthcare related to culture and language. This study suggests gender can influence healthcare providers, bilingual staff who interpret, and LEP patients during an interpreted medical visit. The ways gender may influence the interpreted medical visit are examined within the context of the NCIHC national standards for interpreting in healthcare.

NCHIC Standards Category 1: Accuracy

The six standards within the Accuracy category describe practices that will ensure that parties assisted by an interpreter "know precisely what each speaker has said." Practices within this category include rendering all messages accurately and completely, without adding, omitting, or substituting, replicating the register, style, and tone of the speaker, and managing the flow of communication.

Gender may influence practices related to accuracy indirectly and directly. Accuracy may be affected indirectly due to nondisclosure of information by the patient, as when a male patient does not wish to say something to their provider through a female interpreter. This may be more likely when the topic of the visit regards gender-sensitive issues, such as sexual health and reproductive issues including family planning and malfunction of sexual organs. Accuracy may be influenced directly if the interpreter changes something that is said (through omission, addition, or other alteration) because they do not feel comfortable or may not know how to translate something. This may be because something is said in gender-specific manner (e.g., masculine or feminine slang) or regarding gender-specific anatomy and physiology (e.g., unfamiliarity with the prostate by female interpreters). On the basis of the emphasis on appearing professional among participants within this study, there may be times when the interpreter may change the words and meaning of what is said in order to appear more professional, such as by changing slang words for reproductive organized into their medical equivalents.

NCHIC Standards Category 2: Confidentiality

The two standards with this category explain that the interpreter must maintain all information interpreted in confidence (not discussed outside of the medical visit) and to protect private written information. The intent of these standards is to maintain trust among all parties. There was nothing explicit within our findings that indicated gender would influence confidentiality during an interpreted visit. However, concerns among male patients about not revealing certain information through a female interpreter suggest that nondisclosure may influence confidentiality. Overall results from interpreters, LEP patients, and providers indicated that professional conduct and appearance may be more important than gender regarding confidentiality.

NCHIC Standards Category 3: Impartiality

The two standards within this category aim "to eliminate the effect of interpreter bias or preference." First, one standard says "The interpreter does not allow personal judgments or cultural values to influence objectivity." Second, "The interpreter discloses potential conflicts of interest, withdrawing from assignments if necessary." The goals of these standards are clear, but the methods to attain them are not, especially when regarding gender. There is an assumption that patients and staff can readily detect their biases and act to prevent or reduce the influence of these biases in their interactions. In this study's findings, the female interpreters and male patients reported discomfort and embarrassment in discussing issues regarding prostate screening; some developed techniques to overcome these factors in their interpreting (e.g., thinking of something else). Overall, our focus group findings did not directly indicate a gender role in impartiality during an interpreted medical visit. However, attention to gender-related cultural values and preferences may be important in interpreted visits regarding family planning and reproductive care, as with a male interpreter and female patient from a culture where males are the decision makers for reproductive issues (COSMOS Corporation, 2003).

NCHIC Standards Category 4: Respect

Three standards reflect the need to "acknowledge the inherent dignity of all parties in the interpreted encounter." The standards indicate that the interpreter must use "culturally appropriate ways of showing respect," promote "direct communication across all parties" in the interpreted encounter, and promote "patient autonomy." In some ways, the embarrassment reported by male patients and female interpreters in the study's focus group on prostate cancer screening was respectful in a culturally appropriate manner – although it interfered with the interpreted communication. Other gender-specific circumstances in interpreted visits may be in greetings and introductions and how interpreters intervene to deflect or encourage more direct communication with the provider. In our study with Latino men, there were times that the patients explained their medical history or situation using longer stories rather than direct responses. In such situations, an interpreter would need to use a gender-appropriate manner to respectfully request that the patient answer more directly and avoid stories when possible. Age-dependent gender responses may be important regarding respect, as in how a younger interpreter may address and communicate on behalf of an older patient. As with our study, female interpreters younger than their male patients may find ways to modify what is being said in order to ensure a respectful conversation while maintaining accuracy of what is being communicated.

NCHIC Standards Category 5: Cultural Awareness

Two standards in this category explain that interpreters must aim "to facilitate communication across cultural differences." Often, there is an assumption that the main cultural differences are between the provider and the patient (as through the different languages they speak). However, there are cases when the interpreter may speak the language of the patient and provider but not be the same ethnicity as the patient. This is common with Spanish as there are many different ethnicities in the United States that speak Spanish. With regard to gender, attention to cultural differences between interpreters and providers may be related to differences in professional power, as might be the case with male physicians and female interpreters. Such differences may influence if the female interpreter avoids asking the male provider for clarification of something that was said in order to avoid looking less competent or inferring that the provider was not clear. The issues of respect discussed earlier also point to the importance of gender in cultural awareness. For example, our focus group results suggest that a female and male interpreter would need to be culturally aware of how to best discuss and communicate issues of sexuality other gender-specific topics with male and female patients, respectively. Cultural awareness may also be important regarding traditional medicines and cultural beliefs regarding health and illness. It is possible that if these are gender specific (e.g., menstruation and erectile dysfunction) that an interpreter of a given gender who is not familiar with these practices and terms would have challenges in communicating them appropriately.

NCHIC Standards Category 6: Role Boundaries

Three standards emphasize that an interpreter must "clarify the scope and limits of the interpreting role, in order to avoid conflicts of interest." These standards recommend that the interpreter "limits personal involvement with all parties during the interpreting assignment, limits his or her professional activity to interpreting within an encounter, and that the interpreter with an additional role adheres to all interpreting standards of practice while interpreting." The experiences within this study did not indicate that the interpreter's role was never acknowledged or made clear during the medical visit. Generally, it was assumed that the bilingual staff in the room that was not the provider was going to help the patient and provider to communicate with each other. Issues of personal involvement, professionalism, and interpreting to standards were not formally discussed. One issue regarding role boundaries did occur, but it is not clear it was related to gender. Usually after the visit when the provider left the room, Latino patients might ask the interpreter for medical advice for a decision for which the interpreter did not have professional training or authority to inform. Interpreters in our study did not appear to have training on how to address this challenge of role boundaries. Technically, the interpreter would need to search for and ask the provider to address such questions, a potentially difficult task in a busy clinical environment. It is possible that male and female interpreters may differ in their ability to identify and address such role boundaries with providers and patients.

CONCLUSION

The gender of the interpreter during a medical visit with a patient who does not speak English may influence the interactions between the provider and the patient in important ways. Professional standards and general habits of clinical practice tend to place the interpreter as a neutral party that aims to remain unaffected by and not affecting the interactions between the patient and the provider. The gender of the interpreter may not need to interfere with impartiality, cultural awareness, respect, and other aspects of professionalism within the interpreting encounter. However, patients, providers, and interpreters are likely to react differently because of the visibility of gender. Interpreting training should attend to these differences by teaching interpreters to be more aware of their own gender-related beliefs and practices and how to address gender issues specific to their culture and to medical culture (both Western and of their target ethnicity). Providers serving LEP patients should be educated on how to identify and address potential influences of gender in interpreted medical visits, possibly by selecting an interpreter that is the same gender as the patient when appropriate. Research on the role of gender in interpreted medical encounters may clarify the interactions of gender with other cultural factors (e.g., ethnicity, age, education, and socioeconomic status) and offer interventions to improve provider–patient communication through an interpreter. Increasing our understanding of the role of gender in interpreted medical visits can help improve future efforts to eliminate cultural and linguistic disparities in health and healthcare.

ACKNOWLEDGMENT

This study is supported by grant 63830 from the Robert Wood Johnson Foundation, S. Roussos, PI.

REFERENCES

Angelelli, C. V. (2004a). *Medical interpreting and cross-cultural communication.* New York: Cambridge.
Angelelli, C. V. (2004b). *Revisiting the interpreter's role: A study of conference, court, and medical interpreters in Canada, Mexico and the United States.* Philadelphia: Benjamins.
Bird, C. E., & Rieker, P. P. (2008). *Gender and health: The effects of constrained choices and social policies.* New York: Cambridge University Press.
Chen, A. H., Youdelman, M. K., & Brooks, J. (2007). The legal framework for language access in healthcare settings: Title VI and beyond. *Journal of General Internal Medicine, 22*(Suppl. 2), 362–367.
COSMOS Corporation. (2003). Limited English proficiency as a barrier to family planning services. Prepared for US Department of Health and Human Services. Available at http://029c7c0.netsolhost.com/Docs/FR-DHHS_FamilyPlanning.pdf. Retrieved on November 5, 2009.

Flores, G. (2005). The Impact of medical interpreter services on the quality of health care: A systematic review. *Medical Care Research and Review, 62*(3), 255–299.

Institute of Medicine. (2003). *Unequal treatment: Confronting racial and ethnic disparities in health care.* Washington, DC: National Academies Press.

Karliner, L. S., Jacobs, E. A., Chen, A. H., & Mutha, S. (2007). Do professional interpreters improve clinical care for patients with limited English proficiency? A systematic review of the literature. *Health Sciences Research, 42*(2), 727–754.

National Council on Interpreting in Health Care (NCIHC). (2005). *National standards of practice of interpreters in health care.* Available at http://data.memberclicks.com/site/ncihc/NCIHC%20National%20Standards%20of%20Practice.pdf. Retrieved on November 5, 2009.

U.S. Census. (2000). Available at http://www.census.gov/population/cen2000/phc-t20/tab05.pdf. Retrieved on November 5, 2009.

U.S. Census. (2005). American community survey: Tables S1601, B16001, 16005. Available at http://factfinder.census.gov/servlet/DatasetMainPageServlet?_program=ACS&_submenuId=&_lang=en&_ts. Retrieved on November 5, 2009.

Wooten, B. H. (1997). Gender differences in occupational employment. *Monthly Labor Review* (April), 15–24.

HIDDEN GENDER INEQUALITIES IN OLD AGE: EQUAL TREATMENT DOES NOT MEAN EQUAL RESULTS

Sally Bould

ABSTRACT

Inequalities in health and health care by gender for older adults are often hidden because much data concerning the older adult are not disaggregated by gender. Older women are more likely to have chronic diseases that disable but do not kill. Older men are more likely to have chronic diseases that kill but do not disable for long periods of time. A gender analysis is used to elaborate inequalities by gender in two situations. The first is that of post-hospital care under Medicare. The second is a detailed analysis of living arrangements men and women over 85 years in the community based on the U.S. Census data for 2000. Combined with a population health model, a gender analysis indicates unequal access to health care and well-being by gender as well as unequal control over the provision of necessary care.

A form of treatment of others is equal numerically when it treats all persons as indistinguishable, thus treating them identically. That is not always just. In contrast, a form of treatment of others or distribution is proportional or relatively equal when it treats all relevant persons in relation to their due. The latter produces adequate equality.
— Aristotle

INTRODUCTION

Gender-neutral approaches to health and health care, including service delivery for older adults, overlook the evidence that older women have different health problems and different healthcare needs than men. Aging for women entails different risks than for men. These risks occur not only in physical and mental health but also in access to medical care, services, housing, and income. This is why a population health model (Kindig & Stoddart, 2003) with a gender analysis is necessary to understand the hidden gender inequalities. The biomedical model has been based on an assumption of gender neutrality; if women are given the same health care as men, the result will be the same (Helman, 2001). In truth, gender-neutral approaches to aging issues often disadvantage elderly women, although many of these disadvantages are not obvious.

At the same age older adult women living in the community are more likely to be disabled in performing tasks requiring mobility and strength than older adult men (Wray & Blaum, 2001). Overall her risk of having two or more conditions between the ages of 70 and 79 was 61%, whereas a man's risk in this age group is 47% (Satariano & Popa, 2007). Furthermore, older adult men with a disability are more likely to be living with a spouse who may be able to provide help; only 44% of women over the age of 65 are married in contrast to 75% of men over 65 (Reynolds, 2007). In addition to a higher risk of disability older adult women are less likely to have someone to share household expenses and more likely to be living in poverty. All these factors negatively impact on the overall health and well-being of older women in comparison with men. How these key factors affect the overall health and well-being will be documented in two ways. First is a detailed examination by gender of the impact of Medicare, the public health insurance program covering persons aged 65 and over in the United States. In the example, the focus is on post-hospital care. The second is a detailed examination of the situation of oldest old men and women in the U.S. Census microdata of 2000. Special attention is to be paid to the role of disability as opposed to disease in the overall health and well-being of older adults. A gender analysis provides a detailed focus on the issues of women as distinct from men, and a population health model provides a context for understanding broad aspects of health and well-being (cf. Kindig & Stoddart, 2003), including income and living arrangements.

A GENDER ANALYSIS OF MEDICARE SERVICES

Current Medicare (public) and Medigap (private) health insurance in the United States is able to ensure better care for men than for women because the model of care is more appropriate for men's health needs than for women's. Medicare and Medigap policies are focused on acute care, and for the typical 75-year-old man with only a heart condition, this acute healthcare approach can provide what he needs. He is hospitalized for an acute heart condition, but he has no other disease or disability. After the allowed length of hospital stay for his condition, he is sent home where his wife can take care of him and make sure that he takes his heart medication. He is soon up and around and can get to the bathroom safely on his own. If the house or apartment has stairs, she can help him climb up and down. If his wife cannot manage his care, they are likely to have the economic resources to hire help in the home.

In contrast, a 75-year-old woman, who is hospitalized for an acute heart condition is also likely to have at least one chronic condition, usually arthritis. She typically lives alone, and when she is sent home, arrangements have to be made with neighbors and/or family members who often do not live nearby. She needs help getting to the bathroom because of her arthritis. Without help she risks falling and if there are stairs, the risk is even greater. There is no one in the home to make sure she takes her heart medication regularly, and she is not likely to have the economic resources to hire help. Thus, there is a difference between older men and older women aged 75 in their ability to recover from a hospital stay for an acute heart condition despite their receiving equal treatment for their acute heart condition. She is more likely to suffer a chronic condition and a disability; 51% of women over the age of 70 report mobility limitations, whereas only 36% of men report such limitations (Wray & Blaum, 2001).

Her recovery will depend a lot on the situation post-hospitalization. Family, friends, and neighbors will be critical elements of post-hospital care. In contrast to a man, she has a much higher risk of placement in a nursing home in the month following her hospitalization (Mason, Auerbach, & LaPorte, 2009). The man can usually be provided adequate rehabilitation at home with the help of Medicare in-home help as well as his wife. He usually does not need a nursing home placement because of his lower risk of two or more conditions as well as in-home support. Her rehabilitation will likely be complicated by other conditions, and the availability of in-home support is often limited. For her often the better option is rehabilitation care provided in rehabilitation hospitals, but Medicare specifically restricts her access to rehabilitation hospitals. She must instead go to a "nursing home" where she will be provided rehabilitation services but often in an atmosphere where those around her are not candidates for rehabilitation; an atmosphere of depression and defeat. In a one-year follow-up of surviving patients of hospitalization for congestive heart failure, Chin and Goldman (1998) found that the health-related quality of life was lower for women than men.

Living alone puts her post-hospitalization care at risk, including the supervision of taking medication. The latter is often critical because it is all too likely that she is taking medications for her other conditions as well. A possible side-effect of multiple medications is confusion and/or unstable gait. The danger of falling is even greater if there are safety issues in her home. Osteoporosis and osteoarthritis put older persons at risk for falls and limit the ability of bones to heal. These are diseases that are much more prevalent among women than men. For persons over 65 who had a fall accompanied by an injury, over 70% were women (Warner, Barnes, & Fingerhut, 2000). Falls, even without any serious injury, are a high risk for older adults living alone because lying on the floor for a couple of hours presents a danger itself.

The access to Medicare benefits for acute health care is more or less equal now (cf. Hawkins et al., 2009), but these benefits generally are more protective of the man's health and well-being than the woman's because her out-of-pocket costs are likely to be much higher; she is more likely to be suffering from a chronic disease that results in a disability such as arthritis (Kind & Carnes, 2007, p. 581; Butler, 1996). Recently enacted changes to provide long term in home care insurance under Medicare, the Community Living Assistance Services and Supports program (CLASS) could help, but the amounts provided for are better suited to the situation where there is a live in spouse or caregiver. Although this benefit will certainly be of use to many older persons who live alone, the proposed amounts are more suited to provide for respite care. Thus, at a high level of need, a woman is more likely to find this new long-term care insurance inadequate to meet her needs while living in the community.

DISABILITY AND GENDER

The biomedical disease model in healthcare research not only excludes issues like living arrangements and income but also is usually focused on a single disease or disorder, not on the combined effects of two or more diseases. A single disease is often the focus of health research; for older populations the focus in both research and service delivery needs to be more on the combination of diseases or disorders. A biomedical approach focusing on a single disease is generally insufficient to deal with older populations, especially very old women (Von Strauss, Fratiglioni, Viitanen, Forsell, & Winblad, 2000).

There is another important flaw in the biomedical model of research: the focus is often on the disease and not the disability. A limited biomedical model may even define disability as not a health issue; "disability does not necessarily equate with poor health" (Center for Disease Control, 2004, p. 10). This model of health reflects the narrow focus often found in the current health paradigm. Poor health is defined in terms of disease so that a healthy older woman who cannot go out of the house because her broken hip has not quite healed properly is still defined as healthy and not needing "health care" (cf. Iezzoni, 2003, Chap. 8 & 9). Not being able to get out of the house is a serious population health issue for aging populations. An older person who has cancer certainly has ill health, but cancer is not likely to be seriously disabling (1982 National Long-Term Care Survey quoted in Manton, 1986) except for a short period before death. The concept of active life expectancy or "disability-free life expectancy" or Health Life Years (HLY) is a critical concept not only for understanding aging but also for a gender analysis. A gender distinction is often overlooked in this discussion (cf. Robine, 2007; Crimmins, 2007).

Fries (1980) had been optimistic that the extension of life would be followed by a compression of morbidity such that disability would be limited to the months before death. This he calls the rectangularization of the life span. Thus far, however, the results have been mixed in part because life expectancy, especially among the oldest old, has increased along with increases "in the proportions of the population with chronic conditions" (Crimmins, 2007, pp. 114–115). A gender analysis indicates that it is the women who are most likely to get the long life, with limited compression of morbidity and greater risk of disability. Men have the advantage that their morbidity is compressed and their lives are more active until the end. However, they are missing out on the longevity dimension with a much greater risk of premature death. So the policy focus on achieving a long and healthy life would be very different for older men in contrast to older women. Current evidence indicates that disability prevention for women needs to take place before the age of 50 as almost one-third of the women aged 51–61 already have some form of mobility limitation (Wray & Blaum, 2001, Table 1).

Table 1. Living Arrangements of the Disabled Oldest Old by Gender for the United States in 2000[a].

	Disabled Men (%)	Disabled Women (%)
Living with spouse	58.9	22.1
Living alone	28.4	55.8
Living with other family	10.2	20.0
Living with nonfamily	2.5	2.0

[a]U.S. Census (2000) excluding institutionalized population. Data analyzed by author from the public use microsample of the U.S. Census (2000).

The evidence of Wray and Blaum (2001) indicates that the gender differences in disability may be more complex for the 70 and over population as gender continues to have a significant impact even after the major diseases that cause disability are taken into account. This is in contrast to the results for race. African Americans overall report more mobility disability and more activity of daily living (ADL) difficulties than whites, but once the major disabling diseases and disorders are entered into the equation, the significance of race disappears (Wray & Blaum, 2001). At similar ages, diseases that disable but do not kill more typically occur in women, for example, arthritis, hip, and other fracture, whereas diseases that kill but do not disable more typically occur in men, for example, cancer and ischemic heart disease (Manton, 1986; Rieker & Bird, 2005).

GENDER, DISABILITY, AND THE OLDEST OLD: 85 AND OVER

This very old population illustrates the most dramatic differences between the sexes. This is the population where the "male model of aging" is least applicable because of very skewed sex ratios (Tomassini, 2005; Bould, Sanborn, & Reif, 1989; Bould, 2007; Dunkle, Roberts, & Haug, 2001; Femia, Zarit, & Johansson, 2001; Smith, Borchelt, & Jopp, 2002). The U.S. Census (2000) provides detailed information on the living arrangements and extent of disability for persons 85 and over living in the community; those who live in nursing homes or group quarters are not included in this analysis. In the Public Use Microdata Sample (PUMS) of the U.S. Census (2000), there are four different questions referring to disability. Sensory disability covers "blindness, deafness, or a severe vision or hearing impairment." This disability is usually the result of the age-related increased risk of vision or hearing impairment. The second form of disability, which is common among the very old, is a mental disability that affects "learning, remembering or concentrating." This may be due to depression, but more commonly its cause is some form of dementia. In terms of a physical disability, there are two questions. A milder form of physical disability makes it difficult to go outside the home alone to shop or visit a doctor's office. The more severe form of physical disability is a self-care disability where the person needs help dressing or getting around inside the home.

In the microdata, there is a composite measure reflecting a response of "disabled" to any one of the four measures mentioned earlier. This composite measure results in the highest rates of disability. Women are more likely to report a disability. Of the 61,439 men over 85 in this sample, 64% report at least one form of disability including sensory impairment, mental disability, and/or physical disability. For the women, 72% report at least one form of disability. In understanding disability, it is important to understand the role of sex. Women report more disability not only because they are older but also because they are more likely to be disabled at the same ages as men. As this data covers only the noninstitutional population, it excludes most of the very disabled who reside in nursing homes or group quarters. This population is predominantly women (Bould & Longino, 1997).

Oldest old women are not only more likely to report at least one of the disabilities reported in the Census 2000 than men, they are also more likely to report a severe disability. A composite measure was developed to indicate an overall level of disability among oldest old men and women who reported a disability. At the highest level of functioning are those without any mental disability who do not have any difficulties in self-care or getting around outside of the house. Fifty-four percent of these individuals are women. Half of this high functioning group reports a sensory disability that does not appear to interfere with their activities of daily living.

A lower level of functioning is defined as a person who has neither a mental disability nor a self-care disability but is not able to go out of the house alone. Nearly half of the 85 and over group (47%) have this limitation ($N = 85{,}916$). For 18% of them poor eyesight plays a role. These individuals need either public services or extra income. In this group 60% are women. A similar level of need is defined by those who are able to go out of the house by themselves, have no mental disability but need a little help in self-care; usually this means help taking a bath. Often this service is available through the local public health authorities, although it may be means tested.

Although the level of functional disability is minimal, if the person does not get help, she is at risk of a fall that could very likely create a permanent disability. Only 7% of those have this level of disability ($N = 13,577$). In this group 76.7% are women. At 85 these women are also likely to be at risk because of osteoporosis.

Among the 85 and over, there are a significant number who have some form of mental disability, usually cognitive impairment. At a minimal level, these individuals need supervision to go out of the house ($N = 7,656$). There are also those with mental disability without any physical limitations, but who are likely to need help with managing money or medication ($N = 11,307$). The total ($N = 18,963$) is 10.4% of all those 85 and over. Of this group 65.2% are women. Although these individuals may be coping well at their current state of disability, their mental disability is likely to get worse.

The most severe level of disability are those who need both help in the home and help to go out ($N = 8,476$) and those with a mental disability who also have a self-care disability ($N = 23,049$). These 31,525 individuals have the highest level of need of those living in the community (17.2% of the total). In this group 73.7% are women.

Living with a spouse is usually the culturally preferred family arrangement in the United States (Chipperfield & Havens, 2001; Umberson, Wortman, & Kessler, 1992). There are many individuals who have a mental disability and are living with a spouse. A live-in spouse can often provide adequate care and supervision for the mentally disabled partner especially when all that is needed is help managing money and taking medications. A spouse can also prevent accidents due to forgetfulness such as leaving the stove on. For persons who have only the difficulty of getting out of the house, a spouse can often supply most of the assistance necessary. Even the most disabled may be able to live at home with a spouse. But while men with a disability are most likely to be living with a spouse, women with a disability are most likely to be living alone. Table 1 shows that disabled women aged 85 and over are twice as likely to be living alone as disabled men.

Although many of these very old individuals may get along fine, it is very likely that their disability, such as a hearing impairment, can result in a need for extra expenditure. There are excellent hearing aids but these devices usually require high out-of-pocket expenditures. Limited out-of-home mobility also generally requires out-of-pocket expenditure for transportation and assistance with shopping although groceries or drugs can be delivered for a small charge in some communities. A mental disability and a self-care disability require even more services. But women are much more

Table 2. Risk of Poverty among the Oldest Old Living as Married Couples or Living Alone[a,b].

	Men	Women	Total
Married couple household	9.2	7.9	8.6
N	(37,727)	(28,786)	(66,513)
Living alone	24.3	35.4	33.3
N	(16,693)	(68,478)	(85,171)
Total	54,420	97,264	151,684

[a]U.S. Census (2000) excluding institutionalized population. Data analyzed by author from the public use microsample of the U.S. Census (2000).
[b]Eighty-three percent of the 85 and older live either alone or with a spouse. A woman is more likely to live with other family members than a man. Very few of the 85 and over live with nonfamily members in the community ($N = 3,724$).

likely to have low income than men. Furthermore, it is the woman over 85 years living alone who has a very high probability of having a near-poor income, an income which is below 125% of the U.S. Official Poverty Line. This measure is roughly equivalent to the relative measure of poverty of less than 50% of the average income, which has been used in the European Union (Smeeding, 2008). Table 2 shows the proportion of those married and those living alone over 85 years who have below a near-poor income. Both men and women who are married are at less than 10% risk of near-poverty, but both men and women who live alone face a high risk of near-poverty, with women living alone at the highest risk. Women, however, are disadvantaged because they are the ones most likely to live alone and risk near poverty. Furthermore, the near-poverty budget does not allow for any extra expenditure to pay for devices and services that a disabled woman or man may need, especially when living alone.

THE NEED FOR A GENDER ANALYSIS

The gender analysis of Medicare services and the oldest old presented earlier represents an approach that requires three elements (cf. Overholt, Cloud, Anderson, & Austin, 1991). The first element is to clearly identify gender differences. For older adults this means a specific focus on physical and mental health, diseases and disorders as well as disabilities by gender. The second element is access by gender. Although access to acute care may be equal for men and women, access to long-term care is not; older men are more likely to have a wife to provide such informal care, more likely to have private insurance and/or cash available for such care; they are less likely to need a nursing home. The third element is control over resources by gender. This is a critical aspect of a gender analysis. For example, older adults who must use the means tested Medicaid program are extremely limited in the amount of assets they can keep. In addition, like all programs for the poor, this program puts the individual in a vulnerable situation. First, access to doctors is limited by the doctors' willingness to accept low levels of payment for services. Second, because each state must contribute significantly to this federal–state program, funding is often reduced due to state budgetary requirements. States like California that provided good Medicaid in-home care find that this is an area that they can cut in the current recession. Women, however, are more likely to need help from Medicaid; men are more likely to live in households that have more income available to pay for the health services they need. Control is now recognized as an important aspect of health care in the efforts to provide "consumer directed services;" the new long-term care public insurance plan (CLASS) provides cash, not services, to give the recipient more control over who is hired for in-home care.

The issue of cash is especially important in market-friendly countries like the United States (cf. Myer & Herd, 2007). Income to pay for out-of-pocket health care provides the older adult with some control. For example dental care is not covered by Medicare and is most likely to require out-of-pocket costs. In the *State of Aging and Health* (Center for Disease Control, 2004, www.cdc.gov/aging), there is a call to action on improving oral health for the elderly, including the need for professional oral health care. But the cost of dental visits is very high. Older unmarried women are likely to need dental care but not able to pay for it out-of-pocket. Even if they are eligible for assistance under Medicaid, there will be very few dentists willing to provide the service. Persons who can pay for health services are able to exert some control over those services. For example, older adults with higher income and at least one IADL or ADL difficulty are more likely to receive paid in-home services (Johnson, 2008).

Increasing life expectancy results in older adults from poorer backgrounds living longer. When life expectancy at birth was low, primarily individuals of a high social class lived to a ripe old age (cf. Wilkinson, 1999). This did not create a problem of "old age" because these persons had the economic resources to provide for their own care, and the time of disability was limited. Furthermore, these economic recourses of the well-off or even middle-class families were adequate to hire low-cost in-home help, if needed (cf. Judt, 2010). The increase in life expectancy of the past 50 years means that more and more persons with limited economic resources are living into their 80s; at the same time their risk of disability is high and the cost of private in-home help is beyond the reach of most very old adults and their children.

Income, of course, is only one determinant of population health. The population health model outlines the multiple determinants of health and well-being outcomes. These multiple determinants "include medical care, public health interventions, aspects of the social environment (income, education, social support, culture) and the physical environment, genetics and individual behavior" (Kindig & Stoddart, 2003, p. 282; see also Boufford & Lee, 2001; Maclean, Plotnikoff, & Moyer, 2000; McCubbin & Labonte, 2002; Lee & Paxman, 1997). The importance of income, however, is increased by the extent that market-based services are critical aspects of a nation's policy for assisting older adults (cf. Myer & Herd, 2007) and by the extent to which older women's income past age 65 is lower relative to men's (Bould, Longino, & Worley, 1997).

BRINGING GENDER INTO THE POLICY ANALYSIS

To develop more appropriate healthcare policies for older adults, it is important to begin to understand the need for data disaggregated by gender. The approach of geriatrics and gerontology must move from the concept of "the older adult" to the older man or the older woman. The lack of gender disaggregation results in misleading or inaccurate statements. For example a 2004 report on the *State of Aging and Health in America* (Center for Disease Control, 2004, p. 10, www.cdc.gov/aging/pdf) discusses increasing mental distress with age; although the figure for distress is broken down by race and ethnicity, there is no breakdown by gender. In fact, it is women, not men, who are reporting much higher levels of depressive symptoms, and these symptoms increase with age as well as disability (Bould, 2005; Penninx, 2006; Zeiss, Lewinshon, Rohde, & Seeley, 1996).

The critical mental health issue of suicide provides an example of how the gender neutral model of aging results in misplaced policy emphasis. Consider the statement "Adults over 65 have the highest suicide rate, and among those elders who commit suicide 73% use a gun" (Yoder, 2003). This gender-neutral statement suggests a gender-neutral approach of looking for the presence of guns in the homes of elders. Elderly women, however, would generally be shocked if one asked the question, "do you have a gun in the house?" Individual suicide data in the United States show that over 86% of all elderly suicides are by men, and the suicide rate for men rises throughout old age (Coren & Hewitt, 1999; for Denmark see Erlangsen, Bille-Brahe, & Jeune, 2003). The vast majority of elderly suicides are white men; the men also have the guns (Osgood & Malkin, 1997). Age-adjusted rate of suicide for men over 65 in 2002 in the United States was "nearly 3 times higher than the national rate, whereas the rate for older women was less than half the national rate" (Cohen & Kim, 2007, p. 545). The development of appropriate suicide prevention policies requires the careful examination of the situation of elderly men separately from the situation of elderly women.

An additional problem in understanding the role of gender is that with increasing age a random sample of older adults becomes disproportionately female. Although random samples of 60- to 65-year olds usually contain similar proportions of men and women, this is not the case for samples of 85- to 90-year olds. It follows that part of the changes in the overall situation of the elderly during these years may not be due to aging, but due to the population of older adults becoming predominantly female. The rates of disability and depression increase with age partly because men who are less likely to report these disorders are more likely to have died. What is attributed to "aging" may more accurately be attributed, in part, to the higher mortality rates among men. It should also be noted that random samples of the 70 years and over population generally exclude the institutional population. A significant minority of those 85 years and over live in institutions.

One example of the problems created by a gender-neutral approach is the interpretation of evidence that the elderly lose strength as they age. This musculoskeletal problem is often put in terms of growing old and growing weak. A measure of strength appropriate to the elderly is the measure of being able to lift 10 pounds and to push a piece of furniture across the room. According to this measure, 20 percent of men aged 51–61 have problems with these activities [Health and Retirement Survey (HRS)] but for men over 70 only 28 percent have problems with these activities [Asset and Health Dynamics Among the Oldest Old (AHEAD)] (Wray & Blaum, 2001). These results indicate that the vast majority of men are not losing this minimal strength as they grow older.

The picture, however, is very different when women's strength is examined. Forty-four percent of women aged 51–61 already have difficulty with either lifting 10 pounds or pushing a piece of furniture (HRS survey) and by age 70 and over half (57%) of women have difficulty in this area

(AHEAD survey) (Wray & Blaum, 2001). Unlike men, women do lose a significant amount of strength as they grow older such that in the 70 and older group a majority of women may need help with everyday tasks such as laundry.

A gendered understanding can produce a more sophisticated policy approach. But the process of losing strength for women begins before age 50; many women have already lost this strength before reaching midlife. Without careful attention to gender it appears that there is a large loss of strength with age, but this is, in part, an artifact of the fact that men who are less likely to lose strength as they grow order are less likely to live into advanced old age. Furthermore, for women but not men, strength limitations are correlated with a high body mass index (Wray & Blaum, 2001). That older women need to lose weight, of course, is widely recognized, but what may be overlooked is their need for upper body strengthening exercise before midlife.

CONCLUSION

Women have a different pattern of diseases and disorders than men and are more likely to have two or more diseases and more severe disabilities at similar ages than men. Women are more likely to need long-term care but are less likely to have access to long-term care services in the community provided by a spouse, an insurance company, or a paid caregiver. In addition, the woman's control of the services she gets is likely to be limited because she is more likely to be dependent on publicly provided services for low-income older adults. These issues all come together in the examination of the situation of those 85 years and over.

A population health model with a gender analysis is necessary to understand not only the diseases, disorders, and disabilities of the older population but also the factors that can ease or exacerbate these conditions. Using this approach it is possible to identify hidden gender inequalities in current policies in addition to a tendency to combine results into the category of gender-neutral older adults. A long life with greater risk of many disabled years, while living alone on a limited income, is not an encouraging prospect for women or for governments. There are projections that men's life expectancy will increase over the next 40 years bringing the ratio of women to men over 85 years down to 1.7 to 1.0 from 2.4 to 1.0 in 2000 (Reynolds, 2007). But for women's high risk of disability, there are no optimistic projections (cf. Crimmins, 2007; Thorpe, Ogden, & Galactionova, 2010).

A population health model indicates that for older women the focus should be on disability alleviation and long-term care in the community. New provisions for community long-term care provided by CLASS, however, are not likely to be adequate for very disabled older women living alone. For women, furthermore, disability prevention needs to be targeted at midlife or earlier. The promise of longevity for women should not turn into more years in a nursing home.

ACKNOWLEDGMENT

The author thanks Daniel M. Fox for his helpful comments.

REFERENCES

Boufford, J. I., & Lee, P. R. (2001). *Health policies for the 21st century* (p. 36). New York: Milbank Memorial Fund.

Bould, S. (2005). A population health perspective on disability and depression among elderly men and women. *Journal of Aging and Social Policy, 17*, 7–25.

Bould, S. (2007). Oldest old. In: K. Markides (Ed.), *Encyclopedia of health and aging* (pp. 436–438). Thousand Oaks, CA: Sage Publications.

Bould, S., & Longino, C. F., Jr. (1997). Women survivors: The oldest old. In: J. M. Coyle (Ed.), *Handbook on women and aging*. Westport, CT: Greenwood Press.

Bould, S., Longino, C. F., & Worley, A. (1997). Oldest old women: Endangered by government cutbacks? *International Journal of Sociology and Social Policy, 17*, 223–237.

Butler, R. N. (1996). On behalf of older women. *New England Journal of Medicine, 334*, 794–796.

Bould, S., Sanborn, B., & Reif, L. (1989). *Eighty-five plus: The oldest old*. Belmont, CA: Wadsworth.

Center for Disease Control. (2004). *The state of aging and health in America 2004* Atlanta. Available at http://www.cdc.gov/aging/pdf/State_of_Aging_and_Health_in_America

Chin, M. H., & Goldman, L. (1998). Gender differences in 1-year survival and quality of life among patients admitted with congestive heart failure. *Medical Care, 36*(7), 1033–1046.

Chipperfield, J. G., & Havens, B. (2001). Gender differences in the relationship between marital status transitions and life satisfaction in later life. *Journal of Gerontology: Psychological Sciences, 56B*(3), 176–186.

Cohen, D., & Kim, S. H. (2007). Suicide and the elderly. In: K. Markides (Ed.), *Encyclopedia of health and aging* (pp. 545–548). Thousand Oaks, CA: Sage Publications.

Coren, S., & Hewitt, P. L. (1999). Sex differences in elderly suicide rates: Some predictive factors. *Aging and Mental Health, 3*, 112–118.

Crimmins, E. M. (2007). Compression of morbidity. In: K. Markides (Ed.), *Encyclopedia of health and aging* (pp. 114–115). Thousand Oaks, CA: Sage Publications.

Dunkle, R., Roberts, B., & Haug, M. (2001). *The oldest old in everyday life*. New York: Springer Publishing Co.
Erlangsen, A., Bille-Brahe, U., & Jeune, B. (2003). Differences in suicide between the old and the oldest old. *Journal of Gerontology: Social Sciences, 58B*(5), S314–S322.
Femia, E. E., Zarit, S. H., & Johansson, B. (2001). The disablement process in very late life: A study of the oldest-old in Sweden. *The Journals of Gerontology, Series B, 56*(1), P12–P23.
Fries, J. F. (1980). Aging, natural death, and the compression of morbidity. *The New England Journal of Medicine, 300,* 130–135.
Hawkins, K. R., Hamilton Escoto, K., Ozminkowski, R. J., Bhattarai, G. R., Marshall, J. K., Harbin, H. T., & Migliori, R. J. (2009). Disparities in coronary artery disease care among insureds with AARP Medicare supplement coverage. *Newsletter of the Gerontological Society of America*, December.
Helman, C. (2001). *Culture, health and illness*. London: Arnold, Hodder Headline Group.
Iezzoni, L. I. (2003). *When walking fails*. Berkeley: University of California Press.
Johnson, R. W. (2008). Choosing between paid elder care and unpaid help from adult children. In: M. E. Szinovacz & A. Davey (Eds), *Caregiving contexts*. New York: Springer Publishing Company.
Judt, T. (2010). Bedder. *The New York Review of Books*, February 11, pp. 41–42.
Kind, A. J. H., & Carnes, M. (2007). Women's health. In: K. S. Markides (Ed.), *Encyclopedia of health and aging* (pp. 579–581). Thousand Oaks, CA: Sage Publications.
Kindig, D., & Stoddart, G. (2003). Models for population health: What is population health? *American Journal of Public Health, 93*(3), 380–383.
Lee, P., & Paxman, D. (1997). Reinventing public health. *Annual Review of Public Health, 18,* 1–35.
Maclean, L. M., Plotnikoff, R. C., & Moyer, A. (2000). Transdisciplinary work with psychology from a population health perspective: An illustration. *Journal of Health Psychology, 5,* 173–181.
Manton, K. G. (1986). Past and future life expectancy increases at later ages. *Journal of Gerontology, 41*(5), 672–681.
Mason, S. E., Auerbach, C., & LaPorte, H. H. (2009). From hospital to nursing facility: Factors influencing decisions. *Health and Social Work, 34*(1), 8–15.
McCubbin, M., & Labonte, R. (2002). Toward psychosocial theory for an integrated understanding of the health and well-being of populations. *Ethical Human Sciences and Services, 4,* 47–61.
Myer, M. H., & Herd, P. (2007). *Market friendly or family friendly? The state and gender inequality in old age*. New York: Russell Sage Foundation.
Osgood, N. J., & Malkin, M. J. (1997). Suicidal behavior in middle-aged and older women. In: J. M. Coyle (Ed.), *Handbook on women and aging* (pp. 191–209). Westport, CT: Greenwood Press.
Overholt, C. A., Cloud, K., Anderson, M. B., & Austin, J. E. (1991). Gender analysis framework. In: A. Rao, M. B. Anderson & C. A. Overholt (Eds), *Gender analysis in development planning*. West Hartford, CT: Kumarian Press.
Penninx, B. W. J. H. (2006). Women's aging and depression. In: C. L. M. Keyes & S. H. Goodman (Eds), *Women and depression* (pp. 129–144). New York: Cambridge University Press.
Reynolds, S. L. (2007). The demography of aging. In: K. S. Markides (Ed.), *Encyclopedia of health and aging* (pp. 140–145). Thousand Oaks, CA: Sage Publications.

Rieker, P. P., & Bird, C. E. (2005). Rethinking gender differences in health: Why we need to integrate social and biological perspectives. *Journal of Gerontology: Social Sciences, 60B*(Special Issue II, October), 40–47.

Robine, J. (2007). Active life expectancy. In: K. Markides (Ed.), *Encyclopedia of health and aging* (pp. 2–4). Thousand Oaks, CA: Sage Publications.

Satariano, W. A., & Popa, M. (2007). Multiple morbidity and comorbidity. In: K. Markides (Ed.), *Encyclopedia of health and aging* (pp. 393–395). Thousand Oaks, CA: Sage Publications.

Smeeding, T. M. (2008). The U.S. still has much poverty, far more than comparable countries, like the U.K. *Pathways* (Winter), 3–5. Center for the Study of Poverty and Inequality, Stanford University, Stanford, CA.

Smith, J., Borchelt, M., & Jopp, D. (2002). Health and well-being in the young old and the oldest old. *Journal of Social Issues, 58*(4), 715–733.

Thorpe, K. E., Ogden, L. L., & Galactionova, K. (2010). Chronic conditions account for rise in Medicare spending from 1987 to 2006. *Health Affairs*, Available at http://content.healthaffairs.org/cgi/content/full/hlthaff.2009.0474v1. Retrieved on February 18, 2010.

Tomassini, C. (2005). The demographic characteristics of the oldest old in the United Kingdom. *Population Trends, 120*, 15–22.

Umberson, D., Wortman, C. B., & Kessler, R. C. (1992). Widowhood and depression: Explaining long-term gender differences in vulnerability. *Journal of Health and Social Behavior, 33*(1), 10–24.

United States Census. (2000). 5-percent public use microdata sample (PUMS) files. Available at http://www.census.gov/census2000/PUMS5.html

Von Strauss, E., Fratiglioni, L., Viitanen, M., Forsell, Y., & Winblad, B. (2000). Morbidity and comorbidity in relation to functional status: A community-based study of the oldest old (90+ years). *Journal of the American Geriatrics Society, 48*(11), 1462–1470.

Warner, M., Barnes, P. M., & Fingerhut, L. A. (2000). Injury and poisoning episodes and conditions: National Health Interview Survey, 1997. *Vital and Health Statistics, 10*(202), 1–38.

Wilkinson, R. G. (1999). Income distribution and life expectancy. In: I. Kawachi, B. P. Kennedy, & R. G. Wilkinson (Eds), *The society and population health reader* (Vol. 1, pp. 28–35). New York: The New Press.

Wray, L. A., & Blaum, C. S. (2001). Explaining the role of sex on disability. *The Gerontologist, 41*(4), 499–510.

Yoder, G. (2003). Firearm suicide among older adults: A sociological autopsy. Paper presented at the 56th annual scientific meeting of the Gerontology Society of America, San Diego, CA, November 21–25.

Zeiss, A. M., Lewinshon, P. M., Rohde, P., & Seeley, J. R. (1996). Relationship of physical disease and functional impairment to depression in older people. *Psychology and Aging, 11*(4), 572–581.

SECTION V
LIFE COURSE FACTORS IN DIFFERENCES IN HEALTH AND HEALTH CARE

MOTHERS' PERSPECTIVES ON ENHANCING CONSUMER ENGAGEMENT IN BEHAVIORAL HEALTH TREATMENT FOR MATERNAL DEPRESSION

Sandraluz Lara-Cinisomo, Ellen Burke Beckjord and Donna J. Keyser

ABSTRACT

Purpose – *Despite growing efforts to treat depression, engaging low-income and minority mothers continues to challenge providers. To address this issue, we conducted focus groups to identify responsive strategies for improving engagement of low-income and racially diverse mothers at high risk for depression.*

Methods – *Three focus group discussions (one prenatal, two postpartum) with 21 low-income and racially diverse mothers were held to determine*

This research was supported by UPMC for You, Highmark Foundation, Eden Hall Foundation, FISA Foundation, and Staunton Farm Foundation, with matching support provided by the Centers for Medicare and Medicaid Services.

their definition of depression, attitudes about depression treatment, and perceived barriers to treatment. Discussions took approximately 60 minutes and were audio-recorded. Detailed notes were taken during the discussions. The notes and audio recordings were analyzed using qualitative methods.

Results – *Identification of the source of distress, assessing women's perception of treatment and their related costs and benefits, and addressing cultural and financial barriers to treatment emerged as key themes for improving engagement among participants.*

Conclusion – *To be responsive to women's depression care needs, treatments should be informed by patient perceptions and needs, while addressing barriers to care.*

INTRODUCTION

Untreated maternal depression, particularly for women who have low incomes or are members of minority populations, is an increasingly important public health issue. Maternal depression, alone or in combination with other risk factors, can have adverse consequences for the individual woman and her family, including negative effects on parenting and early childhood health and development outcomes (e.g., Bonari et al., 2004; Field, Johnson, Hayes, Schneiderman, & McCabe, 2000; Huang & Freed, 2006; Moore, Cohn, & Campbell, 2001; Murray & Cooper, 1997; Paulson, Dauber, & Leiferman, 2006; Whitaker, Orzol, & Kahn, 2006). Approximately 12 percent of all women experience depression in any given year (Isaacs, 2004); for low-income women, the estimated prevalence doubles to at least 25 percent (Lanzi, Pascoe, Keltner, & Ramey, 1999; Miranda & Green, 1999; Onunaku, 2005; Riley & Broitman, 2003; Siefert, Bowman, Heflin, Danziger, & Williams, 2000). Estimated rates of depression among pregnant, postpartum, and parenting women in general range from 5 to 25 percent (Gaynes et al., 2005); low-income mothers of young children, pregnant, and parenting teens report depressive symptoms in the 40–60 percent range (Administration for Children and Families, 2003; Kahn et al., 1999; Siefert et al., 2000). Although research has demonstrated that evidence-based care for depression is effective for both the general population and the ethnically diverse and impoverished groups (Miranda et al., 2003), for many reasons, women with maternal depression are not identified, and even when they are identified, they are not effectively engaged in treatment (Swartz et al., 2005). This is especially true for racial and ethnic minorities who have less access to mental health services and are less likely to receive high-quality mental health care (Agency for Healthcare Research and Quality, 2004).

A number of significant barriers to engaging low-income or minority women at risk for depression in treatment have been identified at the local community level (Anderson et al., 2006; Brown, Taylor, Lee, Thomas, & Ford, 2007). These barriers are rooted in conceptual and cultural issues, structural issues, and financing issues. In recognition of these barriers, efforts to modify standard treatments to promote improvements in engagement and retention relative to usual care for depressed mothers on low incomes and others are currently under way (Grote, Swartz, & Zuckoff, 2008; Swartz et al., 2008; Swartz et al., 2007). Nevertheless, effective broad-based engagement of this population remains challenging.

To address this challenge, researchers from the RAND-University of Pittsburgh Health Institute (RUPHI), in collaboration with maternal and child healthcare stakeholders in Allegheny County, Pennsylvania, are currently implementing a quality improvement initiative designed to bridge the silos of Medicaid-managed care (Pincus et al., 2005). The overarching goals of the Allegheny County Maternal Depression Initiative are to increase screening rates and improve access to and engagement in evidence-based treatment for maternal depression among women who are enrolled in Allegheny County's HealthChoices Program, one of Pennsylvania's mandatory managed care programs for Medical Assistance recipients. To ensure that these goals are attained and that initiative components are undertaken in a manner that addresses the needs and preferences of the target population, a series of three consumer focus groups was conducted with prenatal and postpartum women in the community. In this chapter, we present the methodology and results of these focus groups and describe how the lessons learned can be used to improve ongoing and future-related efforts to effectively engage women at high risk for maternal depression in behavioral health treatment.

METHODS

A focus group is "a group of individuals selected and assembled by researchers to discuss and comment on, from personal experience, the topic that is the subject of the research" (Powell & Single, 1996, p. 499).

Focus group research has been used at the preliminary stages of a study, for example, to explore or generate hypotheses; during a study, perhaps to develop or evaluate a particular program or to identify questions for a survey; and after a study has been completed to assess its impact or to direct future research (Gibbs, 1997). The generally recognized parameters for focus group development include ensuring that participants have a specific experience of or opinion about the topic under investigation; using an explicit protocol; and exploring the subjective experiences of participants in relation to predetermined research questions (Merton & Kendall, 1946).

In April 2008, the RUPHI project team conducted three focus groups with prenatal and postpartum women in Allegheny County. The groups were designed to learn more about consumers' perspectives on key issues that are likely to impact engagement of women at high risk for maternal depression in behavioral health treatment.

Eligibility

To be eligible to participate in the focus groups, women had to be pregnant or have delivered 12 months before the focus group date. Most of the participants were enrolled in Allegheny County's HealthChoices Program, one of Pennsylvania's mandatory managed care programs for Medical Assistance recipients.

Recruitment Procedures

Participants were recruited through one of two existing professional networks. The first network involved healthcare providers who are partners in the Allegheny County Maternal Depression Initiative and nursing staff at Allegheny County's HealthChoices Program. These "recruiters" shared with eligible consumers a one-page, color flyer about the focus groups (developed by the RUPHI project team), which explained why they were being asked to meet (i.e., to talk about the stress mothers experience, share their thoughts about the consequences stress has on mothers, and provide suggestions for how to improve care for mothers under stress), and what they would receive for participating (i.e., a snack before the group discussion, a $75.00 gift card to a local supermarket chain, and transportation to the meeting if needed). Women who expressed interest in participating were asked to provide their contact information to the health providers and nursing staff, who then followed up with them by phone to provide further details on the date, time, and location of the focus group discussions.

The second network involved mental health providers who are partners in the Allegheny County Maternal Depression Initiative and provide care for with women with depression. This second group of recruiters approached eligible consumers in the same way as the first group. However, in this case, the women who expressed interest in participating were asked permission to share their contact information with the RUPHI project team, which then followed up with them by phone to provide the relevant details.

Organization and Conduct of the Focus Groups

The focus group discussions took place in a private space provided by two Southwestern Pennsylvania clinics that offer primary and obstetric care to women insured by Medicaid. One prenatal ($N = 10$) and two postpartum ($N = 4$, $N = 7$) focus groups were convened. Separate groups were organized for pregnant and postpartum women because, if a group is too heterogeneous with respect to their experiences or perspectives, the quality of the interaction can be adversely affected. Participants' availability required that the postpartum group be organized as two separate sessions.

Participants gave verbal consent before the start of the discussions. Each focus group discussion was conducted in English and took approximately one hour. One female project team member, with proven levels of group leadership and interpersonal skill, led the discussion, and a second project team member took notes. The discussions were also audio-recorded for verification of notes and for selecting relevant quotes. Following the focus group discussions, participants were asked to complete an anonymous demographic survey. The survey asked about the participant's racial/ethnic background, marital status, age, history of antidepressant use, and history of mental health treatment.

Sample Characteristics

A total of 21 racially and ethnically diverse women participated in the three focus groups. On the basis of data collected using the demographic surveys, the majority of participants were black, non-Hispanic (67 percent); 27 percent of participants were white, non-Hispanic. The mean age was

Table 1. Descriptive Statistics of Focus Group Participants ($N = 21$).

	Percent	Mean (SD)
Race/ethnicity		
White, non-Hispanic	27	
Black, non-Hispanic	67	
Bi-racial	5	
Education		
Less than high school	9	
High School	29	
Some college	33	
Associates degree/vocational training	5	
College degree	9	
Refused/missing	14	
Marital status		
Married	14	
Widowed	5	
Cohabitating	5	
Separated	71	
Never married	5	
Age		23.67 (6.03)
Children		1.38 (1.53)
Prior antidepressant use	38	
Prior behavioral health service use	48	

23.67 ($SD = 6.03$). Forty-eight percent of the women had a history of mental health treatment, and 38 percent had a history of antidepressant use. Table 1 provides complete descriptive statistics for the sample.

Measures

A standard protocol was used to guide the focus groups, covering six primary areas of inquiry: (1) defining depression and postpartum depression; (2) attitudes about depression; (3) treatment paths; (4) treatment attitudes and preferences; (5) benefits and consequences of depression treatment; and (6) strategies for addressing barriers to treatment. These areas were identified based on recognized gaps in the literature relevant to engaging low-income or minority women at risk for depression in behavioral health treatment, with the intention of uncovering concrete and responsive ways that healthcare providers can better engage this population in treatment. Table 2 provides a complete outline of the focus group discussion protocol.

Table 2. Areas of Inquiry Used to Guide the Focus Group Discussions.

Area of Inquiry	Discussion Questions and Probes
Define depression and postpartum depression (PPD)	1. What do you know about stress? *What about depression, what is depression?* 2. Is there a difference between being depressed and "stressed out?" 3. What kinds of things can cause stress on a mother? *(Probe for stress from family, work, economic factors, work, etc.)* 4. How can stress affect a mother? *(Probe for psychological impac.)* 5. What is it like for a woman who is experiencing stress? *(Probe here for specific symptoms.)* 6. What other words would you use to describe a mother who is experiencing a lot of stress? *Probe: Would you describe her as depressed? (Note: Ask this only if the term depression is not mentioned.)* 7. Do women of all races react to stress in the same way?
Attitudes about depression	1. Do you think (term used by group or depression) runs in families? 2. Do you think (term used by group or depression) is a sign of weakness? 3. Can (term used by group or depression) have a bad impact on a woman's child or children? 4. What other types of changes can (term used by group or depression) have on a mother? For instance, can (term used by group or depression) cause changes like pain or headaches? 5. Can a mother who experiences (term used by group or depression) become (term used by group or depressed) again?
Treatment paths, attitudes, and preferences	1. Do you think something that can be done for a mother who is (term used by group or depressed)? 2. What can a (term used by group or depressed) mother do? 3. Where can a (term used by group or depressed) mother go for help? 4. Can (term used by group or depressed) mother be treated by a professional. For instance, if a mother is (term used by group or depressed), should she see a doctor? If so, what type of doctor and why? If none, why? *Probe: Is visiting a doctor when she is depressed helpful? If so, how? Why not?* 5. If a (term used by group or depressed) mother chooses to see a doctor, should medication be used? Why or why not? 5a. Do you think a medication or antidepressants can help a woman who is pregnant or just had a baby? 6. Are medicines good at treating (term used by group or depression)?

Table 2. (Continued)

Area of Inquiry	Discussion Questions and Probes

	7. Do you think a (term used by group or depressed) mother should see a psychologist? Why or why not?
	  7a. Do you think a counselor or psychologist can help a woman who is pregnant or just had a baby?
	8. Do you think counseling is good for treating (term used by group or depression)?
	9. Which would you say is better to use, medication or a counselor/psychologist for treating (term used by group or depression)?
	10. Does a mother who is treated for (term used by group or depression) feel better over time or will she always be (term used by group or depressed)? If so, why?
	11. Can you think of anything else that can be done for a (term used by group or depressed) mother?
	  11a. How can that (approach) help?
	  11b. Can (approach) also help a pregnant woman or a mother who just had a baby?
	12. Is there anything else that can help a (term used by group or depressed) mother that we haven't discussed?
	13. What if we had a counselor/therapist/mental health specialist at the clinic? Let's say your nurse or doctor told you that you had screened at high risk for (term used by group or depression), would you be interested in talking with a counselor/therapist/mental health specialist here in the clinic?

Benefits and consequences of depression treatment	1. We've talked a little bit about the reasons for not using medication when a mother is (term used by group or depressed). Are there other consequences that we haven't discussed? If so, what are they? *Probe for differential effect on pregnant and postpartum mothers. Also probe for external consequences (e.g., partner reaction, criticism by others, and fear of impact on fetus/infant)* 2. Can you think of good reasons for using medicines/antidepressants for (term used by group or depression)? If so, what are those? *Probe for differential benefits to pregnant and postpartum women.* 3. Do you think medication should be continued after a woman feels better? Why or why not? 4. What about seeing a psychologist/counselor, what are some negative consequences? *Probe for differential effect on pregnant and postpartum mothers (e.g., partner reaction, criticism by others, and fear of impact on fetus/infant)* 5. Can you think of other good reasons for a (term used by group or depressed) mother to see a psychologist/counselor? If so, what are they? *Probe for differential benefits to pregnant and postpartum mothers.*

Table 2. (*Continued*)

Area of Inquiry	Discussion Questions and Probes
	6. Should treatment be it medication or counseling be continued after a woman feels better? Why or why not? 7. Are there any negative consequences to (list other approaches mentioned) for a (term used by group or depressed) mother? If so, what are they? *Probe for differential effect on pregnant and postpartum mothers.* 8. Are there benefits to (list other approaches mentioned)? If so, what are they? *Probe for differential benefits to pregnant and postpartum mothers.*
Strategies for addressing barriers to treatment	1. What do you think can keep a (term used by group or depressed) mother from getting the help she needs? *Probe for instrumental barriers (e.g., lack of child care, cost of treatment, and lack of health insurance).* 1a. How can a program help make sure a (term used by group or depressed) mother gets the help she needs? 2. Do you think all mothers have access to the same kinds of help like medication or counseling? Why or why not? 2a. How can a program make sure all (term used by group or depressed) mother get the same kinds of help?

Qualitative Data Analysis

Data analysis was driven by the six areas of inquiry, which served as an initial framework from which to derive themes within and across the focus group discussions. Responses to the discussion items related to each area of inquiry were identified by reviewing the notes of each focus group session and checking for concordance in the audio recordings. First, the focus group leader reviewed the notes along with the audio recording and listed responses to each area of inquiry. Next, a member of the RUPHI project team who did not attend the focus groups either as note taker or discussion leader reviewed the summary report and requested clarification as needed. Using the audio recording, the discussion leader and note takers discussed the reviewer's comments and queries and agreed on a final response. Overall, the team followed recommended techniques for theme identification, including examining text for evidence of word or phrase repetition, for use of metaphors or analogies, and for transitions in discussions (where themes are often revealed) (Ryan & Bernard, 2003).

RESULTS

On the basis of the combined responses to the six areas of inquiry noted earlier, the RUPHI project team identified three themes that were most salient to the participants: (1) sources of distress and coping strategies; (2) attitudes about treatment and treatment options; and (3) barriers and facilitators to engaging in behavioral health treatment. Table 3 provides a summary of the focus group findings organized by these three themes. Below, we provide further detail on the focus group results and include individual quotes from the participants for illustrative purposes only. We note that because focus groups are explicitly designed to elicit a multiplicity of views and emotional processes within a group context, it should not be assumed that individuals in the group are expressing their own definitive individual view (Gibbs, 1997).

Sources of Distress and Coping Strategies

Four common sources of stress were identified by consumers in all three focus groups: (1) meeting family obligations, such as infant care, running the household, and adequately addressing other children's needs; (2) dealing with childhood memories triggered by parenthood, such as abandonment, rejection, exposure to drug and substance abuse, and poor living conditions; (3) lack of financial resources to meet basic needs, such as paying household bills and providing food for the family; and (4) strained romantic relationships, including tension resulting from negotiating "time off" from family obligations with partners. Participants of one postpartum group also noted feelings of guilt when their own needs (e.g., for sleep or time off) competed with their other family obligations.

The prenatal focus group identified additional stressors associated with being pregnant, such as experiencing discrimination at work and when seeking employment, unexpected mood changes, physical limitations that prevent women being as active and mobile as they were before becoming pregnant, and fears of getting pregnant again. One prenatal consumer reported: "Won't nobody hire you they see you're pregnant then they say they'll call you and they never do. I was recently let go because I was pregnant; they claimed that it was because the job made you lift stuff; I went and got cash assistance, which isn't enough."

The most commonly reported, although not always effective, strategy for coping with stress across all three groups was seeking social support

Table 3. Summary of Focus Group Findings.

Sources of Distress and Coping Strategies	Attitudes about Treatment and Treatment Options	Barriers and Facilitators to Engaging in Behavioral Health Treatment
Sources of distress for all groups: • Meeting family obligations • Dealing with childhood memories triggered by parenthood • Lack of financial resources to meet basic needs • Strained romantic relationships *Additional stressors for prenatal focus group:* • Discrimination at work and when seeking employment • Mood changes • Physical limitations • Fears of getting pregnant again *Strategies for coping with stress:* • Social support • Medical advice • Adaptive self-distraction • Substance use	• Acknowledgement of potential benefits of treatment outweighed by common perception that treatment does not help • Primarily negative attitudes of consumers with insurance covering behavioral health care • Mixed perceptions about the pros and cons of using antidepressant medications	*Barriers:* • Lack of insurance coverage or limited coverage • Program requirements • Inappropriate referrals • Previous past experiences not helpful • Perceived disconnect between behavioral health providers and patients *Facilitators:* • Address barriers noted above • Consider alternative approaches to care (e.g., support groups, home visiting programs, peer-to-peer support) • Co-location of behavioral health services in physical health practices • Building trust between providers and patients

from family and friends. Attending church services and spending time with children were also included in this category. Some consumers said that they received harsh criticism when reaching out for help. As one consumer explained: "I tried to go to my mother and she judged me, as did her friends ... I felt alone and was judged ... my husband didn't really understand and he still doesn't."

Consumers who reported seeking medical advice as a way to cope with stress felt they were often negatively judged by their physicians because of their lifestyles. They also believed that their physicians misdiagnosed or failed to diagnose their symptoms until they were quite severe (e.g., suicidal ideation) or were immediately prescribed antidepressants without being screened or consulted about their symptoms: "[Doctors are] too quick to push medication and they don't get to the root of the problem."

Some consumers engaged in constructive, self-distraction coping strategies to deal with their stress, such as writing or keeping a journal, working on crossword or Sudoku puzzles, and shopping. A smaller number of consumers reported coping with their stress through more destructive strategies, namely substance use. One consumer said that when her support system fails, she uses alcohol and marijuana to help her cope because she worries about the side effects of taking antidepressants: "Unfortunately I was self-medicating with alcohol and weed. Smoking a little bit of pot will calm my nerves, but if you take Xanax you're asleep. But I can tell you that I don't need that when I have a support system." Other consumers willingly shared their experiences using drugs during pregnancy and warned of the negative consequences that substance use can have on an unborn child. Some participants were surprised to hear that the "rumors" about fetal alcohol syndrome were true. For others, the need to alleviate their stress outweighed the possible negative consequences: "I smoke marijuana and I know it will hurt my baby and I have to live with that."

Attitudes about Treatment and Treatment Options

While some of the consumers acknowledged the potential benefits of behavioral health treatment ("you do feel better just talking"), the predominant sentiment expressed during the discussions was that treatment does not help. As one participant explained, "I don't mind talking to someone about stress but I don't want to go to therapy or take medicine, this won't do anything, I want *resources*." With regard to antidepressants in particular, another participant asked, "What kind of medication is going to help you pay your rent?"

Participants with insurance that covered behavioral health care were generally dissatisfied with the quality of the care they received. These participants reported that their providers were either poorly trained, unwilling to listen, or unmotivated to provide the necessary care. Two mothers who had specific experiences with a local mental health agency reported extended waiting periods, poor provider training, and limits on the type of insurance coverage they accept.

Focus group participants' views on the use of antidepressants were more diverse. Among the three women who were currently on antidepressants, two said they were happy to be on medication and had plans to continue indefinitely. One of these women explained: "I've accepted that I'm probably going to have to be on [medication] for the rest of my life, I tried to do it naturally, but I realized that I can't do this alone ... It is sad to think that I'll be on Prozac for the rest of my life." Despite her mixed feelings about antidepressant treatment, this same woman also reported that she no longer experiences suicidal ideation and is starting to look forward to her future as a mother. In contrast, another consumer expressed concern about taking antidepressants because she worried it would trigger her drug addiction: "I'm a recovering drug addict, so being on anything is hard. I need to get in a pattern. My preference would be to not be on meds. I think that I need it right now, but I don't want to be on it forever."

Barriers and Facilitators to Engaging in Behavioral Health Treatment

The most common barriers to engaging in depression treatment identified by the focus group participants were lack of (or limited) insurance coverage, along with program requirements and inappropriate referrals. One consumer described how she arrived for a behavioral health appointment only to be told that her insurance was not accepted by that provider: "I go to my appointment and they say, well we don't take your insurance, and we can't help you. I burst into tears, they were like, 'you're on your own now.'" Other barriers to engagement in treatment, such as long wait times for appointments, lack of child care, limited access to providers, inconvenient locations of care, and lack of transportation to get to appointments, were also noted. In one focus group, postpartum consumers with prior outpatient behavioral health experience all reported that their behavioral health providers were unmotivated, overwhelmed, or disinterested. These women regarded their prior experiences as a barrier to seeking outpatient behavioral health care in the future.

Overall, we identified a perceived disconnect between consumers and behavioral health providers. Consumers said that because behavioral health providers have never experienced similar life situations and problems, they cannot have a real understanding of the issues mothers face. Some worried that they would be accused of child abuse if they disclosed their more desperate feelings, such as "I'm about to go over the bridge with my kids." Participants also noted that differences in race, ethnicity, or socioeconomic/ religious background also contribute to this disconnect. As one mother said, "I need someone with a little 'hood' in them."

In addition to addressing the barriers noted earlier, consumers said that approaches other than traditional outpatient treatment, such as professional support groups, home visiting programs, and peer-to-peer support, would be more likely to facilitate their engagement in treatment. Consumers thought that support groups would be most effective if participants were given an opportunity to share their experiences and be listened to and if the facilitators knew "the right questions to ask" so that the participants could talk openly without fear of being judged. Consumers also liked the Healthy Start home-visiting model because it meets their treatment and logistical needs (e.g., lack of transportation), while also providing helpful information and resources (e.g., crib and infant clothing). Peer-to-peer support was especially appealing to consumers, particularly if the peer "coach" was someone who had similar life experiences. As one participant explained: "You have to have a woman who has gone through the muck and is now succeeding who says I know what you're going through, and you can change. You have to know you're strong. Somebody who's already been through it ... no doctor with their condescending attitude is never going to help someone – it's just going to have to be another person who has gone through the muck."

Consumers also liked the idea of co-location, through which they could receive both physical and behavioral health services from providers who know their medical history and understand their needs and preferences. Efforts designed to build trust between consumers and providers were also noted as potential facilitators of treatment engagement. Consumers worry that prescribed medications will hurt them or their unborn child. Whereas one consumer said, "a doctor is not going to give you something that is going to hurt your baby," others noted that they see a number of doctors; so, it is difficult to get to know and trust them. Co-location of behavioral and physical health providers who provide a continuum of care could also help to strengthen consumer-provider trust.

DISCUSSION

The overall aim of organizing the focus groups described earlier was to gather direct feedback from perinatal women insured by Medicaid in Allegheny County on ways to enhance consumer engagement in behavioral health treatment for depression. The recruitment methodology and the organization/conduct of the sessions were ideally suited to ensure high levels of participation, interest, and interaction from a target population that is typically difficult to reach and engage.

Lessons Learned

Several important lessons were learned from the focus groups. First, low-income perinatal women encounter numerous sources of stress in their lives, the experiences of which are often exacerbated by living in poverty and ameliorated, in part, by constructive (e.g., social support) and detrimental (e.g., substance abuse) coping responses. Second, negative attitudes about behavioral health treatment are common and are often based on previous experiences with treatment attempts that did not meet consumers' needs. Third, creative treatment interventions, including peer support, home-based care, and co-located physical and behavioral health, are viewed as more desirable options for behavioral health engagement among low-income perinatal women as compared to traditional outpatient mental health. This feedback is consistent with the conclusions derived from larger scale studies of perinatal women with depression (e.g., Anderson et al., 2006) and includes useful actionable recommendations that maternal and child healthcare stakeholders can use to more effectively engage low-income and minority women at high risk for maternal depression in appropriate behavioral health treatment.

Translating Research into Practice

In any quality improvement initiative, a major challenge is to translate evidence-based research into widely accepted standards of practice and high-quality service delivery that meets the needs of the consumers the system is intended to serve. To address this challenge, ongoing, concerted efforts to understand and respond to consumers' needs and preferences are essential. To this end, consumer focus groups can serve as an efficient and effective tool.

On the basis of the results of the focus groups described herein, partners in the Allegheny County Maternal Depression Initiative are attempting to address consumers' distress regarding their needs for resources by connecting those identified at high risk for depression with a managed care organization (MCO) care manager. These health plan staff are well-positioned to provide both emotional and instrumental (e.g., transportation vouchers and links to financial assistance for food and housing) supports. In addition, by routinely incorporating a care manager into the consumer's treatment team, the Initiative aims to enlist another trusted provider into the consumer's care who can encourage engagement in behavioral health treatment.

The Initiative is also investing significant resources in provider trainings in an attempt to decrease consumers' negative experiences with behavioral health care. These trainings have covered a wide range of topics, from motivational interviewing to perinatal antidepressant use, and each training session emphasizes patient-centered care (consistent with the chronic care model; Coleman, Austin, Brach, & Wagner, 2009) and the importance of actively engaging consumers in needed treatment.

In addition, the Initiative is working to increase the availability and use of behavioral health treatment options other than traditional outpatient mental health. Specifically, home-based service providers in Allegheny County have joined the Initiative, and several efforts are in place to raise awareness of their services and to open communication pathways for referrals to them among the Initiative's physical health providers.

Finally, new co-location strategies (e.g., co-location of a behavioral health provider and a behavioral health case manager in physical health settings) are being tested, also with an eye to increasing consumer engagement in behavioral health treatment.

The Allegheny County Maternal Depression Initiative is now entering its third year of operation, and significant evaluative efforts are under way to track the impact of these interventions. On the basis of the results of the evaluation, the collaborative will recommend universal adoption of those practices/strategies that prove to be effective.

Limitations

As with most focus group studies, our work has several recognized limitations. First, only a small number of participants were included in the study, and those who participated self-selected into the research, thereby limiting the range of responses we could have collected from a larger, randomly selected sample. In particular, a sampling bias may have contributed to the negative views of behavioral health and pharmacological treatments expressed in the focus groups, as women with negative previous experiences may have been more inclined to participate in a focus group study where they could express their feelings and concerns.

Second, respondents represent a select group of mothers who were recruited by clinical staff, which limits the generalizability of the results. Given the background information provided by participants suggesting that 48 percent had a history of behavioral health treatment, it is unlikely that the women who participated in the focus group discussions are representative of the overall population the Initiative aims to serve (women for whom engagement rates are likely considerably lower (Miranda et al., 2003). However, because the findings of the focus groups were intended to inform Initiative strategies for enhancing engagement in behavioral health treatment, it may have been preferable that women with a behavioral health treatment history were overrepresented, as these consumers may have particularly useful insights into the process.

CONCLUSIONS

The perspectives offered by the women who participated in our focus groups reflect the complex and varied barriers encountered by women with perinatal depression (Miranda, Lagomasino, Lau, & Kohn, 2009). Engaging these women in behavioral health is a public health priority, but also a public health challenge (Yonkers et al., 2009). There is now substantial evidence that behavioral health intervention can significantly improve psychological outcomes for prenatal and postpartum women (e.g., Grote et al., 2008). Continued work to understand the most effective ways to facilitate women's engagement in these interventions must be directly informed by the voices of these consumers to effectively meet the needs and preferences of perinatal women.

ACKNOWLEDGMENTS

We extend our sincere appreciation to the partners of the Allegheny County maternal depression initiative who assisted with recruiting the focus group participants and provided the facilities necessary to conduct the focus group sessions. We also thank the focus group participants for sharing their experiences and perspectives. Their insights have been instrumental in guiding our ongoing quality improvement efforts in Allegheny County. In addition, we would like to acknowledge Ray Firth, Policy Initiatives Director, University of Pittsburgh Office of Child Development, and Susan Lovejoy, Project Associate at the RAND Corporation, for their contributions to developing the focus group protocol, coordinating logistics for the focus group sessions, and assisting with the note-taking.

REFERENCES

Administration for Children and Families. (2003). *Research to practice: Depression in the lives of early head start families.* Washington, DC: U.S. Department of Health and Human Services.

Agency for Healthcare Research and Quality. (2004). *National healthcare disparities report: Summary.* Rockville, MD: U.S. Department of Health and Human Services.

Anderson, C. M., Robins, C. S., Greeno, C. G., Cahalane, H., Copeland, V. C., & Andrews, R. M. (2006). Why lower income mothers do not engage with the formal mental health care system: Perceived barriers to care. *Qualitative Health Research, 16,* 926–943.

Bonari, L., Pinto, N., Ahn, E., Einarson, A., Steiner, M., & Koren, G. (2004). Perinatal risks of untreated depression during pregnancy. *Canadian Journal of Psychiatry. Revue Canadienne De Psychiatrie, 49,* 726–735.

Brown, C., Taylor, J., Lee, B. E., Thomas, S. B., & Ford, A. (2007). *Managing depression in African Americans: Consumer and provider perspectives.* Pittsburgh, PA: Mental Health Association of Allegheny County.

Coleman, K., Austin, B. T., Brach, C., & Wagner, E. H. (2009). Evidence on the chronic care model in the new millennium. *Health Affairs (Project Hope), 28,* 75–85.

Field, T. M., Johnson, S. L., Hayes, A. M., Schneiderman, N., & McCabe, P. M. (2000). Infants of depressed mothers. In: *Stress, coping, and depression* (pp. 3–22). Mahwah, NJ: Lawrence Erlbaum Associates Publishers.

Gaynes, B. N., Gavin, N., Meltzer-Brody, S., Lohr, K. N., Swinson, T., Gartlehner, G., Brody, S., & Miller, W. C. (2005). *Perinatal depression: Prevalence, screening accuracy, and screening outcomes.* Rockville, MD: Agency for Healthcare Research and Quality.

Gibbs, A. (1997). Focus groups. *Social Research Update, 19,* Department of Sociology, University of Surrey.

Grote, N. K., Swartz, H. A., & Zuckoff, A. (2008). Enhancing interpersonal psychotherapy for mothers and expectant mothers on low incomes: Adaptations and additions. *Journal of Contemporary Psychotherapy, 38,* 23–33.

Huang, L. N. & Freed, R. (2006). *The spiraling effects of maternal depression on mothers, children, families and communities.* Issue Brief no. 2. Annie E. Casey Foundation, Washington, DC.

Isaacs, M. (2004). *Community care networks for depression in low-income communities and communities of color: A review of the literature.* Submitted to Annie E. Casey Foundation. Washington, DC. Howard University School of Social Work, Washington, DC; the National Alliance of Multiethnic Behavioral Health Associations (NAMBHA), Bethesda, MD.

Kahn, R. S., Wise, P. H., Finkelstein, J. A., Bernstein, H. H., Lowe, J. A., & Homer, C. J. (1999). The scope of unmet maternal health needs in pediatric settings. *Pediatrics, 103,* 576–581.

Lanzi, R. G., Pascoe, J. M., Keltner, B., & Ramey, S. L. (1999). Correlates of maternal depressive symptoms in a national Head Start program sample. *Archives of Pediatrics and Adolescent Medicine*, *153*, 801–807.

Merton, R. K., & Kendall, P. L. (1946). The focused interview. *American Journal of Sociology*, *51*, 541–557.

Miranda, J., Chung, J. Y., Green, B. L., Krupnick, J., Siddique, J., Revicki, D. A., & Belin, T. (2003). Treating depression in predominantly low-income young minority women: A randomized controlled trial. *The Journal of the American Medical Association*, *290*, 57–65.

Miranda, J., & Green, B. L. (1999). The need for mental health services research focusing on poor young women. *Journal of Mental Health Policy and Economics*, *2*, 73–80.

Miranda, J., Lagomasino, I., Lau, A., & Kohn, L. (2009). Robustness of psychotherapy for depression. *Psychiatric Services (Washington, DC)*, *60*, 283.

Moore, G. A., Cohn, J. F., & Campbell, S. B. (2001). Infant affective responses to mother's still face at 6 months differentially predict externalizing and internalizing behaviors at 18 months. *Developmental Psychology*, *37*, 706–714.

Murray, L., & Cooper, P. J. (1997). The role of infant and maternal factors in postpartum depression, mother-infant interactions, and infant outcome. In: *Postpartum depression and child development* (pp. 111–135). New York: Guilford Press.

Onunaku, N. (2005). *Improving maternal and infant mental health: Focus on maternal depression*. Los Angeles, CA: National Center for Infant and Early Childhood Health Policy.

Paulson, J. F., Dauber, S., & Leiferman, J. A. (2006). Individual and combined effects of postpartum depression in mothers and fathers on parenting behavior. *Pediatrics*, *118*, 659–668.

Pincus, H., Thomas, S., Keyser, D., Castle, N., Dembosky, J., Firth, R., Greenberg, M., Pollock, N., Reis, E., Sansing, V., & Scholle, S. (2005). *Improving maternal and child health care: A blueprint for community action in the Pittsburgh region*. RAND, Santa Monica, CA.

Powell, R., & Single, H. (1996). Focus groups. *International Journal of Qualitative Health Care*, *8*, 499–504.

Riley, A. W., & Broitman, M. (2003). *The effects of maternal depression on the school readiness of low-income children*. Baltimore, MD: Annie E. Casey Foundation; Johns Hopkins Bloomberg School of Public Health.

Ryan, G. W., & Bernard, H. R. (2003). Techniques to identify themes. *Field Methods*, *15*, 85–109.

Siefert, K., Bowman, P. J., Heflin, C. M., Danziger, S., & Williams, D. R. (2000). Social and environmental predictors of maternal depression in current and recent welfare recipients. *American Journal of Orthopsychiatry*, *70*, 510–522.

Swartz, H. A., Frank, E., Zuckoff, A., Cyranowski, J. M., Houck, P. R., Cheng, Y., Fleming, M. A., Grote, N. K., Brent, D. A., & Shear, M. K. (2008). Brief interpersonal psychotherapy for depressed mothers whose children are receiving psychiatric treatment. *The American Journal of Psychiatry*, *165*, 1155–1162.

Swartz, H. A., Shear, M. K., Wren, F. J., Greeno, C. G., Sales, E., Sullivan, B. K., & Ludewig, D. P. (2005). Depression and anxiety among mothers who bring their children to a pediatric mental health clinic. *Psychiatric Services (Washington, DC)*, *56*, 1077–1083.

Swartz, H. A., Zuckoff, A., Grote, N. K., Bledsoe, S. E., Frank, E., Shear, M. K., & Spielvogle, H. N. (2007). Engaging depressed patients in psychotherapy: Integrating techniques from motivational interviewing and ethnographic interviewing to improve treatment participation. *Professional Psychology: Research and Practice, 38,* 430–439.

Whitaker, R. C., Orzol, S. M., & Kahn, R. S. (2006). Maternal mental health, substance use, and domestic violence in the year after delivery and subsequent behavior problems in children at age 3 years. *Archives of General Psychiatry, 63,* 551–560.

Yonkers, K. A., Smith, M. V., Lin, H., Howell, H. B., Shao, L., & Rosenheck, R. A. (2009). Depression screening of perinatal women: An evaluation of the healthy start depression initiative. *Psychiatric Services (Washington, DC), 60,* 322–328.

MEDIATING HOSPICE CARE: MAPPING RELATIONS OF RULING IN THE INTERDISCIPLINARY GROUP MEETING☆

Maria DiTullio and Douglas MacDonald

ABSTRACT

A primary impetus of the modern hospice movement was the disparity, during the later 20th century, between the care provided to persons with illnesses considered "curable" and the treatment – or lack of it – accorded the incurably or terminally ill. In its transformation from a reform-oriented, interdisciplinary response to the needs of the dying to an integrated component of the American healthcare system, hospice care's original mission, target population, and modality of service delivery were all significantly altered in ways that generated new disparities in access to "death with dignity." This chapter attempts to trace the political, economic, and institutional dimensions of this transformation as reflected in the experiences of one Northeastern hospice during a 6-month period in 2001. Using an analytic approach known as institutional ethnography (IE),

---

☆This chapter was originally presented at the 5th Annual Carework Conference at the CUNY Graduate Center, New York City, on August 10, 2007.

The Impact of Demographics on Health and Health Care: Race, Ethnicity and Other Social Factors
Research in the Sociology of Health Care, Volume 28, 269–299
Copyright © 2010 by Emerald Group Publishing Limited
All rights of reproduction in any form reserved
ISSN: 0275-4959/doi:10.1108/S0275-4959(2010)0000028015

the authors focus on the work of the Hospice's Interdisciplinary Group (IDG) to uncover the linkages between local problems in the delivery of hospice care and extra-local sites of power and constraint at the mezzo- and macrolevels of the American healthcare system. The significance of these linkages for patients, frontline workers, and other stakeholders are interpreted from several perspectives. Implications for change are discussed.

INTRODUCTION

A primary impetus of the modern hospice movement was the disparity, during the later 20th century, between the care provided to persons with illnesses considered "curable" and the treatment – or lack of it – accorded the incurably or terminally ill. In its transformation from a reform-oriented, interdisciplinary response to the needs of the dying to an integrated component of the American healthcare system, hospice care's original mission, target population, and modality of service delivery were all significantly altered in ways that generated new disparities in access to "death with dignity." This chapter attempts to trace the political, economic, and institutional dimensions of this transformation as reflected in the experiences of one Northeastern hospice during a 6-month period in 2001.

The present study emerged out of a long-term investigation of occupational stress among front-line hospice staff at one Northeastern home care hospice. Our initial findings (DiTullio & MacDonald, 1999) indicated that the stress, demoralization, and "burn-out" experienced by these workers stemmed less from the nature of the work they did, and more from a sense of frustration with the volume and complexity of hospice work demands and the constraints placed on their work by the institutionalization of hospice policy. We therefore decided to focus the next phase of investigation on the linkages between front-line hospice work and the institutional structures – both local and extra-local – that influence how this work actually happens. The regularly scheduled meetings of the Interdisciplinary Group (IDG) offered us a salient point of contact where the work of front-line staff, middle management, and administration routinely came together.

THE INTERDISCIPLINARY GROUP MEETING

The IDG meeting could be considered as the institutional core of hospice, insofar as it constitutes the central mechanism whereby hospice care is translated into an institutionally mediated set of practices that produce, on the one hand, decisions and directives affecting hospice clients – which front-line teams must implement – and on the other, various official documents that "reproduce" the client in abstract, institutional form, as the object of a series of evaluations, interventions, services, and adjudications by the Hospice. However, power within the Hospice often originates elsewhere, in extra-local sites of fiscal and regulatory authority – public and private insurances, accrediting bodies, state and federal entities, and so on – whose interests may not primarily be those of the Hospice, its employees, or its clients. A central aim of our study, as we saw it, was to understand how power operated both within and beyond the institutional reach of the Hospice. This led us to choose the analytic lens offered by institutional ethnography (IE).

INSTITUTIONAL ETHNOGRAPHY

IE is an approach to social research that seeks to reveal linkages between socially organized activities in local settings and larger-scale institutional structures (or "regimes") that coordinate and constrain those activities (Campbell & Gregor, 2002). "Social organization" in IE refers to the systematic but often invisible manner in which the activities of actors in local settings are "concerted" in ways that may be outside their knowledge, and for purposes that are not their own. The data we collected in Phase One of our ongoing study in 1997, and those collected in Phase Two, during the first 6 months of 2001, represent respectively the "two levels of data" required for an IE investigation:

> Beyond the ethnographic accounts that describe experiences [Maria's field notes and interviews of hospice workers during Phase One], the researcher must also work back to see how those experiences happened as they did. Thus second-level data [Maria's field notes of IDG and other meetings] is collected in order to make the social relations explicable ... [IE attempts to show] how knowledge and power come together in the everyday world to organize what happens to people. (Campbell & Gregor, 2002, pp. 8, 12)

Knowledge and power combine to produce what IE terms "ruling relations": the complex, often subtle, yet organized and purposeful ways in which things "happen to people" in an institutional context. Things happen to front-line hospice workers, which they often experience as stress, demoralization, or burnout; things happen also to patients, to middle managers, even to hospice administrators.

Although everyone involved in ruling relations is implicated in "what happens," IE researchers operate from the specific standpoint "of those who are being ruled" (Campbell & Gregor, 2002, p. 16). This means that our objective in Phase Two of our study was to investigate the larger forces at work, in the Hospice and beyond, that generated the front-line worker stress identified in Phase One. The purpose of IE is not to expose heroes or villains, but to locate and study the "problematic" of an organized social setting. Dorothy Smith (1987), the Canadian sociologist who originated the IE approach, used the concept of the problematic

> to direct attention to a puzzle set of questions that may not have been posed, or a set of puzzles that do not yet exist in the form of puzzles but are 'latent' in the actualities of the experienced world. (p. 91)

The "problematic" of an IE study begins to come into view with the identification of "disjunctures" occurring within the social site under investigation. Campbell and Gregor (2002) describe a "disjuncture" as a "moment of recognition that something chafes" (p. 48) in the experiences of local actors in an organized social setting. Disjunctures occur "between different versions of reality – knowing something from a ruling versus an experiential perspective" (p. 48). In the IDG meetings observed during the study period, as well as in other official and unofficial gatherings, participants struggled frequently with procedural dilemmas engendered by the disjunctures between ruling directives – emanating either from local hospice policy or extra-local authorities at the state and federal levels – and experiences at the ground level of day-to-day hospice operations.

HOSPICE: FROM DISCOURSE TO INSTITUTION

In contemporary critical theory, "discourse" is described as "a way of using language that embodies a particular ... set of beliefs and concerns" (Ward, 2003, p. 212). In the language of IE, discourse refers both to institutional "texts" and to the human social actors who "activate" the texts to serve particular institutional objectives (DeVault & McCoy, 2002). Both definitions of discourse can be applied to the hospice movement in America.

The hospice movement emerged from the late modern interest in death and dying as a social and clinical issue, inspired both by influential writings such as Kubler-Ross' (1969) *On Death and Dying* and by the work of early hospice organizers in England. Hospice advocates sought to reform what they saw as the routine medical neglect of the terminally ill within the increasingly technological, cure-oriented model of medical care that prevailed in the late 20th century (Buck, 2007; Stoddard, 1992). Central to the "beliefs and concerns" of hospice discourse were an emphasis on proactive or "preventive" pain management and a concomitant emphasis on attending to the needs of the "whole" person, including the psycho-social and spiritual needs of dying patients. This necessitated a coordinated, interdisciplinary response by a team of professionals and trained volunteers. The IDG thus became a defining difference of the hospice model of terminal care.

In the United States, the efforts of the National Hospice Organization to promote hospice as a cost-effective alternative to traditional care culminated in the creation of the Medicare Hospice Benefit in 1982, which spurred the rapid growth of hospice programs across the United States. To qualify for hospice care, patients were required to have a life expectancy of 6 months or less, as determined by their attending physician, and sign a form which acknowledged their terminal condition and waived their traditional Medicare coverage (which paid for curative medical care) in favor of the palliative (non-curative) care offered by hospice. The Medicare Benefit reimbursed hospices by means of a standard "per diem" rate of payment per patient, which was presumed to cover the costs of all goods and services provided to patients. However, the per diem rate formula was based on faulty cost assumptions and overly optimistic projections of patient enrollment and average lengths-of-stay in hospice. This tended to result in chronic fiscal vulnerability and recurrent periods of organizational restructuring for many hospices, including our study Hospice. Other features of the Medicare legislation placed strong emphasis on medical supervision of patient care, thus diminishing somewhat the original interdisciplinary character of hospice in America (Buck, 2007). The integration of hospice into the bureaucracy of American healthcare resulted in various disjunctures – between the original "discourse" of hospice care and its "textual," institutional functions – that comprise the focus of the present study.

ANALYTICAL METHODOLOGY

The analysis set forth in this chapter looks at data collected in field notes at IDG meetings held during a 6-month period in 2001. Four different dimensions or "levels" of analysis are presented:

- *Level One – Procedural Phenomena:* close observation and explication of formal procedures in the IDG meeting, the sequences of activities performed, who performs them, and what is accomplished.

- *Level Two – Extra-Procedural Phenomena:* a description of verbal and nonverbal interactions among IDG members that reveal "latent" functions and elements of the IDG process.
- *Level Three – Disjunctures and Disempowerment:* examples of case reviews from the Nursing Home Team that highlight some of the issues and problems that typically arise in the course of an IDG meeting.
- *Level Four – Fault Lines:* data from ad hoc meetings held immediately before or after IDG meetings that illuminate wider systemic challenges affecting the Hospice.

OBSERVING THE IDG

For the purposes of our analysis, it is helpful to conceptually picture the IDG and its activities as situated within a wider institutional environment that includes not only the structural hierarchy of hospice (e.g., clerical, front-line, middle management, and administration) but also various parties involved at the level of the local community (e.g., attending physicians, nursing homes, etc.) as well as pertinent entities operating at the macrolevel of American society, such as healthcare funding and regulatory authorities (Fig. 1).

The IDG meetings that Maria attended for each of the Hospice Teams always included the Medical Director (or another physician acting in that capacity), as well as the Team social worker, chaplain, and primary nurses. Normally, one nurse would report current data for each case, based on information from patient charts, whereas another performed the task of writing down the information presented – as well as any action planned regarding the case – on a special IDG form. Sometimes a middle management nurse, whose title was Clinical Director, would also be present. One primary nurse on each Team held the newly created position of "Team Leader," but did not appear to have any specialized role or function within the IDG.

Level One: Procedural Phenomena

Case presentation followed a simple procedural format, generally consisting of three components:

a. Objectified, "textual" data on the patient's medical condition, using jargon related to standard indicators of health status, such as the Karnovsky Scale (a standardized measure of a patient's ability to

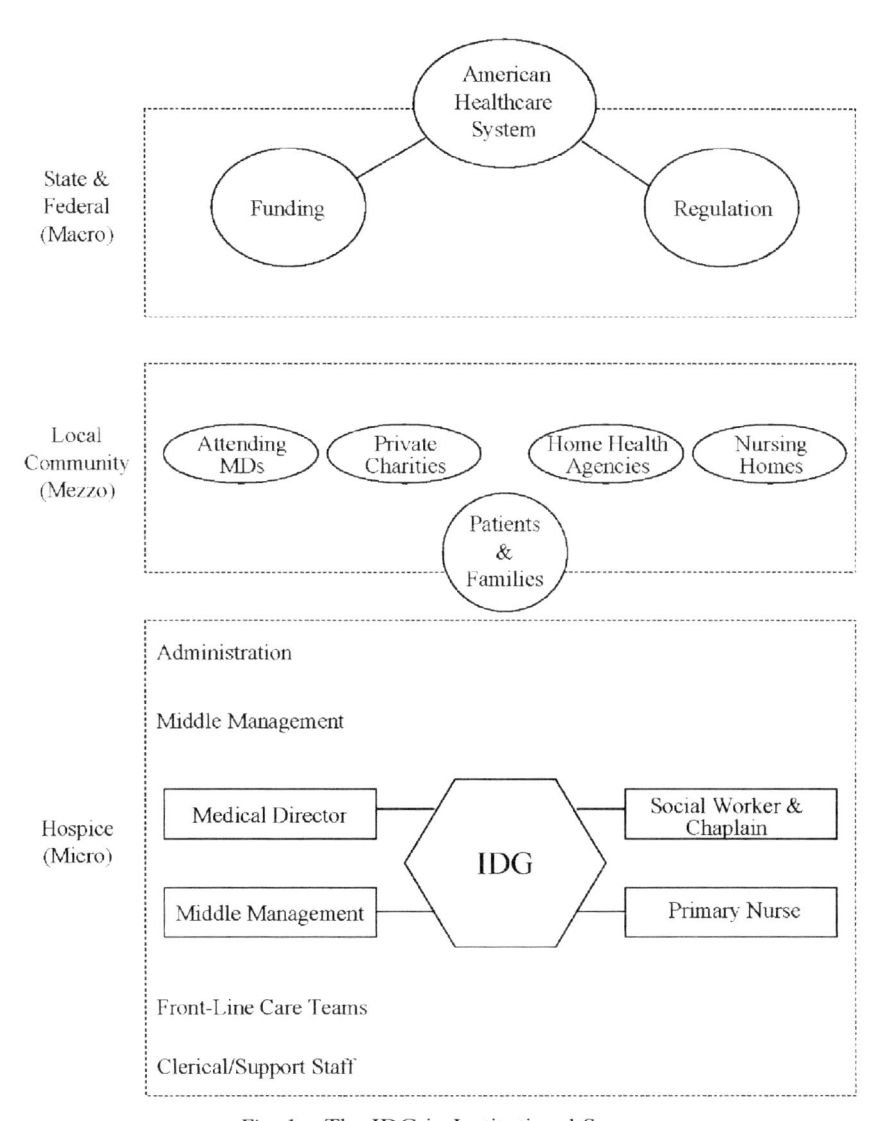

Fig. 1. The IDG in Institutional Space.

perform activities of daily living), or terms related to advance medical directives, such as DNR (a "do not resuscitate" order) or Healthcare Proxy (a document designating someone to make healthcare decisions on behalf of the patient).

b. Discussion of the case by the Medical Director and other Team members, sometimes including a recommendation, an order, or a decision regarding recertification.
c. "Humanizing" or individualizing commentary on the patient and family, in which a particular "person" was allowed to emerge from beneath the "textual" patient data.

Often the sequence of the components varied: for example, "a" might be followed by "c," or the two combined in a presentation that alternated between objectified data and humanizing description of the patient or family. Occasionally "a" and "c" would occur without any input or comment from the Medical Director. Fairly frequently, the "missing" component in a presentation was the humanizing commentary. And at times, although rarely, only the textual, objectified data would be recited, "for the record," without comment or discussion of any kind.

Discussions between nurses and the Medical Director tended to focus on medications, clinical procedures, and authorization of various consults or re-examinations of patients for purposes of verifying a 6-month-or-less prognosis. Authorization of new medications or procedures appeared to be guided primarily by clinical considerations, but issues of cost-containment were sometimes alluded to by statements such as "I think we can justify this because ..." Although there was no evidence that any needed medication or procedure was withheld on the basis of cost, it was clear that budgetary concerns imposed by the hospice per diem rate structure were never far from people's minds during IDG during these meetings. Careful monitoring of resource allocation thus appeared to be a latent if not official function of the IDG.

Two strong impressions arise from observation of the purely structural and procedural dimensions of IDG meetings.

First, "objectified," clinical patient data (component "a") – the "textual" representation of the dying person – was the pre eminent and only indispensable component in the IDG process. In the absence of interdisciplinary discussion, Medical Director input, or humanizing commentary, the intertextual "conversation" between the patient chart and the IDG form, and the transmission of data from one to the other, was sufficient. However, while textual data appeared to form the basis of recertification discussions, they were not – as will be shown later in our analysis – by any means decisive.

Second, the "interdisciplinary" quality of the IDG meeting appeared in practice to be largely a dialogue between nurses and the Medical Director.

Discussion of physical pain and symptom control, or clinical indicators of physical decline or stabilization, predominated in IDG discourse. Input from either social workers or chaplains was minimal, occurring in only a small percentage of the case presentations recorded in Maria's field notes. In those cases in which humanizing or psychosocial commentary did occur, such discourse was as likely to come from nurses as from social workers or chaplains.

These two impressions constituted for us, as researchers, an initial sense of "disjuncture" – a mismatch or contradiction between hospice as discourse and hospice as a site of "ruling." Hospice discourse places great emphasis on the holistic needs of patients – including psycho-spiritual needs – and on the use of an interdisciplinary approach as a means of comprehensively addressing those needs. Yet the actual proceedings observed gave obvious preeminence to physical care and objectified clinical data. Both of the phenomena we observed may be tied to the "textual" basis of IDG proceedings, because, as Campbell and Gregor (2002) have noted:

> In the objectified and ideological version of knowledge being created in organizational records, there is no way back to the client's, or the professional's, own experience. The official version dominates ... The text replaces and 'trumps' competing versions. Officially, the person exists only as an object, just as he appears in organizational documents. (p. 40)

However, this characterization of the IDG, while empirically "real," fails to tell the whole story of what happened in the IDG, partly because objectified, textual data often proved to be unreliable or inconsistent guides to IDG decision making, and partly because Maria observed several instances of IDG members actively resisting, overruling, or otherwise attempting to transcend the strictures placed upon their roles by the "textual" version of reality. Their reasons for doing so were complex and cannot be attributed to a single motive. This will become evident in the examples that appear later in this section.

Level Two: Extra-Procedural Phenomena: Group Interaction in the IDG

In addition to recording information on the structure and procedure of the IDG meeting, Maria noted interactions and other phenomena among team members that occurred parallel to the formal process, which served to deepen our understanding of the disjunctures identified in the preceding section. This examination of nonprocedural activities across all IDG

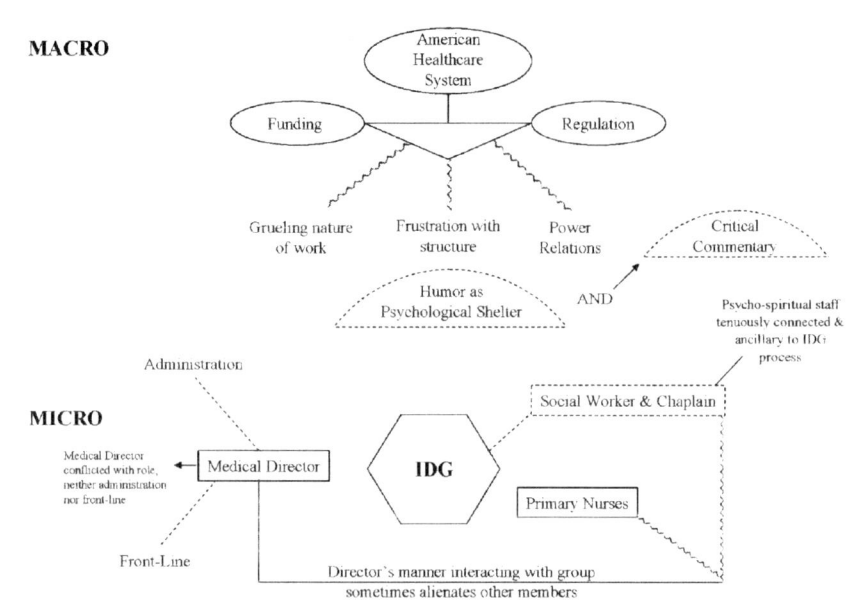

Fig. 2. Nonprocedural Dynamics of the IDG.

meetings Maria attended highlighted three themes: (1) the grueling nature of the IDG process; (2) power relations among the team members; and (3) frustration with the structural realities of hospice. Our attention to these interactions helped to focus and guide our inquiry into how the work of hospice within the IDG meeting happens as it does (Fig. 2).

The Grueling Nature of IDG Process and the Shelter of Humor

The mandate to discuss and document objectified clinical indicators of a patient's disease process has already been established as dictating the form and function of the IDG meeting. This second level of data focused on the abundance of medical information involved (measured in terms of time devoted to medically related discussion and manual documentation) and the tedious, repetitive nature of this process. The volume and complexity of the case presentations routinely generated comments such as "We're never going to get out of here today" and "This won't end today." Less obvious but persistent nonverbal signals included a palpable air of tension and urgency to get through the pile of patient charts, as though they were obstacles to be overcome and disposed of before team members were free to attend to the patient needs that beckoned them from outside the IDG.

Tension was periodically relieved through the use of humor. Humor in the IDG was observed to take many forms but most notable was a type of "gallows" humor expressed with the requisite irony and irreverence. Often, a quip by one team member would become extended and embellished as a "running gag" by other team members throughout the duration of the meeting. This improvisational "play" seemed to provide some respite – however brief – from the time pressure and unrelenting tedium of IDG work.

Power Relations in the IDG

The "medicalization" of hospice under Medicare regulations has altered the interdisciplinary intent of the original IDG model. The consequences resulting from this revision were observed in the form of differential power relations among team members and increased levels of frustration with structural impediments that constrained the work of hospice.

The Medical Director is the central authority around which the work of IDG revolves. The Medicare mandate to document objective clinical data has created an almost exclusive dialogue between nurses and medical directors as they assess, pronounce needed interventions and/or determine recertification status. Psychosocial or spiritual commentary was consistently observed to be infrequent, brief and functioning primarily to "fill in" required psycho-social-spiritual information on Medicare forms. The information provided by social workers and chaplains was respectfully acknowledged and duly noted in most cases. In general, however, input by social workers and chaplains seemed ancillary to the care planning process.

As the meetings proceeded, it was not uncommon for medical staff to ignore humanizing content altogether. According to Maria this did not appear to be intentional, but rather a consequence of side-bar conversation among medical colleagues intent on obtaining or clarifying missing clinical information for the express purpose of documentation. One social worker brought her sense of professional invisibility to the forefront by concluding her psycho-social report to distracted colleagues by joking, "well, let's just get the social side of people right out of the medical picture!"

On rare occasions, social workers interjected psycho-social information into a medical discussion. In these instances, the social worker served as a mouthpiece for the patient in the IDG meeting by helping to place medical issues or problems in psycho-social context. When this psycho-social information was helpful at arriving at a satisfactory medical decision, clinical team members were visibly appreciative. Hence, the ability of nonmedical staff to influence the care plan appeared to be mediated and measured by the perceived usefulness or necessity of their professional input as it bore on medical matters.

Frustration with the Structural Realities of Hospice

The disjuncture between the mission of hospice as a philosophy of care and hospice care as reconstructed by the constraints of Medicare regulations is vividly apparent in the IDG. The group frequently struggled with the consequences of the required 6-month prognosis. Reluctant to attach a definitive end point to a terminal diagnosis, physicians instead choose to continue curative measures, ceasing treatment only when the patient is weeks or days away from death. One team member's response to this common occurrence resonated with feelings of futility and professional devaluation when she said, "it's like the docs can't do *their thing* anymore, so they say 'lets get hospice out here to drain the tank and pronounce this lady dead' ... that's not hospice."

The role of Jake, the Medical Director, emerged in these observations as a complex mixture of conflicting functions and personal impulses. As the principal "decider" and leader of the IDG, it fell to him to act as timekeeper, to mind the agenda, and to rein in discussions. Others at these meetings would occasionally complain about this among themselves. Yet the "person behind the function" often seemed to bridle at the same disjunctures and contradictions of the IDG that frustrated the front-line members. Jake could at times also be disarmingly funny, irreverent, and tender in his responses to cases and to others present. Although nominally associated with Administration in the organizational hierarchy, Jake often seemed uncomfortable with that location and the ruling relations associated with it.

The overriding sentiment gleaned from numerous observations of the IDG meeting is one of frustration regarding the inability to spend sufficient time on developing a care plan that comprehensively addresses the needs of the patient and the patient's family. The processing and documenting of textually driven medical information frequently prevented team members from representing the dying process with the personal richness and dimension of their lived experience. The forms failed to tell the story of the patient's dying experience, as well as the story of the hospice professionals who accompanied them through the process.

Level Three: Disjunctures and Disempowerment in the Nursing Home Team

In 1986, through an act of Congress, states were "given the option of including hospice in their Medicaid programs" (National Hospice and Palliative Care Association [NHPCO], 2007, p. 1), using the same hospice per diem rate structure as the Medicare Hospice Benefit. Hospice care thus became available to patients in long-term care facilities. By 2001, the Hospice in our study had contracts with several area nursing homes, and a designated hospice team to care for nursing home patients. The incorporation of nursing home populations into hospice care introduced a complex range of new and old problems for the Hospice.

New problems included the challenges involved in sharing care responsibilities with nursing home staff and administrators, whose motives, interests, and institutional culture differed sharply in many respects from those of the Hospice, and whose operations were "ruled" by different regulations and funding imperatives. Another significant new problem concerned managing the comfort care of a population of patients with chronic illness and unpredictable "death trajectories" (Buck, 2007). Old problems were those common to hospice work for all teams, and included the challenges of symptom management, the complexity of family situations, and the uncertainty of prognostication.

We have chosen to use examples of IDG processes from meetings with the Nursing Home Team (Team 3) because they illuminate a range of institutional "disjunctures" and ruling relations – some particular to Team 3, others experienced by all teams – that result in various kinds of constraint and disempowerment for both front-line workers and the Hospice as a whole. Moreover, these phenomena can be seen to occur at various local and extra-local sites throughout the "institutional space" in which the IDG is situated.

The disjunctures discussed here can be placed in three general categories: (1) the politics of recertification; (2) relations with nursing homes and other community-level providers; and (3) the vagaries of chronic illness. However, these categories are by no means separate, but instead continually overlap and interpenetrate (Fig. 3).

The Politics of Re-certification

A primary function of the IDG is to adjudicate the continuing eligibility of patients for hospice care at regular intervals prescribed by the Medicare

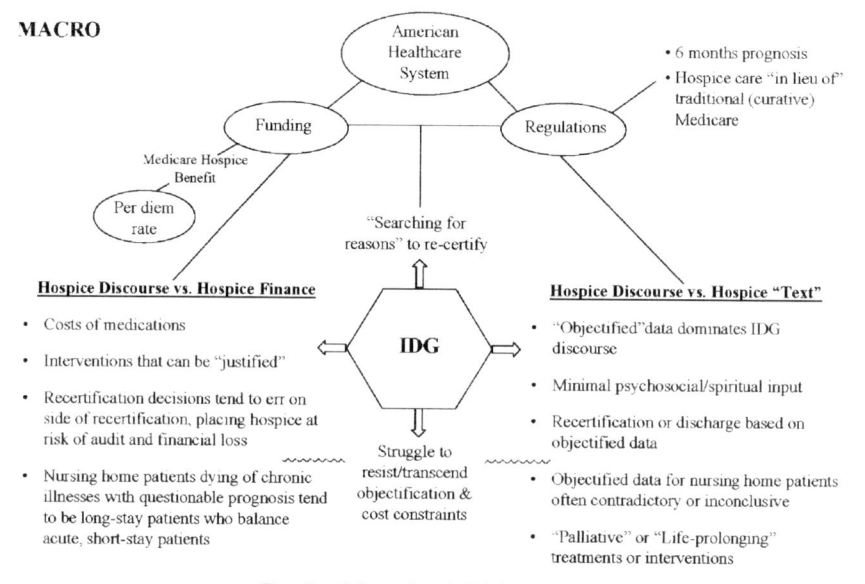

Fig. 3. Macrolevel Disjunctures.

MACRO

- American Healthcare System
  - 6 months prognosis
  - Hospice care "in lieu of" traditional (curative) Medicare
- Funding
  - Medicare Hospice Benefit
  - Per diem rate
- Regulations

"Searching for reasons" to re-certify

IDG — Struggle to resist/transcend objectification & cost constraints

Hospice Discourse vs. Hospice Finance
- Costs of medications
- Interventions that can be "justified"
- Recertification decisions tend to err on side of recertification, placing hospice at risk of audit and financial loss
- Nursing home patients dying of chronic illnesses with questionable prognosis tend to be long-stay patients who balance acute, short-stay patients

Hospice Discourse vs. Hospice "Text"
- "Objectified" data dominates IDG discourse
- Minimal psychosocial/spiritual input
- Recertification or discharge based on objectified data
- Objectified data for nursing home patients often contradictory or inconclusive
- "Palliative" or "Life-prolonging" treatments or interventions

---

Hospice Benefit. If patients are judged to be "still dying," they can be re-certified as hospice-appropriate; if patients appear to have stabilized or improved according to objectified medical indicators, they must be decertified and discharged from hospice. However in the Team 3 IDG meetings that Maria observed, patients were rarely decertified. In the majority of recertification discussions recorded, decisions were either deferred or patients were recertified for reasons that appeared to exceed the logic of purely "textual" data.

Typical examples of these phenomena include the case of a woman whose Karnovsky rating had recently improved, but who had a long history of mental illness and was described as "actively psychotic" by the Team nurse. "There's too much going on with her this week to kick her out," she explained. "Let's keep her and re-assess." The Medical Director agreed and the recertification decision was deferred. In another case, the decision was deferred for a "depressed, suicidal" patient whose physical status had improved but whose emotional instability could have placed his safety at risk if he were discharged from hospice. In a third example, the Team reported on an elderly woman whose functional decline and weight loss had temporarily stabilized:

Nurse: "Karnovsky rating is 30% ... [She is] not losing weight."

Social Worker: "The family is not interested at all in Peggy and [they] rarely visit."

Medical Director: "Tell me, is she sleeping more?"

[*Maria's note: "[Medical Director] is shaking his head in an up and down 'Yes' manner, and the nurse picked this up and said, 'Oh yes, she is really tired and sleeping much more'."*]

Medical Director: "Well, then – we'll keep her for now." [*Patient is re-certified.*]

In these cases, decisions (or deferrals of decisions) appear to be made *in spite of*, rather than pursuant to the textual governance of regulatory guidelines. The motives for these adjudications were likely mixed, and involved disjunctures between the moral and clinical dictates of hospice discourse versus textual ruling, and between hospice discourse and the often treacherous terrain of hospice finance.

Objectified medical indicators are frequently inadequate or contradictory yard – sticks for determining "decline" or "improvement" in elderly or chronically ill nursing home patients. A standard indicator such as weight gain may be contradicted by other indicators, such as a decline in functionality as measured by the Karnovsky scale. The slow but steady deterioration associated with Alzheimer Disease or ALS often does not conform to the more predictable "death trajectories" of cancer patients, on whom textual standards of prognostication were originally modeled. Moreover, the co-morbidity of nonterminal psychiatric conditions further complicate the moral calculus incumbent upon IDG decision-makers, who have an understandable reluctance to withdraw supportive (and possibly stabilizing) services from actively suicidal or psychotic patients.

However, the impulse to "look for reasons" to keep patients on hospice rolls may also be rooted in the problematic financial bind that the ruling structures of hospice funding impose on hospice programs. On the one hand, hospices have a clear financial incentive for retaining the "long stay" patients – both those living at home and in nursing homes – with noncancer illnesses, to offset the "resource drain" of short-stay, service-intensive patients. But on the other hand, hospices may place themselves at grave financial risk by doing so. Beginning in 1995, the federal office of Inspector General announced that Operation Restore Trust (ORT) – "a special program to combat fraud and abuse in Medicare and Medicaid" (NHPCO, 2007, p. 1) – would be expanded to include hospice. A subsequent wave of audits called "Focused Medical Review" began, involving several hospices in different states, and in some cases resulted in Medicare and Medicaid withholding reimbursement from the targeted programs, or demanding sizable "refunds" of monies previously paid. Such audits tended to focus primarily on the kinds of patients Team 3 served in 2001.

Relations with Other Providers

Like every human service organization, the Hospice operates in a physical and institutional community. A complex web of relations at the mezzolevel connects the Hospice to nursing homes, hospitals, home care agencies, physician groups, and other public and private providers of health-related services. As Paradis and Cummings (1986) observed soon after the Medicare era of hospice development had begun

> Early idealism has been tempered by the need to accommodate and negotiate with established medical institutions. Attempts to reform aspects of the American medical care system have been altered as hospice providers recognize the necessity of becoming part of it. (p. 370)

Partly as a consequence of this gradual process of "institutional isomorphism" (DiMaggio & Powell, 1983), by 2001 the Hospice was firmly (if not securely) tied to this web of relations that both constrained its work and made it possible. Each of these other healthcare entities operated by a different set of rules and under a different set of constraints emanating from state and federal authorities, generating periodic problems and tensions between it and the Hospice. Numerous exchanges during IDG meetings alluded to the invisible presence of these other community "players" and revealed some of the disjunctures created by these relations (Fig. 4).

The Case of Mr. D:

> Nurse: " ... 46-year-old man with end-stage AIDS with primary Pneumonia ... went to [the hospital] last night because he had fallen ... Basically, the ER didn't do any blood work. Mr. D went to Dorothy House [a private home that cares for dying AIDS patients] and his significant other, Larry, arrived the next day. Larry is really mad at [the nursing home] because of [Mr. D's] fall and the contusions and abrasions he suffered. [The nursing home] denies the fall and says no injury was documented ... [Another Team 3 nurse] says it was really serious, and he could have broken his nose, and he may have. He is imminent ... Most meds have been discontinued. The family has arrived and are very supportive." [*No comment by Medical Director or other staff.*]

Mediating Hospice Care

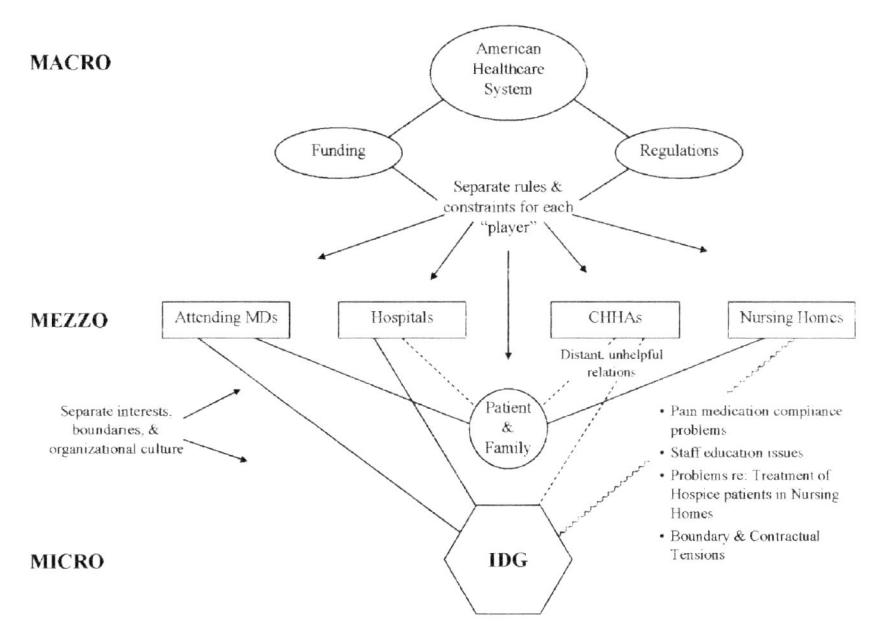

MACRO

```
                    American
                    Healthcare
                     System

         Funding                Regulations
              Separate rules &
              constraints for each
                   "player"
```

MEZZO

Attending MDs   Hospitals   CHHAs   Nursing Homes

Distant, unhelpful relations

Separate interests, boundaries, & organizational culture

Patient & Family

- Pain medication compliance problems
- Staff education issues
- Problems re: Treatment of Hospice patients in Nursing Homes
- Boundary & Contractual Tensions

MICRO   IDG

Fig. 4. Mezzolevel Disjunctures.

The case of Larry D makes visible one aspect of the intricate and constraining relations between the Hospice and one of their "partnering" institutions, nursing homes. The nursing home in this case was the only facility in the area that accepted AIDS patients, whereas concern was expressed in the meeting about this patient's alleged treatment by the facility, there is no pronouncement or recorded action taken by the IDG regarding the incident of Mr. D's injury. Apparently arrangements were made to relocate this patient to Dorothy's House, the private home of two Catholic Worker volunteers who acted as primary caregivers for end-stage AIDS patients as a personal ministry. Dorothy's House is not a "facility" and thus has no formal or "institutional" relationship to the Hospice.

The Case of Phyllis G:

Nurse: "Phyllis has a brain tumor that has decreased in size according to [her doctor]. The tumor is just sitting there and probably has gone into remission, which means this patient probably has more than six months to live."

Medical Director: "I think we'll have to boot her from the program, but I think this will be good news for her."

Nurse: "[Another hospice nurse] will do discharge and talk to her about setting goals for the future, and discussing how she will live at home in her own house."

Medical Director: "This should be doable if she could be downstairs and had a Life-Line [emergency alert device] in case of emergency that she could access."

Nurse: "Yeah, it looks like this tumor may just be in sort of a remission. She has a great social life and neighbors to help, so there's really no need for Home Care [a Certified Home Health Agency]. I'm not sure that she would qualify for it."

Medical Director: "I think Home Care is a big fake ... *Nobody* qualifies for Home Care. You have to literally be catheterized, before someone qualifies for Home Care. Okay, let's discharge Phyllis and then I'll start reading the obituaries ... because every time we do this, they die within a week."

The discharge of Phyllis G, whose tumor has gone into remission, presents a murky picture of what can happen when hospice withdraws its involvement with a patient. Although it appears, in this case, that the patient had adequate supports to get by on her own, the Medical Director's sardonic comments about reading the obituaries "because every time we do this, they die within a week" reflects his ambivalence and sense of powerlessness connected to following the prescribed "rules" of discharge from hospice.

In other models of hospice care operating in other countries, no "6-months-or-less" determinations are required, categories such as "palliative" versus "active" treatment or "home care" versus "institutional care" are less separated and compartmentalized, and patients like Phyllis might continue to have hospice support during the promising but uncertain weeks or months that lie ahead. But within the exceptionalist framework of American healthcare policy, such an option is foreclosed.

The Medical Director's statement about home care agencies introduces another healthcare "player" at the mezzolevel whose relations with hospice are complex. In 2001, Certified Home Health Agencies (CHHAs) were sometimes referral sources for patients, but could also be competitors who felt that they provided palliative care as well as hospices. Occasionally, CHHAs were considered as possible "follow-up" resources for discharged hospice patients. However, CHHAs operated under very different Medicare guidelines and faced their own set of constraints under state and federal regulations. Separate doctor's orders were required for every service, visit, or piece of equipment provided to a patient, and custodial (home-health-aide level) care tended to be quite limited or unavailable in many cases. In practice, discharged hospice patients often could not access adequate support at home from traditional home care agencies, and would end up being hospitalized.

The Vagaries of Chronic Illness

In one of the folksy aphorisms often used to explain what hospice care is designed to do for a terminally ill patient, early hospice brochures would inform readers that "hospice doesn't add days to your life, but life to your days." Helping patients achieve an optimal quality of life through expert pain and symptom management and psychosocial support is thus a central, defining goal of interdisciplinary hospice teams. However, achieving this objective under Medicare can have ironic consequences. Nowhere is this more true than in the case of patients dying of chronic illnesses.

The Case of Margaret H:

Medical Director: "Well, it's anniversary time for little Margaret. We should have a 1-year hospice party for her. Her diagnosis is weight loss with Alzheimer's Disease, a history of stroke, and seizure disorder. Her Karnovsky rating is 30%, And she is out of bed and in a geri-chair from time to time. Her weight in April was 120, and in May 117. Does she need to be re-certified?"

Nurse: "Yes ... she would decline so quickly if we moved her out." [*Patient is re-certified.*]

The Case of Pat M:

Nurse: " ... entered hospice program at 71 pounds, with a diagnosis of multiple sclerosis. She is 87 years of age ... appetite has improved ... no temperatures ... Patient reported no pain ... reports good satisfaction with hospice workers, states, 'This disease is awful', but she is content and relatively accepting of illness ... Patient had dropped to 63 pounds, but since under hospice care has gained 20 pounds."

Medical Director: "She doesn't seem like she will die in six months, and we need to approach this possibility in a positive way. We can ask for a [neurological consult] and explain to her that we want to get an idea of how her disease is progressing."

[*Maria's note: "Nurse and chaplain express their perception that patient is declining."*]

Nurse: She is one patient who is here because hospice is here; she would be dead otherwise." [*Decision is deferred.*]

In the topsy-turvy world of Medicare-certified hospices, decline is "progress" and an improved quality of life may be cause for a discharge. A frequently observed hospice "paradox" is the case in which the extra support, attention, and good care provided by the Hospice to a dying person actually slows his or her observed decline, which places the patient at risk of decertification. In many such cases, the decline resumes after hospice care is withdrawn – hence, the reluctance of IDG members to allow patients to be penalized for successful hospice interventions.

A Perfect Institutional Storm

Occasionally, a complex and clinically challenging chronic illness could pull together all the conditions necessary for a "perfect storm" of disjunctures at the micro-, mezzo-, and macrolevels of hospice work, as illustrated in the case of Kevin L, a patient with ALS who required a ventilator machine to breathe (Fig. 5).

> **Nurse:** " ... a 40-year-old male with ALS. He is taking no breaths on his own, and has to be suctioned [for pulmonary secretions] 5 to 7 times per shift. On admission, he had an increase of the Durogesic patch [a pain medication] to 150 mgs and Roxinol of 40 mgs every two hours. He is given Roxinol before each suctioning because he gets very anxious during this process."

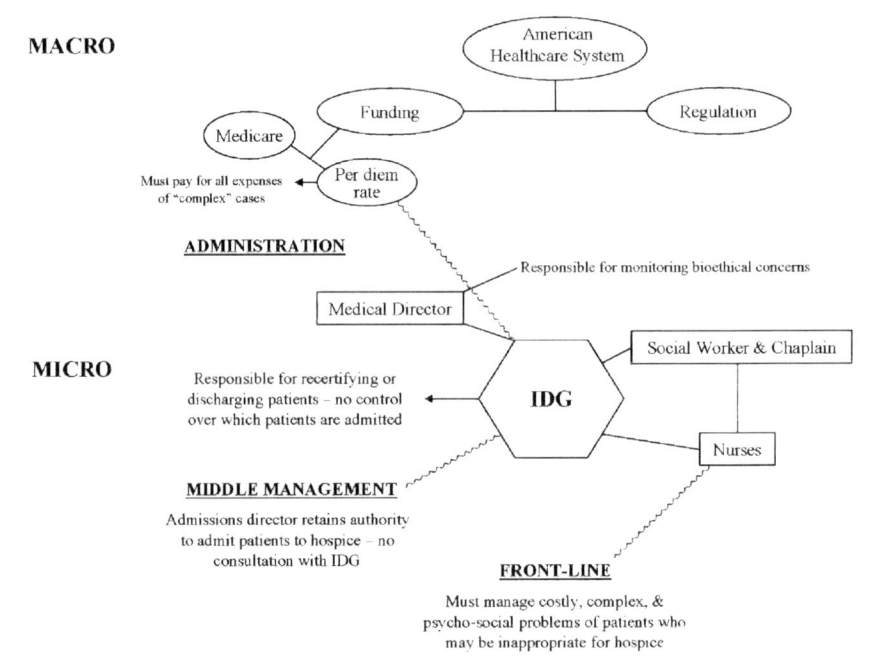

Fig. 5. Microlevel Disjunctures.

[*There follows a discussion between the nurse and the Medical Director concerning a State law regarding the use of "under-the-tongue" medications for ventilator patients. Kevin's lung sounds are described by the nurse as "junky" (meaning congested). The Medical Director suggests an antibiotic be ordered to clear up the congestion.*]

Chaplain: "This is a very difficult situation for the family. They've been back and forth, hoping he'll die and hoping for a miracle."

[*A group discussion ensues about whether the ex-wife should be included in decision-making. The Medical Director asks whether the patient was involved in the decision to have hospice.*]

Nurse: "I think he really understood and was involved, but the whole family has different perspectives on what Kevin understands and what Kevin doesn't ... "

Medical Director: "I have trouble with this ALS patient. We have denied people before with ventilators. There was a meeting here, but we were not involved. He could live another six months or a year. We shouldn't have him in hospice."

Nurse: "Yeah, and we're obligated to pay for the vent and the pulmonary visits. [The nursing home] is making a ton of dollars off of this. This should have been discussed before. We at hospice are going to take a bath on this one."

Medical Director: "This is an issue of justice and fairness as well. We are giving preferential treatment for a vent patient which we don't do for everybody. Why did we take this patient? We really shouldn't have."

Nurse: "I know Admissions struggled with this and eventually said yes, but [the Admissions Director] never really looked at this patient. Our agreement was 'no antibiotics', but it was written as 'no IV antibiotics'. Can we still give him antibiotics via [feeding] tubes?"

Medical Director: I'm going to have the Ethics Committee revisit this case and express our dismay about it. The biggest question here is, did we do the right thing or the wrong thing here by deciding to admit this person in the first place? ... do we prolong life or provide comfort? For this patient we're prolonging life, which theoretically we don't do. Ditto for the feeding tube. I just think it was the wrong decision."

The remarkable IDG discussion of Kevin L's case reveals a dizzying conflation of ethical, legal, fiscal, and teleological concerns, and highlights the limitations of the IDG's "ruling" authority. Although the IDG's ostensible function is to make clinical and recertification decisions for admitted hospice patients, it appears from this case that it had no authority over which patients can be *admitted* to the Hospice – "There was a meeting, but we were not involved." As a result of the Admission Director's decision to admit this patient, the IDG was faced with the problem of whether (and how) to treat his lung infection, concerning which there may be state regulations prohibiting certain procedures.

Moreover, because under the Medicare Hospice Benefit the hospice was required to pay for all medications, equipment and procedures associated with the patient's terminal diagnosis, the extraordinary costs associated with maintaining this patient under hospice were also a concern, as cost-containment is another, "latent" function of the IDG.

The Medical Director invoked bioethical standards of "justice and fairness," alluding to the fact that "we have denied people before with ventilators" but in this case a patient was being given "preferential treatment." The complex nature of many patients' end-stage illnesses appears to result in "case-by-case" decision making in the IDG and elsewhere within the Hospice, which at times may seem inconsistent to observers. This apparent inconsistency was exacerbated by a locus of control concerning admission decisions that was beyond the institutional reach of the IDG as a deliberative body. Finally, there is the teleological question of hospice's primary purpose – the Medical Director asked, "do we prolong life or provide comfort?" As numerous other cases reviewed in the IDG seem to attest, the answer to this question often seems to be "both." Figures 2, 3, and 4 "map" the disjunctures discussed in this section at the macro-, mezzo-, and microlevels of institutional space.

Level Four: "Fault Lines" – Issues and Events Surrounding the IDG

Because the IDG meetings were a central and regularly scheduled event in the institutional life of the Hospice, the occasion of an IDG meeting appeared to serve other, latent organizational functions. One was to bring together members of hospice teams who might otherwise rarely see each other face-to-face, so hectic were their schedules of visits to the many patients and families on their teams' caseloads. Sometimes teams would use the opportunity to tack on an unscheduled meeting immediately following the conclusion of IDG business, in order to check in with each other or discuss issues of concern.

Others in the organization also took advantage of teams being assembled for the IDG and would come in to address the group either immediately before or after the meeting. Topics of discussion on these occasions were generally not directly related to the work of the IDG, but often revealed other sources of institutional strain and disjuncture that broadened our understanding of how things happened in the organization. In this way, the IDG appeared to act as a magnet that drew disjunctures and ruling relations of various kinds toward itself, and into visible form. "Fault lines" of power and relative powerlessness, originating elsewhere, thus ran through the IDG in ways not originally intended or foreseen (Fig. 6).

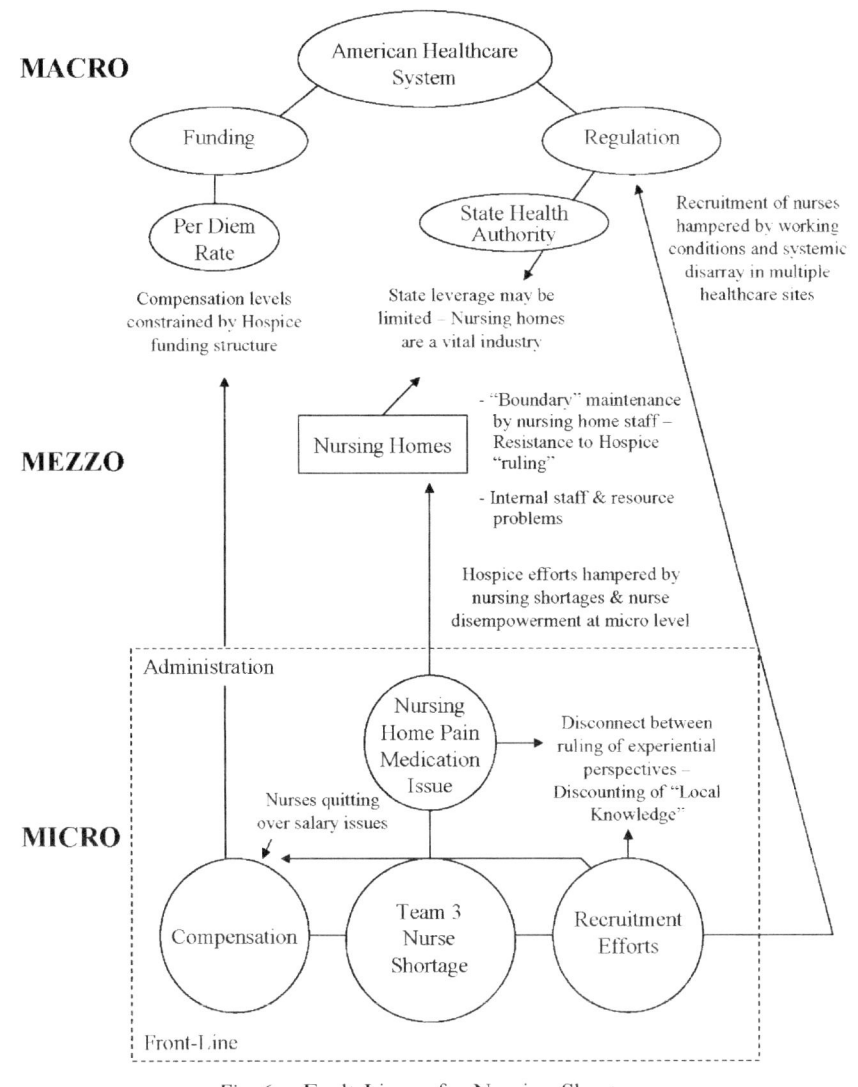

Fig. 6. Fault Lines of a Nursing Shortage.

Here, we focus on one particular item of concern for Team 3 in 2001, namely a shortage of nurses. We will draw from Maria's field notes of impromptu meetings and other interactions during March 2001 and attempt to map the various fault lines that lead from this issue to related issues and disjunctures, both within the Hospice and beyond it. Either job titles or pseudonyms are used for the participants in the following accounts.

In one such meeting that took place on March 8 after the IDG session had concluded and the Medical Director had left the room, the Team discussed the issue of "merit" pay raises and cost-of-living adjustments, which were widely considered unsatisfactory. A new Primary Nurse related her story of being told that she would be given a raise a few months after being hired; however, she continued, "that didn't happen ... Being promised something and not having them follow through makes me feel really betrayed." Another nurse remarked that "they count on us to do this work because they know it's our mission in life, and we won't leave because it's so important to us."

A week later on March 15, the Medical Director initiated a discussion at the conclusion of the IDG case reviews for the purpose of encouraging the nurses present to assist in the Hospice's efforts to recruit new nurses. The Hospice was offering those nurses already employed a $2,000 bonus "for recruiting one of your colleagues to come in and work for hospice." However, those present were reluctant to persuade other nurses to join them because of the pay-cut that working for a hospice could entail. Jake responded to this reluctance by asking, "Isn't there something redeeming about working here at hospice? Isn't this good work that we do?" One of the nurses replied, "Yes, but if you want to pay your mortgage, you can't make the choice to come here."

A third unscheduled discussion occurred on March 29, after the regular IDG meeting had already begun. Madeline, the Hospice Vice President, was reading a letter from the State Capitol aloud to the IDG team, regarding a problem involving the misuse of pain medication for hospice patients residing in nursing homes. This issue was a major concern for the Nursing Home team in 2001. After reading the letter, Madeline commented, "They are hearing our plight, and I believe the issue of educating [nursing home] nurses about morphine is being addressed – and should be addressed – at the physician level."

At this point, the Team Leader for Team 3, Nadine, initiated a tense discussion with Madeline regarding the shortage of nurses in the Nursing Home team, the recent resignation of one of their nurses, and the acute stress felt by the remaining Team members due to the extraordinarily high number of patients currently being cared for by that team. "We just can't handle these additional people," said Nadine, "We do not have the personnel." Madeline replied, "Well, there appear to be two issues: one is resource allocation and the other is internal team dynamics ... I hear your frustration and that's why I've asked Jake and [another hospice physician] to get involved in ... the medication issue because you can't do all that education. You need to do patient care." Nadine retorted, "I need to be a Team Leader!" and added, "That's one of the reasons there's so much concern about the medication incidents in nursing homes – We just can't be there enough to make sure they are appropriately using the pain medications." Madeline responded, "I'm prepared to pull the contracts if nursing home doctors don't get involved with our doctors."

In this series of gatherings and exchanges we see an issue of pressing concern to Team 3 addressed from various situated perspectives – Team 3 members, the Medical Director, and the Vice President – and tied to related issues such as employee compensation, agency recruitment efforts, and a crisis involving the administration of pain medications at nursing homes. Fault lines lead from the central issue – the nurse shortage – to other problems implicated in or exacerbated by the nurse shortage. And at the far end of each fault line lie asymmetries of knowledge and power, ruling versus experiential perspectives, that we have been calling disjunctures.

In the first example, team members shared similar views regarding what they saw as the inadequacy of proposed salary increases, and expressed a sense of betrayal. One member, Beth, theorized a deliberate attempt by Administration to exploit their dedication to hospice and its "mission" (i.e. the hospice discourse), saying, "they know ... we won't leave, because the work is so important to us."

In the second exchange – this time between the Medical Director and Team 3 members – we see an opposition of perspectives that lends some credence to Beth's perception of a calculated appeal to their sense of dedication, as Jake asked, "Isn't there something redeeming about working here at hospice? Isn't this good work that we do?"

Finally, in the dialogue between Nadine and the Hospice Vice President, Madeline, ruling and experiential perspectives literally "talked past" each other, as Madeline maintained an administrative "rational management" viewpoint in the face of Nadine's impassioned explication of the situation on the ground at the nursing homes. Madeline appeared to see the issue under discussion – misuse of narcotic medications by the nursing home staff – as an issue separate from Nadine's "resource allocation" problem, an issue to be addressed by assigning Jake and other hospice doctors to confer with the "nursing home doctors," thus freeing the hospice nurses to concentrate on "patient care." Nadine saw the issue as a staff shortage problem, in that there were not enough hospice nurses to adequately monitor what the nursing home staff were doing with pain medications (a function that would seem to be an integral part of "patient care").

Subtle practices of ruling are visible in this exchange, as Madeline employed the objectifying language of rational management to recast nurses as "resources," whose "allocation" rested in others' hands, and the problems caused by the nursing shortage as a matter of "internal team dynamics," presumably beyond Madeline's purview as an administrator. Language was used, in this instance, to re-inscribe distances and differences in rank and location within the organizational hierarchy rather than to problem-solve. In addition, Madeline's suggestion to Nadine that "you can't do all that education – you need to do patient care" implied an effective diminution of the primary nurses' role within the nursing homes, in favor of an expanded role for the Medical Director and other doctors: a further move toward "medicalization" of hospice and away from an interdisciplinary model. Nadine's response to this implication – "I need to be a Team Leader!" – attempted to counter this notion that an interorganizational problem in patient care could be effectively addressed by disempowering hospice nurses.

The differences in Madeline's and Nadine's analyses of the nursing home medication issue reflect two distinct modalities of organizational ruling. In one, language was used to assert authority and reinforce hierarchical boundaries in response to a perceived challenge. In the other, a top-down solution "at the physician level" was proposed to a problem raised by hospice nurses at the ground level, where the problem was actually occurring. This proposed solution overlooked the nurses' "local knowledge" and potentially disempowered them further.

The concept of "local knowledge" comes from feminist standpoint theory (Swigonski, 1994) and focuses on the validity of the perceptions of marginalized groups about their own lives. The knowledge generated by the lived experience of such groups is usually ignored or discounted by dominant or hegemonic groups in a society. Whether or not it was intentional, Madeline's "marginalization" of Nadine's experience – similar to Jake's earlier discounting of nurses' material circumstances in favor of an ideological appeal – presents a vivid instance of ruling that helps to explain "how knowledge and power come together in the everyday world to organize what happens to people" (Campbell & Gregor, 2002, p. 12).

Neither, however, should analysis be confined to ruling practices within the organization. The fault lines extend from the nursing shortage to related problems and beyond the Hospice to mezzo- and macrolevels of institutional space (Fig. 6).

With respect to the nursing home issue, a number of factors could be considered. Aside from the local disjuncture that disempowered hospice nurses in their efforts to control the misuse of medications, it is likely that nursing home staff were resentful of the Hospice's attempt to impose its own brand of "ruling" on their local practices; moreover, their administrators may have been constrained by staffing and resource problems of their own. Although it appears that hospice administrators had approached authorities at the state level about the issue, it was uncertain in 2001 how much and how effectively state leverage could be exerted against an industry vital to a rapidly aging society.

Hospice staff compensation is of course linked to hospice funding, a primary source of which is revenue from the Medicare Hospice Benefit which, as discussed earlier, can be precarious. The Hospice is a private, not-for-profit agency that actively fund-raises, and in fact had established a Foundation to provide ancillary financial support. However, the vicissitudes of offering competitive professional salaries amid unpredictable, structurally induced fluctuations of census and length-of-stay appeared to constrain hospice administrators, while exacerbating recruitment problems.

Nursing shortages were by no means confined to, or exclusively caused by local conditions at the Hospice, but were a nation-wide phenomenon in 2001 (American Association of Colleges of Nursing [AACN], 2004). During the same Team 3 meeting that Maria observed on March 8, a nurse commented that she left hospital nursing, despite its better pay, because she "couldn't work in the hurried and chaotic way that it demanded. I came to hospice to get away from all that."

It appears that work conditions in multiple healthcare sites were in a state of stress and disarray in 2001, reflecting fundamental disjunctures in the ruling apparatus of American health care as a whole.

SUMMARY OF PHASE TWO FINDINGS

In 2001, front-line hospice workers were visiting dying people, helping to alleviate their physical and psychic suffering, and supporting their families. Many of these patients were close to death, and their families in a state of crisis; they required frequent visits, several kinds of services, and a major investment of staff time and energy during their few days in hospice. Other patients – particularly those who lived in nursing homes – were dying more slowly of a wide variety of ailments that were complex and sometimes difficult to manage. Often, they were cared for by several different people who were not family and were busy with many other patients; so mistakes were sometimes made in their care, and problems often developed that were hard for hospice nurses and social workers to correct or control. Regardless of where patients lived, what was wrong with them, or which kinds of challenges their care presented, there were reasons why it all happened as it did.

Front-line hospice workers spent a great deal of time in 2001 writing about their work with patients and families, and reporting what they had written to others. It often seemed to them, in fact, that the words on the pages counted for more than the actual work they did, and that the "paper" patients were more important to the Hospice than the flesh-and-blood people they had visited every day. As they sat for long hours in IDG meetings and talked about the paper patients, the chaplains and social workers often felt left out of the conversation, because so much of the talk was a dialogue between nurses and doctors. But this was to be expected, because the "paper" patients were mostly constructed of symptoms held together by medications – very little of the fearful, funny, complicated, angry, confused, and thoughtful people they had come to know survived in these versions. Sometimes in these meetings, it was decided that the paper patient had to be discharged from hospice, and everyone would worry about them. Often, the paper person was allowed to stay in hospice, but people still worried because it was hard to know whether they were making the right decision, or what the consequences might be. There were reasons why all this happened as it did.

Although they continued to love the work they did, front-line hospice workers in 2001 often felt over-worked, under-compensated, and generally misunderstood by the Hospice they worked for. In recent memory, several of their co-workers had lost their jobs from the last "restructuring" that occurred, and others had quit because they could not afford to stay. These departures left those who remained short-handed and unable to devote as much time and attention to their patients as they wanted to. When they voiced their concerns to Hospice administrators, the answers they received often seemed unhelpful, irrelevant, or patronizing, and spoken in a different "language" than their own. Again, there were reasons why this happened as it did.

The purpose of Phase Two of our study was to trace the experiences just described to the organizational "reasons" for their occurrence.

Although some of the reasons we discovered were based on the way knowledge and power came together in the local setting of the Hospice, a great deal of what we observed in and around IDG meetings in 2001 appeared to be rooted farther away, in relations with other healthcare providers in the community, and ultimately in structures and practices of ruling at the state and federal levels, where the original "discourse" of the hospice movement had been converted, under Medicare, into a cost-containment strategy.

Despite the many positive aspects of legislation that provided to patients a means of receiving holistic end-of-life care and reimbursement to those who delivered it, the Medicare Hospice Benefit came with many significant "strings" attached that enforced a "ruling relation" between patients and hospices, and between hospices and the funding and regulatory regimes of the American healthcare system. The various disjunctures produced by these relations – between the ideals of hospice "discourse" and the day-to-day realities of hospice "text" – gradually became visible in our study of processes and activities in and around the IDG.

Under the ruling logic of the American healthcare system, there appeared to be no limit to the amount of money, time, and regulatory oversight that could be expended in the interest of controlling the costs of healthcare, and although hospices constituted only a tiny fragment of the system, they were subject to the same relentless scrutiny as other, larger cost-containers, such as hospitals, nursing homes, and so on. Much of the exhaustion, stress, and discontent expressed by hospice workers in both Phase One and Phase Two of our study can be traced to the fundamental disjuncture involved in trying to serve the healthcare system and dying patients at the same time.

CONCLUDING REMARKS

Hospices continue to provide compassionate care and support to many thousands of patients and families throughout the United States. However, the work of hospice exacts a price from the people who deliver the care and try to embody the hospice philosophy on a day-to-day basis. Phase One of our study examined the price paid, in stress and demoralization. Phase Two employed techniques of IE to explicate how this "price" came into being, and why it seemed to persist in 2001. In some ways, it appeared that front-line hospice workers bore the financial and psychic burden of the difference between what hospice promised, in the early reform movement, and what it was able to deliver in its translation to a reimbursable healthcare "benefit."

How those daily sacrifices were linked to structures of institutional power, and how those linkages could be discerned and mapped through observation of the IDG, were the central concern of this chapter. Numerous disparities – between various classes of dying people, between ruling perspectives and local knowledge, and between hospice ideals and institutional realities – emerged in sharp relief in the course of this investigation. These disparities, and their linkage to macrolevel policies and structures, reflect a fundamental dilemma in American health care that defies local or merely technical solutions.

The implications of our findings for change are daunting to consider, because in our view meaningful change would entail a significant reorientation of the ruling logic of contemporary American healthcare, as well as a concomitant overhaul of the institutional grid-work of public and private interests, governance, and delivery systems that serve that logic. Moreover, we are all implicated in the creation and maintenance of that logic and that grid-work. The only reason to commit to such an undertaking would be a widespread recognition – among embodied, local "knowers" everywhere – that change is necessary.

ACKNOWLEDGMENTS

The authors are indebted to Naomi Streeter for her invaluable assistance with the literature review for this chapter and with preparation of the figures that appear in it .We also wish to thank Joy Buck, RN, PhD, for her gracious permission to examine portions of her manuscript for information on Medicare and the early American hospice movement.

REFERENCES

American Association of Colleges of Nursing (AACN). (2004). Nursing shortage fact sheet. AACN website. Available at http://www.aacn.nche.edu/Media/FactSheets/NursingShortage.htm. Retrieved on February 7, 2009.

Buck, J. (2007). *Reweaving a tapestry of care for the dying: A history of Hospice, Medicare, and the translation of an ideal.* Pre-publication manuscript.

Campbell, M., & Gregor, F. (2002). *Mapping social relations: A primer in doing institutional ethnography.* Aurora, Ontario: Garamond Press.

DeVault, M., & McCoy, L. (2002). Institutional ethnography: Using interviews to investigate ruling relations. In: J. Gubrium & J. Holstein (Eds), *Handbook of interview research: Context and method.* Thousand Oaks, CA: Sage Publications.

DiMaggio, P., & Powell, W. (1983). The iron cage revisited: Institutional isomorphism and collective rationalizing in organizational fields. *American Sociological Review, 48*, 147–150.

DiTullio, M., & MacDonald, D. (1999). The struggle for the soul of hospice: Stress, coping & change among hospice workers. *American Journal of Hospice & Palliative Care, 16*(5), 641–655.

Kubler-Ross, E. (1969). *On death and dying.* New York: MacMillan.

National Hospice and Palliative Care Association (NHPCO). (2007). Hospice: A historical perspective. http://www.nhpo.org/i4a/pages/index.cfmNati?pageid = 3285. Retrieved on February 7, 2009.

Paradis, L., & Cummings, S. (1986). The evolution of hospice in America toward organizational homogeneity. *Journal of Health and Social Behavior, 27*(December), 370–386.

Smith, D. (1987). *The everyday world as problematic: A feminist sociology.* Toronto: University of Toronto Press.

Stoddard, S. (1992). *The hospice movement.* New York: Vintage.

Swigonski, M. (1994). The logic of feminist standpoint theory for social work research. *Social Work, 39*(4), 387–393.

Ward, G. (2003). *Postmodernism.* Chicago: Contemporary Books.